Health and Social Research in Multiethnic Societies

Research on ethnicity is of relevance to a wide variety of health, economic and social issues in modern societies. This is reflected in the growing body of research with a focus on ethnicity. Despite this, there are no ready sources of information on the methodological issues facing such research. This volume aims to fill that gap.

Straightforward in its approach and accessible to those who are not specialists in studies of ethnicity, *Health and Social Research in Multiethnic Societies* provides essential and clear guidance on appropriate methods. Topics covered include:

- approaches to conceptualising ethnicity and understanding the context of ethnicity in modern societies
- ethical issues and the political context within which ethnicity research is conducted
- how researchers could engage with communities and with service users in general;
- cultural competence in research
- practical issues faced by both qualitative and quantitative research
- use of secondary and administrative data sources for research.

Using a combination of critical analysis and case studies to illustrate the benefits and pitfalls of particular approaches, this volume provides access to core issues relevant to research with ethnic minority groups. It is a vital resource for those carrying out and using what is a considerable body of research, including students, academics, researchers and research commissioners.

James Y. Nazroo is Professor of Medical Sociology in the Department of Epidemiology and Public Health, UCL. He is author of *Ethnicity, Class and Health* and joint editor of the journal *Ethnicity and Health*. Ethnic inequalities in health have been a major focus of his research. Central to this has been improving our understanding of the links between ethnicity, racism, class and inequality.

Health and Social Research in Multiethnic Societies

Edited by
James Y. Nazroo

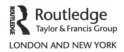

Routledge
Taylor & Francis Group

LONDON AND NEW YORK

First published 2006 by Routledge
2 Park Square, Milton Park, Abingdon, Oxon OX14 4RN

Simultaneously published in the USA and Canada
by Routledge
270 Madison Avenue, New York, NY 10016

Routledge is an imprint of the Taylor and *Francis Group, an informa business*

© 2006 James Y. Nazroo, selection and editorial matter;
individual chapters, the contributors

Typeset in Times New Roman by
Florence Production Ltd, Stoodleigh, Devon
Printed and bound in Great Britain by
MPG Books Ltd, Bodmin

British Library Cataloguing in Publication Data
A catalogue record for this book is available from the British Library

Library of Congress Cataloging in Publication Data
A catalog record for this book has been requested

ISBN10: 0–415–39365–5 (hbk)
ISBN10: 0–415–39366–3 (pbk)
ISBN10: 0–203–96993–6 (ebk)

ISBN13: 978–0–415–39365–2 (hbk)
ISBN13: 978–0–415–39366–9 (pbk)
ISBN13: 978–0–203–96993–9 (ebk)

Contents

Illustrations

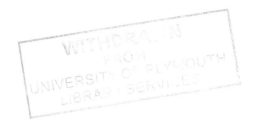

Figures

Tables

Boxes

Contributors

James Y. Nazroo is Professor of Medical Sociology, Department of Epidemiology and Public Health, University College London.

Karl Atkin is Senior Lecturer in Ethnicity and Health, Department of Health Sciences, University of York.

Peter J. Aspinall is Senior Research Fellow, Centre for Health Services Studies, University of Kent.

Madhavi Bajekal is Head of Morbidity Statistics Branch, Office for National Statistics, London.

Sangeeta Chattoo is Senior Research Fellow, Centre for Research in Primary Care, Institute of Health Sciences and Public Health Research, University of Leeds.

Bob Erens is Health Research Group Director, National Centre for Social Research, London.

Ini Grewal is Senior Researcher, National Centre for Social Research, London.

Mark R.D. Johnson is Professor of Diversity in Health & Social Care and Director, Centre for Evidence in Ethnicity Health and Diversity, Mary Seacole Research Centre, De Montfort University, Leicester.

Saffron Karlsen is Senior Research Fellow, Department of Epidemiology and Public Health, University College London.

Sally McManus is Research Director, National Centre for Social Research, London.

Ann Oakley is Professor of Sociology and Social Policy and Founding Director of the Social Science Research Unit at the Institute of Education, University of London.

Irena Papadopoulos is Professor of Transcultural Health and Nursing, Head of Research Centre for Transcultural Studies in Health, School of Health and Social Sciences, Middlesex University.

Jane Ritchie is formerly Director of Qualitative Research Unit, National Centre for Social Research, London.

Graham Scambler is Professor of Medical Sociology, Centre for Behavioural and Social Sciences in Medicine, University College London.

Melba Wilson is Director of Race Equality, London Development Centre, Care Services Improvement Partnership.

Preface

This volume deals with methodological issues relating to research with ethnic minority groups. The intention is to provide guidance that would, by giving a clear indication of the issues that research should address, contribute to improving the quality of research. It is targeted at those familiar with health and social research methods, on which there are several excellent texts, but who seek guidance on how to apply such methods to research involving ethnic minority people. As such, it is of use to researchers, commissioners and users of research, and students.

Research on ethnicity, ethnic relations and the position of ethnic minority groups is of relevance to a wide variety of health, economic and social issues, and, consequently, to a broad range of users in academia, policy and practice, and community groups. This is reflected in the large and growing body of research that is commissioned and conducted with a focus on ethnicity. Coupled with this growth in research is a growing body of expertise on conducting research in a multicultural environment, which has, paradoxically, also revealed shortcomings in the quality of much research on such issues. There is also some evidence that the body of expertise built up by those who conduct research on ethnicity is not adequately disseminated to those involved in 'mainstream' research, partly because of the marginalisation of some of that research and of some of those who conduct it. Not only does this mean that this expertise has to be continually re-created, it also means that experienced researchers who are unfamiliar with methods to include ethnic minority groups in their research do not have ready sources of information illustrating the strategies for doing so. The volume aims to plug that gap, using and building on existing expertise in the research community, from a range of disciplines and methodologies. It is intended to be accessible to members of the research community who are not specialists in studies of ethnic minority groups, so as to illustrate the value of extending their work to cover these groups and issues relevant to ethnic inequalities, and to give clear guidance on methods for doing this.

The first three chapters cover fundamental issues that need to be considered by all research addressing issues related to ethnicity, ethnic relations and multiculturalism. Chapter 1 provides an account of the situation of ethnic minority people in Britain, illustrating the need to consider the impact of ethnic relations and inequalities in health and social research. Chapter 2 illustrates the complexity of ethnicity and ethnic identity, showing the need to be sensitive to issues relating to lay and academic conceptions of ethnicity and how these might influence the direction of research. Chapter 3 deals with ethical issues and the complex political agendas that exist in both research and user communities, by examining the implications of the complex relationships between politics, research and policy. All three chapters are concerned with the interface between theory and practice, and with making explicit the implications of theory to research practice.

Chapters 4, 5 and 6 address broad methodological issues that are relevant regardless of the disciplinary or methodological focus of the research. Chapter 4 is concerned with strategies to engage a variety of users in the research, dealing with their potentially conflicting needs and expectations, and maximising the input of community organisations and community representatives at key stages of the research to ensure the relevance and acceptability of research to ethnic minority communities. Chapter 5 assesses the theoretical basis of, and evidence for, the need for ethnic and language matching of the researcher and researched, often considered to be a necessary strategy in research on ethnic minority groups. Chapter 6 provides an account of culturally competent research and the steps that need to be undertaken to improve the quality of research that is conducted.

Chapters 7 to 10 cover the key methods used in health and social research and how these need to be reconsidered when undertaking research with ethnic minority groups. The intention here is to provide rapid and straightforward access to core issues for research on ethnic minority groups for those already experienced in applying these methods for general population research. The chapters cover qualitative research, the conduct of surveys, evaluation research and a critical review of the use of administrative and routine data. Finally, Chapter 11 provides a review of the volume and its main messages, seen from the eyes of a policy user of research.

Acknowledgements

The work that led to this volume was funded by the Department of Health's Policy Research Programme. The views expressed in the publication are those of the authors and not necessarily those of the Department of Health. I am particularly grateful to Christine McGuire, who managed the work on behalf of the Department of Health. I am also grateful to the advisory group for the work, who played a central role in turning the broad idea for the volume into a balanced final product. Members of the advisory group were: Waqar Ahmad, Bob Erens, Mark Johnson, Christine McGuire and Nicky Vick. And thanks to Sheema Ahmed, who prepared the manuscript for delivery to the publishers.

Finally, I would like to thank the large number of people who have participated in the research conducted by myself and other authors of chapters in this volume.

Chapter 1

Demography of multicultural Britain

James Y. Nazroo

Introduction

This chapter provides an overview of ethnic groups in the UK, their make-up and their social positions relative to each other. It is hoped that this will provide important context for other chapters, and for the reader. Indeed, such context is central to an understanding of ethnicity, ethnic differences in health, and the provision of health and social care. So, even if the reader is conducting, planning or evaluating research conducted outside the UK, the messages contained here are relevant. For those interested in the UK context, more detail can be obtained by following up the references in the text, and in particular Modood *et al.* (1997) and Mason (2003).

Many equate ethnicity with visible, non-White, minority groups. While such an assertion is challenged throughout this volume, with a consideration of White minority groups and an examination of ethnicity in relation to (White) majority groups, much research focuses on non-White minorities. The non-White population of the UK has a relatively recent history. Although some non-White people settled in the United Kingdom prior to the Second World War (mainly in London and the ports on the west coast of the UK – Bristol, Cardiff, Liverpool, Glasgow – and primarily related to the slave trade), most of the non-White migration to Britain occurred after the Second World War. This was triggered by the passing of the 1948 British Nationality Act and was driven by the post-war economic boom and consequent need for labour, a need that could be filled from British Commonwealth countries – primarily countries in the Caribbean and the Indian subcontinent. This 'economic' migration was followed by migration of spouses and children and, sometimes, older relatives, in a climate when the legislation regulating entry into the UK became increasingly restrictive. Immigration from the Caribbean was greatly reduced by the Commonwealth Immigrants Act of 1962, and immigration from the Indian subcontinent was similarly restricted by the Immigration Act of 1971 (Salt 1996). Nevertheless, the post-war period has continued to see a rapid increase in the numbers of non-White people in the UK. Estimates suggest that numbers rose from around 100,000 in 1951, to just over 400,000 in 1961, to 1.2 million in 1971, and 2.1 million in 1981 (Owen 2003). The 1991 Census, the first to directly record ethnicity, estimated the non-White population of the UK to be 3.1 million and the 2001 Census recorded 4.6 million people in non-White groups.

Data from the 2001 Census are shown in Table 1.1, which shows that the 4.6 million non-White people made up almost 8 per cent of the UK population. Focusing

Table 1.1 2001 UK population by ethnic group, country and country of birth

	England	Wales	Scotland	Northern Ireland	UK total	UK %	% UK born
White	44,679,361	2,841,505	4,960,334	1,672,698	54,153,898	92.12	95
British/Scottish	42,747,136	2,786,605	4,832,756	*	n/a	n/a	98
Irish	624,115	17,689	49,428	*	n/a	n/a	34
Other White	1,308,110	37,211	78,150	*	n/a	n/a	21
Mixed	643,373	17,661	12,764	3,319	677,117	1.15	79
White Black Caribbean	231,424	5,996	*	*	n/a	n/a	n/a
White Black African	76,498	2,413	*	*	n/a	n/a	n/a
White and Asian	184,014	5,001	*	*	n/a	n/a	n/a
Other Mixed	151,437	4,251	*	*	n/a	n/a	n/a
Asian or Asian British/Scottish	2,248,289	25,448	55,007	2,679	2,331,423	3.97	47
Indian	1,028,546	8,261	15,037	1,567	1,053,411	1.79	46
Pakistani	706,539	8,287	31,793	666	747,285	1.27	55
Bangladeshi	275,394	5,436	1,981	252	283,063	0.48	46
Other Asian	237,810	3,464	6,196	194	247,664	0.42	31
Black or Black British/Scottish	1,132,508	7,069	8,025	1,136	1,148,738	1.95	50
Black Caribbean	561,246	2,597	1,778	255	565,876	0.96	58
Black African	475,938	3,727	5,118	494	485,277	0.83	34
Black Other	95,324	745	1,129	387	97,585	0.17	79
Chinese or other ethnic group	435,300	11,402	25,881	5,435	478,018	0.81	23
Chinese	220,681	6,267	16,310	4,145	247,403	0.42	29
Other	214,619	5,135	9,571	1,290	230,615	0.39	16
All population	49,138,831	2,903,085	5,062,011	1,685,267	58,789,194	100	92

* Answer category not provided as a tick-box option in this country.

Source: 2001 Census.

more specifically on the England and Wales columns, which had a more detailed ethnic categorisation, overall almost 9 per cent of the English population identified themselves as belonging to one of the non-White ethnic minority groups, with a further 4 per cent identifying themselves as a member of a White ethnic minority group (Irish or Other White). The table also indicates the great diversity of the ethnic minority population in the UK, with those identified as members of non-White groups spread across a range of categories, many of which are, themselves, far from culturally, or ethnically, homogeneous, such as the Black African and Indian groups. For example, 45 per cent of the Indian group are Hindu, 29 per cent Sikh, 13 per cent Muslim and 5 per cent Christian. And the Other White group is similarly heterogeneous. In addition, the table shows the emergence of 'mixed' ethnic groups, another sign of heterogeneity in the non-White population, and just over half of ethnic minority people were born in the UK, though this varies across specific groups reflecting both period of migration and patterns of fertility.

Indeed, migration from the New Commonwealth countries was not evenly spread over time: immigration from the Caribbean and India occurred throughout the 1950s and 1960s, peaking in the early 1960s; from Pakistan, largely in the 1970s; from Bangladesh, mainly in the late 1970s and early 1980s; and from Hong Kong, in the 1980s and 1990s. In addition, there was a notable flow of immigrants from East Africa in the late 1960s and early 1970s, made up of migrants from India to East Africa who were subsequently expelled. After the 1980s, migration to the UK has taken a very different form, including large numbers from the rest of the European Union and numbers from non-European Union and non-Commonwealth countries increasing more rapidly than elsewhere (Owen 2003). This relates to a world-wide growth in the numbers of refugees, but also to economic growth in the UK, with the peaks of migration coinciding with periods of rapid growth (Owen 2003). Figure 1.1 gives an indication of the change in the non-White ethnic minority population between the 1991 and 2001 Censuses, using a subset of the more restricted categories that were used in 1991. It includes a measure of the growth of particular groups (absolute change) and how this growth relates to total population growth (relative change). As can be seen, for all groups growth is greater than for the total population (the darker bars), but it also varied substantially across the ethnic minority groups, with relatively low growth in the Black Caribbean and Indian groups, and marked growth in the Black African and Chinese groups.

Finally, alongside this 'visible' migration, it should be noted that there has been a long history of migration to England from Ireland, which continued during the active recruitment of labour from the Caribbean and the Indian subcontinent. The history of Irish migration to England holds important lessons on the circumstances

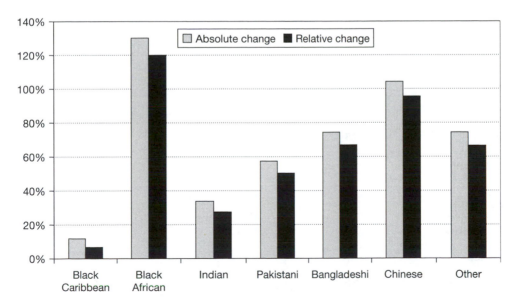

Figure 1.1 Change in the ethnic composition of the English population: 1991 to 2001.*

* 2001 Census figures are calculated using an algorithm derived using data from the 1999 Health Survey for England.

of economic migrants and their descendants, and how far skin colour is a demarcating factor.

Ethnic differences in age and household structure

Table 1.2 shows differences in age profiles across the ethnic categories that were included in the 1999 Health Survey for England (Erens *et al.* 2001). It clearly shows the similarity in age profiles between the White English and White minority groups, and the younger age profiles of the non-White minority groups. This is most notable in the youngest categories and the oldest categories. Data from the 2001 Census show that the mean age of people from minority ethnic groups is about ten years less than

Table 1.2 Age profile of ethnic groups in England (%)*

Age	Caribbean	Indian	Pakistani	Bangla-deshi	Chinese	White minority	White English
2–15	33	29	40	43	29	19	20
16–40	38	39	42	40	34	34	32
41–50	8	15	10	7	20	16	14
51–60	8	8	5	4	9	12	13
61–70	9	7	3	4	6	10	11
Over 70	4	3	1	1	2	10	11

Source: 1999 Health Survey for England.

* In some cases percentages do not add up to 100 because of rounding.

Table 1.3 Ethnicity and family structure in the UK*

	Average household size	Households with dependent children (%)	Lone parent households (%)
White British	2.3	28.3	22.1
White Irish	2.2	20.6	23.1
Other White	2.4	29.3	17.2
Mixed	2.5	40.8	38.9
Indian	3.3	50.0	9.6
Pakistani	4.1	66.2	13.0
Bangladeshi	4.5	74.4	11.6
Other Asian	3.2	49.3	12.2
Black Caribbean	2.3	37.0	47.8
Black African	2.7	47.7	36.0
Other Black	2.4	46.8	52.1
Chinese	2.7	37.0	15.1
Other ethnic groups	2.8	43.5	18.0
All households	2.4	29.4	22.2

Source: 2001 Census.

* In some cases percentages do not add up to 100 because of rounding.

that of White people. In part, the age profile for White people reflects the 'baby booms' of the late 1940s and 1960s and the decline in fertility thereafter. Among minority ethnic groups, Black Caribbean people are oldest on average, followed by Indian, Other Asian and Chinese people. The youngest are people of mixed parentage, with a mean age of just over 20, and Pakistani and Bangladeshi people, with a mean age of around 24 or 25.

Differences in age structure are reflected in differences in household structure, some of which are shown in Table 1.3. The middle column of Table 1.3, showing the proportion of households with dependent children, reflects the larger number of children in the non-White groups, but also shows variability across them. Three-quarters of Bangladeshi people live in households containing dependent children, compared with just over a third of Black Caribbean and Chinese households, with other groups between these. This, in part, is a consequence of higher fertility rates and family sizes for the South Asian groups, which leads to the larger household sizes shown in the first column of Table 1.3. Also notable in Table 1.3 are differences in the proportion of lone parent households, ranging from the low rates found in the South Asian groups to the high rates found in Mixed and Black groups.

Ethnic/racial disadvantage – variation and similarities across groups

There is considerable socioeconomic diversity and inequality between the major ethnic groups in the UK. Some of the main dimensions of this are described below.

Residential segregation

Although analyses of residential segregation are not as developed in the UK as they are, for example, in the US, they do show marked differences between the geographical locations of ethnic minority and White people. Analysis of the 1991 Census (Owen 1992, 1994) has shown that the non-White ethnic minority population is concentrated in particular areas, reflecting their post-migration location in London, Birmingham and the other industrial cities and towns of the midlands and northern England, where jobs in the manufacturing industry and public sector services were readily available. Table 1.4, which illustrates the differences in the location of the White and non-White population at the 2001 Census using a broad geography, supports the conclusions drawn from Owen's analysis of the 1991 Census.

Key conclusions to draw from Table 1.4 are:

- Non-White people are much more likely to live in England than White people.
- More than half of the ethnic minority population live in London and South East England, where less than a quarter of the White population live.
- Greater London contains 44.6 per cent of the ethnic minority population and only 9.4 per cent of the White population.
- The only other broad area where ethnic minority people are more likely to live than White people is the West Midlands.
- Around two-thirds of ethnic minority people live in London, elsewhere in the South East and the West Midlands, compared with about a third of White people.

Table 1.4 Regional distribution of the non-White and White population in the UK in 2001 (%)

	All non-White groups	All White groups
English regions		
North East	1.3	4.5
North West	8.1	11.7
Yorkshire and the Humber	7.0	8.6
East Midlands	5.9	7.2
West Midlands	12.8	8.6
East	5.7	9.5
London	44.6	9.4
South East	8.4	14.0
South West	2.4	8.9
UK countries		
England	96.2	82.5
Wales	1.3	5.2
Scotland	2.2	9.2
Northern Ireland	0.3	3.1

Source: 2001 Census.

- Elsewhere, the North West and Yorkshire and Humber display the highest concentrations of people from ethnic minorities.

Owen's analysis of the 1991 Census suggests that there are even greater differences when smaller areas, enumeration districts, are considered. At that time, more than half of ethnic minority people live in areas where the total ethnic minority population exceeds 44 per cent, compared with the 5.5 per cent national average. And these analyses of smaller geographical areas also show differences in the locations of specific ethnic minorities, with groups concentrated in different areas from each other.

Analysis of the areas where ethnic minority people live in England shows that they are much more likely to live in deprived areas (Karlsen *et al.* 2002). For example, as shown in Table 1.5, 81 per cent of Pakistani and Bangladeshi people, 72 per cent of Caribbean people and 49 per cent of Indian people lived in the bottom quintile of areas using the Townsend area deprivation score. In contrast, only 15 per cent of Indian people, 8 per cent of Caribbean people and less than 3 per cent of Pakistani and Bangladeshi live in the top two quintiles. On the other hand, there is emerging evidence that the establishment of ethnic minority communities in particular geographical areas may carry benefits. For example, in contrast to the high deprivation scores for the areas where they live, ethnic minority people perceive the amenities in the areas where they live more positively than White people do (Karlsen *et al.* 2002). This finding appears to reflect the investment that ethnic minority people have made to establish commercial (such as shops) and civic (such as schools, places of worship, community centres) facilities for their communities, and, importantly, this is related to the quality of life of ethnic minority people (Bajekal *et al.* 2004, Grewal *et al.* 2004).

Table 1.5 Distribution of ethnic groups in England and Wales according to Townsend scores in quintiles (%)

	White	Caribbean	Indian	Pakistani and Bangladeshi
Townsend score				
Highest quintile	20.4	3.3	5.8	1.0
	20.2	5.1	9.5	1.6
	20.1	11.3	9.9	4.0
	19.4	8.0	26.3	12.7
Lowest quintile	19.8	72.3	48.5	80.6

Source: Fourth National Survey of Ethnic Minorities, Karlsen et al. 2002.

Economic position

There are marked economic inequalities by ethnic group in the UK. Some indicators of this are summarised in Table 1.6, which is based on data from the 1999 Health Survey for England (Erens et al. 2001). The first part of the table shows rates of paid employment for men aged 16 to 65 (i.e. men of working age). For the White English group three-quarters of men are in paid employment. Figures are clearly lower for all of the ethnic minority groups, except for the White minority (Irish and other White) and Chinese groups, with particularly low rates in the Caribbean and Pakistani groups, and even lower rates for the Bangladeshi group, for whom less than half are in paid employment. These figures are echoed in the data collected at the 2001 Census, which also show that among women the highest rates of economic participation are found for White and Black Caribbean women (with almost three-quarters economically active), with very low rates of economic activity among Pakistani (just over a

Table 1.6 Ethnic differences in socioeconomic indicators in England (%)

	Caribbean	Indian	Pakistani	Bangla-deshi	Chinese	White minority	White English
Male employment rates aged 16–65	58	69	59	46	67	72	75
Registrar General's class							
I/II	24	34	23	12	40	46	35
IIInm	19	12	10	7	16	13	14
IIIm	28	29	40	39	34	25	32
IV/V	29	26	27	42	11	16	19
Equivalised household income							
Bottom tertile	48	45	69	90	41	27	31
Middle tertile	28	31	20	5	22	30	35
Top tertile	24	24	11	5	36	43	34

Source: Health Survey for England 1999.

quarter) and Bangladeshi (just under a quarter) women. Both these groups also have the highest rates of unemployment for women, at one in six for Pakistani women and one in four for Bangladeshi women.

The second part of Table 1.6 shows occupational class of the head of household. The data suggest that the profiles of White English and Indian people are similar, with White minority and possibly Chinese people better off, and Caribbean, Pakistani and, particularly, Bangladeshi people, worse off. Four out of five Bangladeshi people live in households headed by someone in a manual occupation. Chinese and Indian people are more likely than others to work in managerial and professional jobs. Managers will include people running their own businesses; and a much higher percentage of those (especially men) from South Asian and Chinese ethnic groups are entrepreneurs than White and Black people. People from Black ethnic groups tend to be more likely than other ethnic groups to work in associate professional (e.g. nursing) and administrative occupations.

The third and final part of Table 1.6 shows equivalised household income from all sources, split into tertiles on the basis of the general population distribution. The data suggest that on this measure the two White groups are equivalent, with the Indian and the Caribbean groups worse off, and the Pakistani and the Bangladeshi group particularly poorly off. Two-thirds of the Pakistani group and almost 90 per cent of the Bangladeshi group are in the bottom income tertile. In terms of the top income tertile, the Chinese group is equivalent to the two White groups, but it has substantially more households in the bottom tertile, suggesting greater inequality within the Chinese group.

Finally, Table 1.7 shows differences in level of qualification for those of working age. It reflects the inequalities shown in previous tables. For example, Pakistani and Bangladeshi people are most likely to have no qualifications and least likely to have progressed into higher education. It also shows, however, that White British do not have the best education profile, with several of the other groups doing better. These figures are, of course, complicated by migration history, age profiles and period/cohort effects.

Experiences of racism and discrimination

Experiences of and awareness of racism appear to be central to the lives of ethnic minority people. Qualitative investigations of experiences of racial harassment and discrimination in Britain have found that for many people experiences of interpersonal racism are a part of everyday life, that the way they lead their lives is constrained by fear of racial harassment, and that being made to feel different is routine and expected (Virdee 1995, Chahal and Julienne 1999). Experiences of racial harassment and discrimination were investigated quantitatively in some depth in the British Fourth National Survey (FNS) (Virdee 1997). This suggested that more than one in eight ethnic minority people had experienced some form of racial harassment in the past year. Although most of these incidents involved racial insults, many of the respondents reported repeated victimisation and as many as a quarter of all of the ethnic minority respondents reported being fearful of racial harassment. The FNS also showed that among ethnic minority respondents there was a widespread belief that employers discriminated against ethnic minority applicants for jobs, and widespread experience of such discrimination (Modood 1997). For example, 20 per cent of ethnic

Table 1.7 Highest qualification by ethnic group, people of working age in Britain (%)

	Degree or equivalent	Higher education*	A-Level or equivalent	GCSE grades A–C or equivalent	Other	None
White British	15	9	25	23	12	16
White Irish	23	10	19	12	17	19
White Other	22	5	12	6	42	13
Mixed	18	7	21	24	15	15
Indian	22	5	18	16	20	18
Pakistani	11	3	13	16	23	34
Bangladeshi	8	–	10	15	22	44
Other Asian	21	6	14	10	37	13
Black Caribbean	10	9	23	25	17	17
Black African	21	10	15	12	27	15
Other Black	13	–	23	22	21	15
Chinese	23	6	13	8	30	20
Other	24	5	11	6	41	13
All ethnic groups	16	8	24	22	14	17

* Below degree level.

Source: Annual Local Area Labour Forces Survey, Office for National Statistics, 2001–2002.

minority people reported being refused a job for racial reasons, and almost three-quarters of them said it has happened more than once. And 20 per cent of ethnic minority people believed that most employers would refuse somebody a job for racial reasons, with only 12 per cent thinking that no employers would do this. This is also reflected in the reported attitudes of White people. When White respondents to the survey were asked about their own racial prejudice, in a face-to-face interview, 26 per cent admitted to being prejudiced against South Asian people, 20 per cent to being prejudiced against Caribbean people and 8 per cent to being prejudiced against Chinese people.

Heterogeneity of the ethnic patterning of health

Differences in health across ethnic groups, in terms of both morbidity and mortality, have been repeatedly documented in the UK (Marmot *et al.* 1984, Rudat 1994, Harding and Maxwell 1997, Nazroo 1997a, 1997b, 2001, Erens *et al.* 2001), as they have in the US (Department of Health and Human Services 1985, Rogers 1992, Sorlie *et al.* 1992, 1995, Rogot *et al.* 1993, Krieger *et al.* 1993, Davey Smith *et al.* 1998, Pamuk *et al.* 1998, Williams 2001), Latin America (Pan American Health Organization 2001), South Africa (Sidiropoulos *et al.* 1997), Australia (McLennan and Madden 1999) and elsewhere (Polednak 1989).

In the UK, mortality data are not available by ethnic group. Country of birth is recorded on death certificates and mortality rates have been published by country of birth using data around the 1971, 1981 and 1991 Censuses. The most recent of these analyses is summarised in Table 1.8, which shows variation in mortality rates by

Table 1.8 Standardised mortality ratio by country of birth for those aged 20–64 years, England and Wales 1991–1993

	All causes		Coronary heart disease		Stroke		Respiratory disease		Lung cancer	
	Men	Wom.	Men	Wom.	Men	Wom.	Men	Wom.	Men	Wom.
Caribbean	89*	104	60*	100	169*	178*	80*	75	59*	32*
Indian sub-continent	107*	99	150*	175*	163*	132*	90	94	48*	34*
India	106*	–	140*	–	140*	–	93	–	43*	–
Pakistan	102	–	163*	–	148*	–	82	–	45*	–
Bangladesh	137*	–	184*	–	324*	–	104	–	92	–
East Africa	123*	127*	160*	130	113	110	154*	195*	35*	110
West/South Africa	126*	142*	83	69	315*	215*	138	101	71	69
Ireland	135*	115*	121*	129*	130*	118*	162*	134*	157*	143*

* $p < 0.05$.

Source: Office for National Statistics.

country of birth and gender. However, analysis of these data carries significant problems. First, and most obvious, it ignores the situation of ethnic minority people born in the UK, whose experiences might be quite different. Second, given forced migration patterns and the artificial construction of national borders after the 'fall' of the British Empire, country of birth groupings do not necessarily reflect ethnic groups (e.g. the heterogeneity of those born in South Asia or India, the large South Asian population who migrated to Britain from the Caribbean). Third, British colonial history means that a significant number of White people were born in ex-colonies and migrated back to Britain after the Second World War.

Although the UK does not have mortality data by ethnicity, there has been a growth in data on ethnic differences in morbidity over the last decade. Figure 1.2, drawn from the 1999 Health Survey for England (Erens *et al.* 2001), shows differences in self-reported health across ethnic groups. It charts the odds ratio and 95 per cent confidence intervals, in comparison with a White English group, for reporting health as fair or bad. Immediately obvious is the heterogeneity in experience across ethnic groups. Most notable is the wide variation for the three South Asian groups – Indian, Pakistani and Bangladeshi – who are typically treated as one and the same ethnic group in British data (e.g. McKeigue *et al.* 1988, Gupta *et al.* 1995). Again the diversity in health experience across ethnic minority groups in the UK is paralleled by differences in migration history, patterns of settlement in the UK and economic experiences, as illustrated earlier.

The data in Figure 1.2 are age-standardised, to deal with differences in age profiles shown earlier in Table 1.2. Figure 1.3 shows how ethnic differences in self-reported fair or bad health vary by age group. As expected, for each ethnic group there is an increase in the proportion reporting fair or bad health with age. Interestingly, the figure suggests that the ethnic differences at the youngest ages disappear in late childhood and early adulthood, and then re-emerge in the mid-20s, becoming very large by the mid-30s and continuing to grow with age. For the Bangladeshi people, the

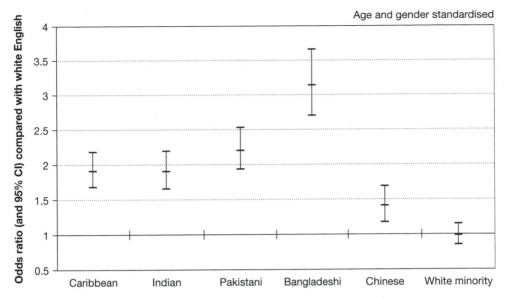

Figure 1.2 Ethnic differences in reported fair or bad general health in England.

Source: Health Survey for England 1999.

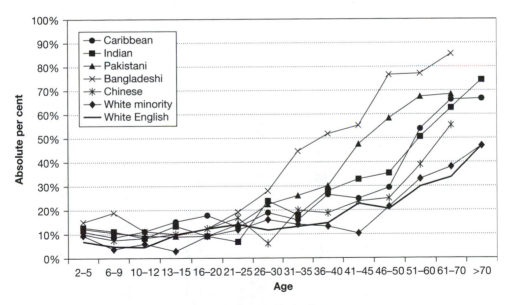

Figure 1.3 Fair/bad health by ethnic group and age in England.

Source: Health Survey for England 1999.

group with the poorest health, from the mid-40s onwards rates are around 50 per cent higher in absolute terms than those for White English people. How far these differences with age are a consequence of differences between cohorts, perhaps as a consequence of migration, or the accumulation of disadvantage with age, is uncertain (Nazroo 2004).

Socioeconomic inequalities in the ethnic patterning of health

Interestingly, the differences in Table 1.8, Figure 1.2 and Figure 1.3, mirror the inequalities in economic position shown in Tables 1.5 and 1.6. However, the factors underlying such differences remain contested. The significance of social determinants, particularly the social inequalities that ethnic minority groups face, remains the subject of considerable debate. Some claim that social and economic inequalities make a minimal, or no, contribution to ethnic inequalities in health (Wild and McKeigue 1997), others suggest that even if they do contribute, the cultural and genetic elements of ethnicity must also play a role (Smaje 1996), and others argue that ethnic inequalities in health are predominantly determined by socioeconomic inequalities (Navarro 1990, Sheldon and Parker 1992).

However, it now seems reasonably clear that a socioeconomic patterning of health is present within ethnic groups in industrialised countries. Figure 1.4 contains data from the Health Survey for England, showing rates of reporting fair or bad health by ethnicity with each of the ethnic groups stratified by income (equivalised tertiles) (Nazroo 2003). It shows a clear relationship between reported general health and

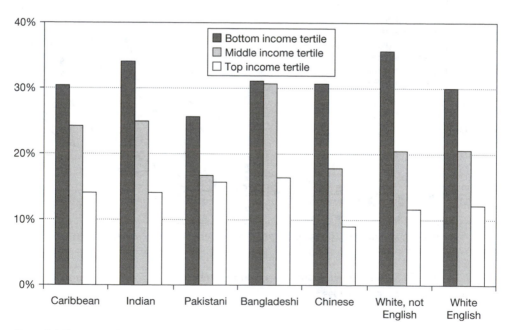

Figure 1.4 Reported fair or bad health by ethnic group and income tertile in England.
Source: Health Survey for England 1999.

economic position for each ethnic group. Important here is that, as for Figure 1.2, the data point to heterogeneity within broad ethnic groupings. It is misleading to consider, for example, Caribbean people to be uniformly disadvantaged in terms of their health; those in better socioeconomic positions have better health. There is nothing inevitable, or inherent, in the link between being Bangladeshi etc. and a greater risk of mortality and morbidity.

However, the figure also raises the possibility that socioeconomic effects do not explain ethnic inequalities in health. For example, Figure 1.4 shows that for the top and middle income groups those in the Bangladeshi group were more likely than those in the White English group to report fair or bad health. Although this might suggest that socioeconomic factors do not contribute to ethnic inequalities in health, it is important to recognise that the process of standardising for socioeconomic position when making comparisons across groups, particularly ethnic groups, is not as straightforward as it might at first sight seem. As Kaufman *et al.* (1997, 1998) point out, the process of standardisation is effectively an attempt to deal with the non-random nature of samples used in cross-sectional population studies – controlling for all relevant 'extraneous' explanatory factors introduces the *appearance* of randomisation. But, attempting to introduce randomisation into cross-sectional studies by adding 'controls' assumes that the available variables adequately capture all of the significant differences in socioeconomic profiles between ethnic group (see also the discussion of this point in Chapter 2). In fact, evidence from the British Fourth National Survey of Ethnic Minorities shows that this is not the case. The first part of Table 1.9 shows the mean equivalised household income for individuals within particular classes by ethnic group. Each ethnic group shows the expected income gradient by occupational class. However, when comparisons are drawn across ethnic groups, the table shows that within each occupational class Caribbean and Indian or African Asian people appear to have similar locations, while White people were better off than them and Pakistani or Bangladeshi people worse off than them. Indeed, comparing the White and Pakistani or Bangladeshi groups shows that within each occupational class band those in the Pakistani or Bangladeshi group had, on average, half the White income, and class I or II Pakistani or Bangladeshi people had an equivalent average income to class IV or V White people. This suggests that using a measure such as Registrar General's class to adjust for socioeconomic status is far

Table 1.9 Ethnic variations in income within occupational classes in England and Wales

	White	Indian or African Asian	Pakistani or Bangladeshi	Caribbean
Mean weekly income by Registrar General's class (£)*				
I/II	250	210	125	210
IIInm	185	135	95	145
IIIm	160	120	70	145
IV/V	130	110	65	120

* Based on bands of equivalised household income. The mean point of each band is used to make this calculation, which is rounded to the nearest 5.

Source: Fourth National Survey of Ethnic Minorities.

from adequate for comparisons across ethnic groups, even if this indicator does reflect socioeconomic differences within ethnic groups.

The overall conclusion, then, is that using single or crude indicators of socio-economic position is of little use for 'controlling out' the impact of socioeconomic position when attempting to reveal the extent of a 'non-socioeconomic' ethnic/race effect. Within any given level of a particular socioeconomic indicator the social circumstances of ethnic minority people are less favourable than those of White people. This leads to two related problems with approaches that attempt to adjust for socioeconomic effects when making comparisons across ethnic groups. The first is that if socioeconomic position is simply regarded as a confounding factor that needs to be controlled out to reveal the 'true' relationship between ethnicity and health, data will be presented and interpreted once controls have been applied. This will result in the impact of socioeconomic factors becoming obscured and their explana-tory role in determining the health of ethnic minority people will be lost. The second is that the presentation of 'standardised' data allows the problems with such data, outlined by Kaufman *et al.* (1997 and 1998) and Nazroo (1997a and 1998) and illus-trated by Table 1.9, to be ignored, leaving both the author and reader to assume that all that is left is an 'ethnic/race' effect, be that cultural or genetic. Nevertheless, if these cautions are considered there are some benefits in attempting to control for socioeconomic effects. In particular, if controlling for socioeconomic effects alters the pattern of ethnic inequalities in health, despite the limitations of the indicators used, we can conclude that at least a part of the differences we have uncovered are a result of a socioeconomic effect.

These conclusions are supported by Figure 1.5, which uses data from the 1999 Health Survey for England to show changes in the odds of reporting fair or bad health for ethnic minority groups compared with White English people before and after the data had been standardised for a variety of socioeconomic factors. Comparing the adjusted and unadjusted figures shows a clear and large reduction in odds ratios for most ethnic groups (to give an accurate visual impression of the size of the change in odds, the natural logarithm of the odds ratio compared with White English people is used). Exceptions are the White minority (predominantly Irish) and Indian groups. This impression is strengthened if the process is repeated across outcomes, as has been shown using data from the British Fourth National Survey (Nazroo 2001, 2003).

The significance of socioeconomic effects is illustrated by analysis presented by Davey Smith *et al.* (1998) of US mortality data. They show that standardising for mean household income in area of residence reduces the relative risk for Black compared with White men for all causes of mortality from 1.47 to 1.19. Conversely, adjusting the Black–White mortality differential for a number of medical risk factors – diastolic blood pressure, serum cholesterol, cigarette smoking, existing diabetes and prior hospitalisation for coronary heart disease – only decreased the relative risk from 1.47 to 1.40. This demonstrates that socioeconomic position – as indexed by income of area of residence in this case – is a considerably more important determinant of Black–White differentials in mortality than biological markers of risk and behavioural factors, such as cigarette smoking or diet (to the extent to which the diet influences serum cholesterol and blood pressure).

Of course such analyses do not account for another element of social disadvan-tage experienced by ethnic minority people, racial discrimination and harassment.

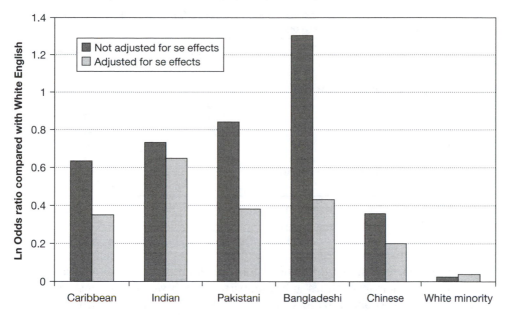

Figure 1.5 Reduction in (Ln) odds ratio of reporting fair or bad health compared with White English after adjusting for socioeconomic effects.

Source: Health Survey for England 1999.

In the few studies that have been conducted, experiences of racial harassment and discrimination appear to be related to health. Laboratory studies reveal that experiences of discrimination are stressful and produce acute physiological effects (Harrell *et al.* 2003, Clark *et al.* 1999). Population-based studies from the US and elsewhere have shown a relationship between self-reported experiences of racial harassment and a range of health outcomes, including hypertension, psychological distress, psychiatric disorders, poorer self-rated health and days spent unwell in bed (Krieger 2000, Williams and Neighbors 2001, Williams *et al.* 2003). In the UK, analyses of the Fourth National Survey of Ethnic Minorities also suggested a relationship between experiences of racial harassment, perceptions of racial discrimination and a range of health outcomes across ethnic groups (Karlsen and Nazroo 2002a, 2002b). Table 1.10, drawn from these analyses, shows that reporting experiences of racial harassment and perceiving employers to discriminate against ethnic minority people are independently related to likelihood of reporting fair or poor health, and that this relationship is independent of socioeconomic effects. Elsewhere, it has also been shown that fear of racism per se also increases risk of reporting fair or poor health by about 60 per cent after adjustments for age, gender and class (Karlsen and Nazroo 2004). It may be that these findings represent three dimensions of social and economic inequality operating simultaneously: economic disadvantage (as measured by occupational class), a sense of being a member of a devalued, low status, group (British employers discriminate, fear of racism), and the personal insult and stress of being a victim or potential victim of racial harassment.

Table 1.10 Racial harassment, racial discrimination and risk of fair or poor health in England and Wales (all ethnic minority groups)

	Odds ratio*	95% confidence intervals
Experience of racial harassment		
No attack	1.00	–
Verbal abuse	1.54	1.07–2.21
Physical attack	2.07	1.14–3.76
Perception of discrimination		
Fewer than half of employers discriminate	1.00	–
Most employers discriminate	1.39	1.10–1.76

* Adjusted for gender, age and occupational class.

Source: Fourth National Survey of Ethnic Minorities.

So, these data suggest that differences in social and economic position make a key contribution to ethnic inequalities in health, particularly if we take seriously Kaufman *et al.*'s (1997, 1998) and Nazroo's (1997a, 1998) cautions on the difficulties with making effective adjustments for socioeconomic inequalities. It is also worth emphasising that the analyses shown here simply reflect current socioeconomic position, data on the life-course and data on other forms of social disadvantage were not included and are almost universally not available in existing studies of ethnic inequalities in health, although some resources, such as the Millennium Birth cohort and the ONS longitudinal study, are being developed in the UK.

Conclusion

This chapter has detailed the ethnic composition of the UK population and differences in the demographic profiles, social and economic position, and health of ethnic groups. A key point to bear in mind, which is also relevant in other country contexts, is the great heterogeneity within and across ethnic groups. This is relevant to the ethnic categories that we typically use in analysis and policy development, which combine diverse ethnic groups and perhaps merit more thought and some disaggregation. And it points to the need to consider differences in age, family and household structure, geographical location, economic position, etc. when considering data on ethnic differences and policy responses to inequality. Most important is the extent of socioeconomic inequality across ethnic groups, and the difficulty of dealing with this in our analyses. In many studies socioeconomic data are either not collected at all, or collected at very crude levels that are plainly inadequate for drawing comparisons across ethnic groups. The evidence presented here shows the importance of collecting high quality information on economic, social and demographic characteristics when conducting research on ethnic differences in health and social outcomes.

References

Bajekal, M., Blane, D., Grewal, I. *et al.* (2004) 'Ethnic differences in influences on quality of life at older ages: a quantitative analysis', *Ageing and Society*, 24(5): 709–728.

Chahal, K. and Julienne, L. (1999) *"We Can't all be White!": racist victimisation in the UK*, London: YPS.

Clark, R., Anderson, N.B., Clark, V.R. and Williams, D.R. (1999) 'Racism as a stressor for African Americans: a biopsychosocial model', *American Psychologist*, 54: 805–816.

Davey Smith, G., Neaton, J.D., Wentworth, D. *et al.* (1998) 'Mortality differences between black and white men in the USA: contribution of income and other risk factors among men screened for the MRFIT', *The Lancet*, 351: 934–939.

Department of Health and Human Services (1985) *Report of the Secretary on Black and Minority Health*, Washington, DC: US Department of Health.

Erens, B., Primatesta, P. and Prior, G. (eds) (2001) *Health Survey for England: the health of minority ethnic groups 1999, (Volume 1: Findings, Volume 2: Methodology and Documentation)*, London: The Stationery Office.

Grewal, I., Nazroo, J., Bajekal, M. *et al.* (2004) 'Influences on quality of life: a qualitative investigation of ethnic differences among older people in England', *Journal of Ethnic and Migration Studies*, 30: 737–761.

Gupta, S., de Belder, A. and O'Hughes, L. (1995) 'Avoiding premature coronary deaths in Asians in Britain: spend now on prevention or pay later for treatment', *British Medical Journal*, 311: 1035–1036.

Harding, S. and Maxwell, R. (1997) 'Differences in the mortality of migrants', in F. Drever and M. Whitehead (eds) *Health Inequalities: decennial supplement series DS no. 15*, London: The Stationery Office.

Harrell, J., Hall, S. and Taliaferro, J. (2003) 'Physiological responses to racism and discrimination: an assessment of the evidence', *American Journal of Public Health*, 93: 243–248.

Karlsen, S. and Nazroo, J.Y. (2002a) 'The relationship between racial discrimination, social class and health among ethnic minority groups', *American Journal of Public Health*, 92: 624–631.

Karlsen, S. and Nazroo, J.Y. (2002b) 'Agency and structure: the impact of ethnic identity and racism in the health of ethnic minority people', *Sociology of Health and Illness*, 24: 1–20.

Karlsen, S. and Nazroo, J.Y. (2004) 'Fear of racism and health', *Journal of Epidemiology and Community Health*, 58: 1017–1018.

Karlsen, S., Nazroo, J.Y. and Stephenson, R. (2002) 'Ethnicity, environment and health: putting ethnic inequalities in health in their place', *Social Science and Medicine*, 55: 1647–1661.

Kaufman, J.S., Cooper, R.S. and McGee, D.L. (1997) 'Socioeconomic status and health in blacks and whites: the problem of residual confounding and the resiliency of race', *Epidemiology*, 8: 621–628.

Kaufman, J.S., Long, A.E., Liao, Y., *et al.* (1998) 'The relation between income and mortality in U.S. Blacks and Whites', *Epidemiology*, 9: 147–155.

Krieger, N. (2000) 'Discrimination and Health', in L. Berkman and I. Kawachi (eds) *Social Epidemiology*, Oxford: Oxford University Press, pp. 36–75.

Krieger, N. and Sidney, S. (1996) 'Racial discrimination and blood pressure: the CARDIA study of young black and white adults', *American Journal of Public Health*, 86: 1370–1378.

Krieger, N., Rowley, D.L., Herman, A.A. *et al.* (1993) 'Racism, sexism, and social class: implications for studies of health, disease, and well-being', *American Journal of Preventive Medicine*, 9 (suppl): 82–122.

McKeigue, P., Marmot, M., Syndercombe Court, Y. *et al.* (1988) 'Diabetes, hyperinsulinaemia, and coronary risk factors in Bangladeshis in East London', *British Heart Journal*, 60: 390–396.

McLennan, W. and Madden, R. (1999) *The Health and Welfare of Australia's Aboriginal and Torres Strait Islander Peoples*, Commonwealth of Australia: Australian Bureau of Statistics.

Marmot, M.G., Adelstein, A.M., Bulusu, L. and OPCS (1984) *Immigrant Mortality in England and Wales 1970–78: causes of death by country of birth*, London: HMSO.

Mason, D. (2003) *Explaining Ethnic Differences: changing patterns of disadvantage in Britain*, Bristol: The Policy Press.

Miles, R. (1982) *Racism and Migrant Labour*, Routledge & Kegan Paul.

Modood, T. (1997) 'Employment', in T. Modood, R. Berthoud, J. Lakey *et al.*, *Ethnic Minorities in Britain: diversity and disadvantage*, London: Policy Studies Institute.

Modood, T., Berthoud, R., Lakey, J. *et al.* (1997) *Ethnic Minorities in Britain: diversity and disadvantage*, PSI Report 843, London: Policy Studies Institute.

Navarro, V. (1990) 'Race or class versus race and class: mortality differentials in the United States', *The Lancet*, 336: 1238–1240.

Nazroo, J.Y. (1997a) *The Health of Britain's Ethnic Minorities: findings from a national survey*, London: Policy Studies Institute.

Nazroo, J.Y. (1997b) *Ethnicity and Mental Health: findings from a national community survey*, London: Policy Studies Institute.

Nazroo, J.Y. (1998) 'Genetic, cultural or socio-economic vulnerability? Explaining ethnic inequalities in health', *Sociology of Health and Illness*, 20: 710–730.

Nazroo, J.Y. (2001) *Ethnicity, Class and Health*, London: Policy Studies Institute.

Nazroo, J.Y. (2003) 'The structuring of ethnic inequalities in health: economic position, racial discrimination and racism', *American Journal of Public Health*, 93: 277–284.

Nazroo, J. (2004) 'Ethnic disparities in aging health: what can we learn from the United Kingdom?' in N. Anderson, R. Bulatao and B. Cohen (eds) *Critical Perspectives on Racial and Ethnic Differentials in Health in Late Life*, Washington, DC: National Academies Press, 677–702.

Owen, D. (1992) *Ethnic Minorities in Great Britain: settlement patterns, National Ethnic Minority Data Archive 1991 Census Statistical Paper No. 1*, Centre for Research in Ethnic Relations University of Warwick.

Owen, D. (1994) 'Spatial variations in ethnic minority groups populations in Great Britain', *Population Trends*, 78: 23–33.

Owen, D. (2003) 'The demographic characteristics of people from minority ethnic groups in Britain', in D. Mason (ed.) *Explaining Ethnic Differences: changing patterns of disadvantage in Britain*, Bristol: The Policy Press, pp. 21–52.

Pamuk, E., Makuc, D., Heck, K. *et al.* (1998) *Socioeconomic Status and Health Chartbook. Health, United States*, Hyattsville, MD: National Center for Health Statistics.

Pan American Health Organization (June 2001) *Equity in Health: from an ethnic perspective*, Washington, DC.

Polednak, P. (1989) *Racial and Ethnic Differences in Disease*, New York: Oxford University Press.

Rogers, R. (1992) 'Living and dying in the USA: sociodemographic determinants of death among blacks and whites', *Demography*, 29: 287–303.

Rogot, E., Sorlie, P.D., Johnson, N.J. and Schmitt, C. (1993) *A Mortality Study of 1.3 million Persons by Demographic, Social and Economic Factors: 1979–1985. Follow-up, US national longitudinal mortality study*, Washington, DC: NIH.

Rudat, K. (1994) *Black and Minority Ethnic Groups in England: health and lifestyles*, London: Health Education Authority.

Salt, J. (1996) 'Immigration and ethnic group', in D. Colman and J. Salt (eds) *Ethnicity in the 1991 Census. Volume One: demographic characteristics of the ethnic minority populations*, London: The Stationery Office, pp. 124–150.

Sheldon, T.A. and Parker, H. (1992) 'Race and ethnicity in health research', *Journal of Public Health Medicine*, 14: 104–110.

Sidiropoulos, E., Jeffery, A., Mackay, S. *et al.* (1997) *South Africa Survey 1996/97*, Johannesburg: South African Institute of Race Relations.

Smaje, C. (1996) 'The ethnic patterning of health: new directions for theory and research', *Sociology of Health and Illness*, 18: 139–171.

Sorlie, P.D., Backlund, E. and Keller, J. (1995) 'U.S. mortality by economic, demographic and social characteristics: the National Longitudinal Mortality Study', *American Journal of Public Health*, 85: 949–956.

Sorlie, P., Rogot, E., Anderson, R. *et al.* (1992) 'Black-white mortality differences by family income', *Lancet*, 340: 346–350.

Virdee S. (1995) *Racial Violence and Harassment*, London: Policy Studies Institute.

Virdee, S. (1997) 'Racial Harassment', in T. Modood, R. Berthoud, J. Lakey *et al.*, *Ethnic Minorities in Britain: diversity and disadvantage*, London: Policy Studies Institute.

Wild, S. and McKeigue, P. (1997) 'Cross sectional analysis of mortality by country of birth in England and Wales', *British Medical Journal*, 314: 705–710.

Williams, D.R. (2001) 'Racial variations in adult health status: patterns, paradoxes and prospects', in N.J. Smelser, W.J. Wilson and F. Mitchell (eds) *America Becoming: racial trends and their consequences*, Washington, DC: National Academy Press.

Williams, D.R. and Neighbors, H.W. (2001) 'Racism, discrimination and hypertension: evidence and needed research', *Ethnicity* and *Disease*, 11: 800–816.

Williams, D.R., Neighbors, H.W. and Jackson, J.S. (2003) 'Racial/ethnic discrimination and health: findings from community studies', *American Journal of Public Health*, 93: 200–208.

Chapter 2

Defining and measuring ethnicity and 'race'

Theoretical and conceptual issues for health and social care research

Saffron Karlsen and James Y. Nazroo

Introduction

> *The choice of an analytical perspective or 'research hypothesis' is not an innocent act. If one goes out to look for ethnicity, one will 'find' it and thereby contribute to constructing it.*
>
> (Eriksen 2002: 177)

The exploration of ethnicity and 'race' raises a number of definitional and measurement issues about what 'ethnicity' and 'race' are, how they relate to each other and how they relate to wider social and economic circumstances and experiences. In particular, there are debates as to how far the characteristics ascribed to particular 'ethnic'/'race' groups signify group differences in innate biological or genetic ability, culture, social and economic power, or a combination of these, and even how far these may be considered 'groups' at all. This chapter seeks to explore the range of approaches to the definition of 'ethnicity', the theories underpinning them and their implications for measurement, analysis and interpretation.

As the quote above suggests, there are a number of different ways of 'finding', or constructing, ethnicity, and each will have different consequences for the research undertaken, the conclusions drawn and, ultimately, for those under study (as well as those who are not). Research findings may directly influence attitudes towards members of ethnic minority (and majority) groups. The policy implications of identifying a genetic/biological or behavioural basis for the differences we see are, for example, very different from those where ethnic inequality is identified as a consequence of the limited opportunities following on from ethnic or racial disadvantage. Our view of 'ethnicity' may, then, directly influence the extent to which this disadvantage continues. We have a responsibility, therefore, to be thoughtful and thorough in our approaches to research.

A starting point must be to acknowledge the socially contingent nature of ethnicity. By this we mean both that ethnicity is strongly related to social circumstances and economic position, in both developed and less developed countries, and that the significance of one's ethnicity is a consequence of how ethnic signification reflects and influences social relationships between groups and individuals. It is common in health research for genetic factors or a stereotyped culture to be alluded to as causally import-ant once potential economic and social 'confounders' have been statistically controlled for (Marmot, Adelstein and Bulusu 1984, Harding and Maxwell 1997). But the com-plex social and contingent nature of ethnicity and ethnic relations means that the social and economic inequalities faced by people from ethnic minority groups cannot be fully captured by the simple measures of, for example, socioeconomic position that are used in health research, such as class or education. The assignment of residual effects in a statistical model to unmeasured factors, such as cultural or genetic effects, is, there-fore, even more unjustified than usual (Kaufman *et al.* 1997, 1998, Nazroo 1998, 2001).

There are also aspects of the relationship between ethnicity, social position and health that are generally ignored in empirical health research. In particular, measures of social position often fail to account for the accumulation of disadvantage over the life course – measuring socioeconomic status only at one time point – and they typi-cally ignore the role of ecological effects resulting from the concentration of ethnic minority groups in particular residential areas. Perhaps surprisingly, the effects of racism on social identity, social status and economic position are also often ignored (Bonilla-Silva and Baiocchi 2001). As a consequence, the investigation of the way in which social and economic disadvantage may structure the experiences of different ethnic groups has remained relatively superficial (Nazroo 2003).

As this brief introduction to the complexity of the meaning of ethnicity suggests, producing meaningful data and analyses of ethnicity in health and social research requires a careful consideration of conceptual issues. There are a range of concepts that are of potential relevance to those conducting research on ethnicity and health and social issues, something to which we now turn. We will later discuss how these concepts might be operationalised.

Concepts

'Ethnicity'

According to Weber (1922) and others, the concept of *ethnicity*, and an *ethnic group*, implies:

- members of a group, which in turn requires recognition of who is, and who is not a member of that group; a categorisation which may be defined by personal choice by 'members' of that group (internally) and/or by an external audience;
- the establishment of a common identity on the part of group members; and
- the development of perceived stereotypes related to that group which are imposed on them by other (external) social groups.

Bolaffi *et al.* state that: 'it is preferable not to refer the concept of ethnicity to stable groups, but to groups which share certain economic, social, cultural and religious characteristics at a given moment in time' (2003: 94). An ethnic group should not, then, be seen as something static, or grounded in anything as inflexible as particular genes or historical or linguistic ancestry, although the common identity *may* be expressed as such. People *choose* what characteristics with which to define themselves, which may or may not have recourse to ideas of colour, language, history or ancestry.

> The features that are taken into account are not the sum of 'objective' differences, but only those which the actors themselves regard as significant ... some cultural features are used by the actors as signals and emblems of differences, others are ignored, and in some relationships radical differences are played down and denied.
>
> (Barth 1969: 14)

But, as Weber (1922) argues, such choices are also influenced by the stereotypes that other social groups impose and by the (ethnic and other) group identities of those around them (Smaje 1996, Gilroy 1987). The experience of being a member of any particular ethnic group will also be affected by an individual's other social identities (relating to gender, age, social class etc.); being 'African American' may mean different things to young African American males than to older African American females, for example. And these definitions will also change over time and circumstance.

Ethnic groups, then, rather than being definitive, timeless entities existing independent of the world around them, are entirely historically and spatially located, defined from the outside as well as within. Considering, and therefore exploring, them as if they were otherwise is, therefore, potentially meaningless. The process of ethnic identification is a means of defining yourself as part of an 'us' in opposition to a 'them', or an 'other'. An ethnic 'minority', obviously, requires an ethnic 'majority', even if that ethnic majority has sufficient power to ignore the ethnic dimension to its associations. Being 'White' is as much a definition of ethnicity as being 'non-White'. But ethnic affiliations are mobilised in response to a particular need (for social integration or economic support, for example) which may be considered more apparent in certain (particularly threatening) circumstances, situations that are likely to occur more frequently among 'minority'/less powerful groups. And differing circumstances may promote the mobilisation of different forms of 'ethnic' identification. Indeed, individuals may define themselves as 'Black' in some circumstances, 'British', (south) 'Asian', 'Bangladeshi' and 'Sylheti' in others (or as 'female', 'young' or 'old'), depending on the criteria considered salient. This creates obvious problems for the collection of meaningful quantitative single-response data to ethnically categorise participants in research.

'Race' and the evolution of ideas of 'racial difference'

In contrast to an understanding of *ethnicity* which might contain elements of a chosen cultural identity, the concept of *race* may be considered to be more externally motivated, stemming more from the apparent need of human beings to categorise, identify and control others than the need to form inclusive social groups. To an extent, the concepts of 'ethnicity' and 'race' are similar; both require the maintenance of group boundaries/identification based on perceived similarities between members of a group. However, 'race', rather than ethnicity, places emphasis on the process of stereotyping/exclusion by others, a process that inherently contains a judgement of value.

In much the same way as members of an ethnic group are 'free' to choose that with which they identify themselves, the characteristics emphasised in racial stereotyping are opportunistic; their wider significance, mythical. As discussed above, Weber's (1922) definition of ethnic groups allows for the imposition of stereotypes by an external 'other'. While a role for power is not necessary to a definition of ethnicity, though, the concept of 'race' is in some senses dependent on the ability of certain social groups to exploit science, the media and education to promote stereotypes relating to the 'natural' inferiority of certain social groups compared with others, which become perceived as 'common sense', 'rational' and therefore unquestioned attitudes regarding differences between them. Not only for those who may potentially gain from such negative stereotyping, but also potentially among those whom they stereotype. Research suggests that the negative stereotyping of a 'racial' group has a significant effect on the self-perceptions of people considered (by themselves and others) part of that group. Further, being a victim of racist stereotyping has been found to be one dimension along which people may define their 'ethnic identity' (Nazroo and Karlsen 2003, Karlsen 2004). Discrimination on the grounds of 'race', then, provides us with a more convincing explanation for the persistence of inequalities between different ethnic/'racial' groups, than that based on ethnicity (Omi and Winant 1994). The continued assumption that 'race' has a clear, unambiguous, neutral and meaningful definition stems from this desire to categorise: the particular reasons for the pervasiveness of these ideas requires an exploration of early interactions between 'Europeans' and non-Europeans.

The idea of the existence of distinct 'races' was used from the sixteenth and seventeenth centuries, to explain the appearance and behaviour of the (supposedly) 'uncivilised' and 'immoral' people 'discovered' by early European explorers. Colour symbolism – where white was seen to be associated with all things good, and black, all things undesirable – had been evident at least since medieval times. This symbolism was exaggerated further, 'Blackness' coming to be associated with an inversion of everything European, Christian and civilised (Jordan 1982).

> The Europeans who travelled in pursuit . . . of trade, military advantage, religious mission and curiosity carried with them expectations about what and whom they might meet . . . A negative representation of the Other . . . [which] served to define and legitimate what was considered to be the positive qualities of the author and reader.
>
> (Miles 1989: 20–21)

During the sixteenth century, 'race' was perceived of as a consequence of lineage or descent, rather than biology, with differences a product of ignorance rather than inability; an idea that prompted the 'civilising mission' of Christianity from Europe around this time. From the end of the eighteenth century, however, ideas of the basis of perceived ethnic or racial differences became increasingly narrow and precise. Phrenology brought arguments that such differences were innate and that, in fact, certain 'races' could not be 'civilised' due to their limited brain capacity. Certain groups were argued to be inherently more suited to carrying out certain tasks, such as heavy labour, an argument used to justify the systems of slavery that had been introduced to exploit the natural resources available in the newly 'discovered' colonies.

So, the beginning of the nineteenth century saw a growing acceptance of science and its ability to explain the basis of nature and society. Ideas of biological determinism, which saw differences between human beings as natural and unchangeable, rather than environmental and therefore adaptable, became increasingly popular. Human beings were argued to be a species made up of a number of races of differing capacity and temperament – recognisable by group differences in appearance (phenotype). Western Europeans identified a 'great chain of being' (Miles 1989) that organised the different groups they recognised into a supposedly biological hierarchy, with White people from western Europe (with a few exceptions (Curtis 1968, 1971, Mosse 1978)) at the top.

> Before the slave trade in Africa there was neither a Europe nor a European. Finally, with the European arose the myth of European superiority and separate existence as a special species or 'race' . . . the particular myth that there was a creature called a European which implied, from the beginning, a 'white' man.
>
> (Jaffe 1985: 46)

It followed that people could only be understood in the light of their 'racial' characteristics, which 'explained' why some groups were naturally inferior to others. In essence, though, as mentioned above, rather than being based on any scientific fact, these arguments were part of an ideological process to justify the exploitation of the less powerful by the more powerful, both by the colonial empires (both before and after the abolition of slavery) and in Nazi Germany, Apartheid South Africa, post-slavery southern USA and elsewhere.

In research terms, though, attempts to use scientific, particularly genetic, exploration to lend support to the existence of systematic relationships between phenotype and behaviour have proved unproductive. As Krieger puts it: 'the fact that we know what "race" we are says more about our society than it does our biology' (2003: 195). Sadly, this has not always meant an end to the prejudice that such arguments have justified.

Nation

Arguments about inherent 'racial' differences also played a central role in the creation of conceptions of *national* origin during the twentieth century, and still do today (Miles 1989, CCCS 1982). Labour shortages in Western Europe between the 1940s and 1970s saw the development of a contract migrant worker system that encouraged workers from Africa, the Caribbean and Asia to move to the UK for employment. But this migration was met with concern regarding a potential disruption of 'national unity'. However, rather than returning to the biological or cultural superiority/ inferiority arguments of previous centuries, the 1960s and 1970s saw the development of ideas suggesting that it is 'natural' for people to live among their 'own kind' and that, as a result, discrimination towards migrants – those not of this 'common community' – was to be expected (Barker 1981). The British Conservative politician Enoch Powell, for example, was concerned with the destruction of cultural homogeneity caused by the influx of immigrants. British Prime Minister Margaret Thatcher also voiced concern regarding the potential for immigrants to 'swamp' the culture of England's 'own people'. So while nations were not explicitly seen to be hierarchical, they were argued to be natural and the promotion of ethnic boundaries was therefore unavoidable (Miles 1989). It has been argued more recently that the supposed need for the 'dispersal' of asylum-seekers arriving in the UK at the turn of the twenty-first century, as promoted by the British Labour government under Tony Blair, is similarly motivated by ideas relating to the existence of a 'threshold of tolerance' of 'outsiders' among 'British' people (Kundnani 2000).

In as far as a *nation* indicates a geographically based community, it may be seen simply as a particular form of ethnic group. It is described as having a collective name, a common myth of descent, a distinctive shared culture and a sense of solidarity, as well as an association with a specific territory (Smith 1986). Defining a nation is as problematic as defining an ethnic group, and the idea of the existence of a national character, or *folk*, is as potentially ethnocentric and racist as ideas of racial difference. In essence, the promotion of ideas of who is (and who is not) part of a nation can be considered one of a number of examples of the 'rebranding' of racist motivations into more acceptable forms. Lack of access to resources, mistrust and mistreatment can be justified along national, as well as 'biological' lines, and minority groups can continue to be associated, and blamed, for unwanted social change, or for any lack of resources among those seen to be more 'entitled' (Miles 1989, Eriksen 1993). People who wish to continue to hold a xenophobic standpoint can do so without feeling obliged to also label themselves *racist*.

Race relations and racialisation

This blaming of ethnic minority, or migrant, groups for unwanted social change, increased social tension/reduced social stability and economic (housing, employment etc.) shortage, where 'racial' meanings are attached to non-racial social relations, is termed *racialisation*. This concept is used by authors wishing to discuss *race relations* – relations between different racialised groups – while emphasising the socially constructed nature of 'race'. Racialisation allows a refocus of social problems from those of inadequate supply to those of demand and is the principal justification for racist discourse by individuals, social organisations, political parties and governments today, such as the supposed need to control immigration, which has tended to employ an ethnically/'race'-specific focus to related policies and panic.

Racism, racial discrimination and racial harassment

> The distinguishing content of *racism* as an ideology is, first, its signification of some biological characteristic(s) as the criterion by which a collectivity may be identified. In this way the collectivity is represented as having a natural, unchanging origin and status, and therefore being inherently different. . . . Second, the group so identified must be attributed with additional, negatively evaluated [biological or cultural] characteristics and/or must be represented as inducing negative consequences for any other . . . it is represented ideologically as a threat.
>
> (Miles 1989: 79)

The unequal treatment or exploitation of social groups stemming from the racialisation of a social relationship, with its associated assumptions of the inherent superiority/inferiority of different social groups, is described as *racial discrimination*:

> . . . institutions and individual practices that create and reinforce oppressive systems of race relations whereby people and institutions engaging in discrimination

adversely restrict, by judgement and action, the lives of those against whom they discriminate.

(Krieger 2003: 195)

Racial discrimination is often, particularly in the UK, assumed to refer solely to the exclusion of non-White, by White, groups; largely in response to the negative treatment of Black and Asian groups migrating to the UK during the second half of the twentieth century. In reality, though, White migrants have also been, and still are (Fekete 2001, Hickman and Walter 1997), victims of racial discrimination and, as such, a broader focus is often taken when using this term.

Racial discrimination is sometimes divided into intentional (or direct) and unintentional (or indirect) discrimination (Krieger 2000). Direct discrimination occurs when someone is treated unequally as a consequence of his/her 'racial group'. Indirect discrimination occurs when a person is either unable to comply with a requirement that cannot be justified on other than racial grounds, or is less likely to be able to do so compared with people from other 'racial groups'. In this way, it is possible for someone who is non-prejudiced to be discriminatory, often as a consequence of *institutional racism*. Institutional racism refers to the continued adherence of large-scale enterprises to racially discriminatory policies, assumptions, or procedures, without consideration of how they may disadvantage certain 'racial groups' (Macpherson 1999).

Racial harassment is often used to denote demeaning, derogatory, threatening, violent, or other forms of offensive racially motivated behaviour, by individuals from one ethnic group towards those of another. Research suggests that simply the awareness of such behaviour may affect ethnic minority communities, regardless of the actual experience (Karlsen and Nazroo 2004, Virdee 1995, 1997, Chahal and Julienne 1999), and partly as a consequence of a failure to condemn such behaviour by the wider community (including institutions with a responsibility to deal with complaints of victimisation) (Sibbitt 1997, Virdee 1995). Racial harassment and institutional racism are not, as this would suggest, unrelated experiences.

The individual acts of bias and interpersonal discrimination that grow out of racism represent its latter-day, or surface (Williams 1997: 328), manifestations. They are salt in wounds previously inflicted by a host of negative life events whose relationship to racism is often cloaked. Indeed, it is likely that, at the point at which people encounter these individual forms of racism, other racist forces already have encroached on their lives.

(Harrell *et al.* 2003: 243)

A large body of research has shown discrimination and harassment to occur in almost every facet of public and private life – from the 'daily hassles' experienced when going about your normal life, to major events, such as being the victim of a racist physical attack. For example, there is widespread evidence of intolerance towards immigrants and asylum seekers and the United Nations Committee on Racial Discrimination has severely criticised race-relations in the UK (United Nations 2000). Responses to the British Social Attitudes surveys suggest that between a quarter and two-fifths of people in the UK are racially prejudiced (Rothon and Heath 2003). But this is not a problem only apparent in the UK. Oakley concludes that: 'there is prima facie (if often anecdotal) evidence that racial violence and harassment occur in all countries of Europe in which visible minorities of post-war immigrant origin are settled' (Oakley 1992: 40).

This can be seen in the growth of far-right electoral parties across some countries of Europe during the 1990s, particularly France, Italy, Belgium, Germany, the Netherlands and some parts of Eastern Europe (Oakley 1992, Bjorgo and Witte 1993). Similarly, 80 per cent of Black respondents to a US study reported having experienced racial discrimination at some time in their lives (Krieger and Sidney 1996). Such experiences of racism and discrimination have been shown to be associated with poor health outcomes (Brown *et al.* 2000, Karlsen and Nazroo 2002, 2004, Krieger 2000, 2003), and are considered to account for at least part of the socioeconomic disadvantage in which many people from ethnic minority groups are situated (Krieger 2000, Nazroo 1998, 2001).

Implications for measurement

The discussion of the complex and contextual nature of ethnicity, and the range of concepts that might be relevant to research in a multiethnic society, has implications for measurement. First, it highlights the need to think carefully about the historical and social context within which the research is conducted. Second, it indicates that researchers need to be clear about the theoretical basis of their research; which dimensions of ethnicity, 'race' and ethnic relations might be relevant to the research questions that they are addressing. Finally, how might these dimensions be operationalised, or empirically covered, in the research, rather than being simply assumed? Below, we briefly introduce some of the dimensions that might be operationalised in research, and indicate how this has been done in existing research.

The need to classify participants in research

A starting point is the need to code respondents into ethnic categories. Although this process might seem straightforward, there exist a number of pitfalls in relation to this. Researchers may, for example, use broad categories that do not reflect the specific groups they study (for example, studies of 'South Asians' in Tower Hamlets when the dominant South Asian group is Bangladeshi), or invent labels that reflect only one specific domain (or ethnic marker) of those under study (for example, studies of 'Urdus', used to describe people whose primary language is Urdu). Several papers have been written on this topic in relation to health research and these all contain useful advice (Bhopal 1997, Bradby 1995, 2003, McKenzie and Crowcroft 1994, 1996, Senior and Bhopal 1994). But, perhaps the best advice is to start with an official category, such as that used in the Census, or in government surveys. As discussed in Chapter 8, using an 'official' classification offers a number of benefits, most notably standardisation across surveys, or other data sources, which can then be compared with each other. In addition, considerable time will have been devoted to ensure that such questions reflect the population profile. In England and Wales, the 2001 Census used the question in Box 2.1 to identify the ethnic profile of the population.

Respondents are expected to first select the main category that applies to them (the bold items: White, Mixed, Asian or Asian British, Black or Black British, Chinese or other ethnic group), and then to choose from the subcategories. It is immediately obvious that such a categorisation reflects a number of aspects of ethnicity (nationality,

---

Box 2.1 England 2001 Census question on ethnicity

What is your ethnic group? Choose ONE section from A to E, then tick the appropriate box to indicate your ethnic group.

A White

British

Irish

Any other White background, please write in _____

B Mixed

White and Black Caribbean

White and Black African

White and Asian

Any other Mixed background, please write in _____

C Asian or Asian British

Indian

Pakistani

Bangladeshi

Any other Asian background, please write in _____

D Black or Black British

Caribbean

African

Any other Black background, please write in _____

E Chinese or other ethnic group

Chinese

Any other, please write in _____

---

country of birth, geographical origin, skin colour). And that it contains compromises, for example all individuals from sub-Saharan Africa are covered by a single category. This highlights the need for some studies to use more detailed classifications to reflect the population in the locality under study. So, while people from Somalia might not be a large enough group to warrant their inclusion as a category in the 2001 Census, a local study in East London, where they make up a significant part of the ethnic minority community, might include such a category.

The other, perhaps obvious, issue with such classifications is that they are simply that, means of classifying the population under study. They do not in themselves carry explanation, despite a common assumption that they directly reflect economic, genetic or cultural risk. These issues need to be explored separately. One way forward is to include more 'objective' measures of cultural origins or migration history. Simple questions can be asked around family origins, as in the Fourth National Survey of Ethnic Minorities (FNS) (Modood *et al.* 1997). Similarly, respondents to the National Survey of American Life (NSAL) (Jackson *et al.* 2005) were asked their, and their parents', racial group(s), their state or country of birth and those of their parents and grandparents, their age and reason for migration, and their skin colour and that of any partner.

Measuring ethnic identity

Relying on ethnic classifications alone encourages the use of crude and inflexible assessments of ethnicity that treat the categories as undifferentiated groups, even when such schemes carry an implicit acknowledgement of this by the inclusion, for example, of 'mixed' categories. In fact, as mentioned earlier, 'ethnicity' is in no way predetermined, objective or absolute. It is a form of identity, and as such our measures should reflect the strength and nature of that identity. It certainly is important to recognise that this will vary across time, context and according to other socio-demographic characteristics, such as: age, gender, age at migration, religion, occupational class, housing tenure, economic activity, education and residential area (Nazroo and Karlsen 2003, Karlsen 2004, Phinney 1992).

A starting point to a deeper investigation of ethnic identity is to ask respondents to choose, from a range of descriptors, those that they would apply to themselves. For example, in the NSAL (Jackson et al. 2005) respondents were asked: 'In addition to being American, what do you think of as your ethnic background or origins?.' Those giving more than one response to this question were then asked: 'Which do you feel best describes your ethnic background or origins?'. Phinney (1992) and others (Kuhn and McPartland 1954, Saeed et al. 1999) have used forms of the Twenty Statement Test, where respondents are asked to respond to the question 'Who am I?' using a sheet containing ten blanks. This is sometimes followed by a request to complete ten statements beginning 'I am not . . .'. Respondents are then asked what they consider to be the three most important statements from each set. This can allow important insight into the importance of ethnic identity in itself and also the dimensions along which this is defined – using national, religious, ancestral or phenotype criteria, for example. More simply, the 2002/2003 New Zealand Health Survey (NZHS) asked respondents 'How often do you think about your ethnicity?' (Ministry of Health 2004).

As implied by these questions, one purpose is to assess the centrality of ethnicity to an individual's identity. The FNS (Modood et al. 1997) asked respondents: 'Suppose you were describing yourself on the phone to a new acquaintance of your own sex from a country you have never been to. Which of these would tell them something important about you . . . And which would be the two most important things?'

- Your age?
- Your job?
- Your father's job?
- Your nationality?
- Your education?
- Your level of income?
- Your religion?
- Your height?
- Whether you are White, Black, Asian, Chinese or mixed?

- The country(s) your family came from originally?
- The colour of your hair and eyes?
- The colour of your skin?

They were then asked: 'If a white person who knew and liked you was describing you to another white person, would they think it important to mention . . .' in relation to the same criteria. A similar question in the Belgium General Election Survey (ISPO 1998) included gender, class and language in the categories offered. And the Home Office Citizenship Survey (HOCS) (Attwood *et al.* 2005, HORDSD 2004, Murphy, Wedlock and King 2005) additionally included: 'your family', 'your ethnic group or cultural background', 'any disability you may have', 'your sexuality' and 'your interests', as well as offering a 'something else' category.

It is also possible to explore how close respondents feel towards a particular group, as an indication of group identification and membership. For example, respondents to the NSAL (Jackson *et al.* 2005) were asked: 'Do you think what happens generally to Black people in this country will have something to do with what happens in your life?'. And they were also asked: 'How close do you feel in your ideas and feelings about things to':

- Black people in this country?
- White people in this country?
- Spanish-speaking groups in this country like Puerto Ricans, Cubans or Mexican-Americans?
- American Indians?
- Asian Americans – like Chinese or Japanese – in this country?
- Black people from the Caribbean, like people from Jamaica, Bermuda or Haiti?
- Black people in Africa?

As well as asking questions about perceived identity and group affiliation, it is also possible to ask about behavioural markers of identity. Areas that have suggested fruitful avenues for exploration in earlier research include:

- social networks, support and interaction;
- community involvement;
- language use;
- attitudes towards ethnically mixed marriage;
- attitudes towards parental involvement in marriage decisions;
- preferences in terms of the ethnic (and religious and gender) mix of children's schools.

In considering the dynamic evolving nature of ethnic identities, it is worth considering Hutnik's (1991) suggestion that there may be four strategies that people use in ethnic self-definition: assimilative, dissociative, acculturative and marginal. Assimilative strategies are used by people from ethnic minority groups who see themselves as belonging *only* to the majority ethnic group, and not to any ethnic minority group. People who use dissociative strategies see themselves as belonging only to the ethnic minority group. Acculturative strategists identify with both majority and minority groups, while those with marginal identities identify with neither. Hutnik

(1991) hypothesises that these four categories can also be explored in terms of cultural adaptation or the maintenance of cultural 'traditions'. Those employing assimilative processes of cultural adaptation would, it follows, wholly reject the customs of an ethnic minority group, while those employing dissociative strategies would adhere to the customs of the ethnic minority group, rejecting those of the majority. Acculturative strategists would include aspects of the minority and majority culture in their lifestyle; either fusing the two cultures together (Bhangra music, for example), allowing the two cultures to coexist and integrate, or alternating between the two as appropriate. Those with marginal identities, on the other hand, are argued to employ a more idio-syncratic person-based adaptation strategy.

To tap into these possibilities, respondents to both the FNS (Modood *et al.* 1997) and the NSAL (Jackson *et al.* 2005) were asked how strongly they identified with their minority identity and to their British/American identity. Other questions can be used to investigate 'traditional', as opposed to 'assimilative', behaviours and attitudes. Two items in the Multigroup Ethnic Identity Measure (Phinney 1992) explore partici-pating in 'ethnic' behaviours – 'being active in organisations or social groups that include mostly members of my own ethnic group' and 'participating in cultural prac-tices of my own ethnic group, such as special food, music or customs'. And one of the dimensions of ethnic identity determined using principal components analyses of a range of questions appeared to be summarising the maintenance of customs and attitudes that could be perceived to be 'traditional' to an ethnic (minority) group (Nazroo and Karlsen 2003, Karlsen 2004). These included how often, and under what circumstances, the respondents wore 'Asian' clothes or something that was meant to show a connection with the Caribbean or Africa; whether and to whom respondents spoke a language other than English; attitudes towards ethnically mixed marriage; and how far the respondent agreed with the statements:

- 'In many ways I think of myself as being Asian/Caribbean/Irish.'
- 'People of Asian/Caribbean/Irish origin should try to preserve as much as possible of their culture and way of life.'

Similar questions in that work appeared to relate to a factor summarising attitudes towards cultural assimilation (Karlsen 2004). These included responses to the state-ments:

- 'In many ways I think of myself as being British.'
- 'People of Asian/Caribbean/Irish origin should adopt more the culture and way of life of white/English people.'*
- 'People of Asian/Caribbean/Irish origin are seeing their way of life and culture being replaced by the culture of white/English people.'

The measurement of racial discrimination, harassment and prejudice

Perhaps the major problem associated with measuring incidents of racial harassment and discrimination concerns the recognition of events as racially motivated. Defining exactly what does, and does not, constitute racism is complex, and this often leads

* For Irish people, the term 'English' was used.

to inconsistencies in the definitions used for data collection. Studies exploring self-reports of actual experiences of interpersonal racism, for example, may collect information on criminal incidents, or those reported to and recorded by the police, or may include coverage of 'low-level' experiences, such as racial abuse or insulting behaviour. The FNS (Virdee 1997), for example, when covering racial harassment asked respondents whether they had been verbally abused, or experienced a physical attack, to either their person or their property, for reasons that they perceived related to their race or colour (see also the CARDIA study, Krieger and Sidney 1996). The NSAL (Jackson *et al.* 2005), extended coverage to experiences of a variety of forms of disrespect, including:

*   being treated with less courtesy/respect than other people;
*   receiving a poorer service compared with other people;
*   people acting as if they think you are not smart;
*   people acting as if they are afraid of you;
*   people acting as if they think you are dishonest;
*   people acting as if think they are better than you are;
*   being called names or insulted;
*   being threatened or harassed; and
*   being followed while shopping.

(See also the 'Daily Life Experiences' and 'Racism and Life Experiences' scales, Harrell 1997, Scott 2003.)

Similar questions have been used to measure experiences of discrimination in domains such as employment and access to public services. For example, the NSAL (Jackson *et al.* 2005) asks questions exploring experiences of:

*   ever having been unfairly fired, not hired or denied promotion;
*   ever having been unfairly stopped, searched, questioned, physically threatened or abused by the police;
*   ever having been unfairly discouraged by a teacher or advisor from continuing education;
*   ever having been unfairly prevented from moving into a neighbourhood because the landlord or a realtor (estate agent) refused to sell or rent you a house or apartment;
*   ever having moved into a neighbourhood where neighbours made life difficult for you or your family;
*   ever having been denied a bank loan; and
*   ever having received a poorer service, compared with others, from a plumber or car mechanic.

Respondents are then asked whether the main reason for this was related to ancestry or national origins, gender, race, age, height or weight or skin shade. The NZHS asked respondents if they had 'ever been treated unfairly (e.g. treated differently, kept waiting) by a health professional (e.g. doctor, nurse, dentist, etc.) because of your ethnicity?' (Ministry of Health 2004). The HOCS asked respondents about their contacts with a variety of organisations, and if they felt they employed racially discriminatory practices (Attwood *et al.* 2005, HORSD 2004, Murphy, Wedlock and

King 2005). These organisations included health and social services, commercial services, police and judiciary, and local governments.

These examples illustrate a second measurement issue, they rely on the respondent attributing racist motivations to others involved in an incident. The likelihood of such an attribution being made clearly depends on a number of factors that will vary from incident to incident, including the characteristics of the individuals involved. Research suggests, for example, that the perception or reporting of racism may be associated with gender, with women reportedly more likely to under-report experiences compared with men (Armstead *et al.* 1989), social class, with more under-reporting occurring among those with fewer socioeconomic resources (Krieger 2000, Ruggiero and Taylor 1995), or particular historical cohorts, with those coming of age during or after the civil rights movement of the 1960s more likely to report racism than older cohorts (Essed 1992, Davis and Robinson 1991).

In order to reduce these measurement problems, it is argued that when collecting data, questions should be direct and address the multiple facets of discrimination; asking about distinct types of unfair treatment, in particular situations and locations, and avoiding global questions about experiences or awareness (Krieger 2000). Also important are assessments of the domain in which the racism occurs, the magnitude and temporal characteristics of the event, the associated threat, and the impact of other individual characteristics and stressors (Williams *et al.* 2003). At the same time, it has been argued that:

> approaches to the assessment of discrimination that involve long lists of questions in which a respondent is repeatedly asked whether a particular event occurred 'because of your race' can produce demand characteristics that lead to either overreports or underreports of exposure.
>
> (Williams *et al.* 2003: 204)

Studies have also suggested that, unlike other criminal acts, racism need not have been experienced personally for it to produce a sense of threat (Virdee 1995, Oakley 1992). This may be seen in findings that suggest that those living with the threat of, or in fear of, racism are more numerous than those reporting actual personal experience of racism (Virdee 1995, 1997). To explore this, some studies also ask about respondent knowledge of other people's (in this case, family members') experiences of racism (Noh and Kaspar 2003). Others have asked more general or abstract questions, exploring whether respondents feel the amount of racial prejudice (in Britain, for example) has changed, or will change in the future (Attwood *et al.* 2005, HORDSD 2004, Murphy, Wedlock and King 2005); whether people felt British employers employed inclusive (recruitment and other) policies (Attwood *et al.* 2005, HORDSD 2004, Modood 1997, Murphy, Wedlock and King 2005); or whether people living in New Zealand are generally treated differently by health professionals because of their ethnicity (Ministry of Health 2004). Other studies have asked more directly about people's concerns about being the victim of racism (Virdee 1997). As with direct experiences of racism and discrimination, perceptions of discrimination against one's ethnic group, and fear of racism, have been shown to correlate with health (Karlsen and Nazroo 2002, 2004). It is also suggested that how one responds to racism may be important in determining its effects (Jackson *et al.* 2005, Krieger and Sidney 1996, Noh and Kaspar 2003).

Socioeconomic measures

There is considerable evidence demonstrating the concentration of people from ethnic minority groups in socioeconomic, residential and occupational disadvantage, in the US, UK and elsewhere (Lillie-Blanton and Laveist 1996, Massey and Denton 1989, Modood *et al.* 1997, Navarro 1990, Nazroo 2001, Williams and Collins 2001). Despite this, the impact of socioeconomic position on the relationship between ethnicity and health is often ignored in favour of more biological approaches (Nazroo 2003). Often, as mentioned earlier, this is done implicitly, through the statistical adjustment of models exploring the relationship between ethnicity and health for the effects of socio-economic status, in the expectation that this will uncover any core 'ethnic' effect. As Kaufman *et al.* (1997, 1998) point out, the process of adjustment is, in essence, an attempt to deal with the non-random nature of samples used in cross-sectional popu-lation studies. Of course, such an approach does not contain either the theoretical or empirical work needed to demonstrate what the remaining 'ethnic' effect in a model might be (Nazroo 1998).

In addition, while adjusting for all relevant 'extraneous' explanatory factors intro-duces the *appearance* of randomisation, attempting to introduce randomisation into cross-sectional studies by adding 'controls' has a number of problems:

> When considering socioeconomic exposures and making comparisons between racial/ethnic groups . . . the material, behavioral, and psychological circumstances of diverse socioeconomic and racial/ethnic groups are distinct on so many dimen-sions that no realistic adjustment can plausibly simulate randomization.
>
> (Kaufman *et al.* 1998: 147)

For example, close inspection has suggested serious problems associated with the use of occupational class measures (the most common socioeconomic measure used in health research in the UK) when adjusting for socioeconomic position, because the apparent homogeneity of class groupings masks the concentration of people from ethnic minority groups in lower income occupations compared to White people in the same class. Data from the FNS shows that within each class group Pakistani and Bangladeshi people have around half the income of White people and Pakistani and Bangladeshi people in the most affluent classes have average weekly incomes similar to that of White people in the least affluent classes (Nazroo 1998, 2001). Similarly, in the US there are not only pay disparities between Black-dominated and White-dominated occupations, but Black workers are on average paid less than White workers in occupations in both of these categories (Huffman 2004). These problems are aggravated when cruder measures, such as area-level rather than individual-level indicators, are used. Perhaps not surprisingly, more sensitive measures of social position have been shown to have significant effects on the relationship between ethnicity and health (Krieger 2000, Nazroo 1998, 2001). And here it is worth revisiting the quote from Kaufman *et al.* (1998) above, which indicates that socio-economic data need to be collected across a range of dimensions (for example, economic activity, housing, wealth, consumption, area of residence, etc.). Although moving in this direction involves the collection of a wider array of data, the 'easy' option of collecting crude individual level measures, or using external area-based measures, would not be accepted when measuring other domains in health research, so should not be here.

Conclusions

We ought to be critical enough to abandon the concept of ethnicity the moment it becomes a straitjacket rather than a tool for generating new understanding.

(Eriksen 2002: 178)

In order to fully understand 'ethnicity', both in itself – as an identity and experience – and in its relationship with other experiences, we have argued that it is important to be clear about theory, concepts and measurement. This includes recognising the influence of external factors on the experience of being a member of an ethnic minority group – covering racism and socioeconomic position – and the importance of ethnicity as a form of identity. Each ethnic group contains individuals who vary according to 'culture', religion, migration history and pre- and post-migration geographical and social location. Different individuals are likely to experience differing levels and types of racism (Essed 1992, Krieger 2000). And, as mentioned earlier, the experience of being a member of an ethnic group will be influenced by the other aspects of who you are. For some people, ethnicity will be a fundamental part of how they see themselves and how they interact with others. For others, ethnicity will have little or no salience. All of these aspects need to be reflected in our approaches to the classification and measurement of ethnicity.

We require methods that have meaning, not only in research and policy terms, but also for those whom we wish to study. Measures that allow people to classify themselves meaningfully according to whichever criteria they choose. We also need measures that can allow flexibility in these assessments, so that people's definitions of who they are can change over time, and enable an exploration of how, under what circumstances, and with what implications, people's definitions change. Perhaps the most important issue is that, as with other meaningful social categorisations, you cannot have only one ethnic group. Recognition of difference in itself requires comparison. In order to have a minority, there must be a majority. Ethnic identity development is both motivated and influenced by the identities and reactions of people around you. This means that the conclusions we draw in this chapter apply equally to the ethnic majority groups we study. Finally, as Erikson (2002) suggests in the quote above, in order to satisfactorily measure ethnicity, like anything, we must first be mindful of what we seek to explore and why.

References

Armstead, C., Lawler, K., Gordon, G. *et al.* (1989) 'Relationship of racial stressors to blood pressure responses and anger expression in black college students', *Health Psychology*, 8: 541–556.

Attwood, C., Singh, G., Prime, D. *et al.* (2003) *2001 Citizenship Survey: people, families and communities. Home Office Research Study 270*, London: Home Office.

Barker, M. (1981) *The New Racism*, London: Junction Books.

Barth, F. (1969) *Ethnic Groups and Boundaries: the social organisation of culture difference*, Oslo: Universitetsforlaget.

Bhopal, R. (1997) 'Is research into ethnicity and health racist, unsound, or important science?' *British Medical Journal*, 314: 1751–1756.

Bjorgo,T. and Witte, R. (1993) *Racist Violence in Europe*, London: Macmillan Press.

Bolaffi, G., Bracalenti, R., Braham, P. and Gindro, S. (2003) *Dictionary of Race, Ethnicity and Culture*, London: Sage.

Bonilla-Silva, E. and Baiocchi, G. (2001) 'Anything but racism: how sociologists limit the significance of racism', *Race and Society*, 4: 117–131.

Bradby, H. (1995) 'Ethnicity: not a black and white issue. A research note', *Sociology of Health and Illness*, 17(3): 405–417.

Bradby, H. (2003) 'Describing ethnicity in health research', *Ethnicity and Health*, 8: 5–13.

Brown, T.N., Williams, D.R., Jackson, J.S. *et al.* (2000) 'Being black and feeling blue: the mental health consequence of racial discrimination', *Race and Society*, 2: 117–131.

Centre for Contemporary Cultural Studies (CCCS) (1982) *The Empire Strikes Back: race and racism in 70s Britain*, London: Hutchinson.

Chahal, K. and Julienne, L. (1999) *"We Can't all be White!": racist victimisation in the UK*, London: YPS.

Curtis, L.P. (1968) *Anglo-saxons and Celts*, Bridgeport, CT: University of Bridgeport Press.

Curtis, L.P. (1971) *Apes and Angels: the Irishman in Victorian caricature*, Washington, DC: Smithsonian Institution Press.

Davis, N.J. and Robinson, R.V. (1991) 'Men's and women's consciousness of gender in-equality: Austria, West Germany, Great Britain and the United States', *American Socio-logical Review*, 56: 72–84.

Eriksen, T.H. (1993) *Ethnicity and Nationalism: anthropological perspectives*, London: Pluto Press.

Eriksen, T.H. (2002) *Ethnicity and Nationalism: anthropological perspectives (expanded version)*, London: Pluto Press.

Essed, P. (1992) *Understanding Everyday Racism: an interdisciplinary theory*, London: Sage.

Fekete, L. (2001) 'The emergence of xeno-racism', *Race and Class*, 43: 23–40.

Gilroy, P. (1987) *There Ain't No Black in the Union Jack: the cultural politics of race and nation*, London: Routledge.

Harding, S. and Maxwell, R. (1997) 'Differences in the mortality of migrants', in F. Drever and M. Whitehead (eds) *Health Inequalities: decennial supplement series DS no. 15*, London: The Stationery Office.

Harrell, S.P. (1997) *The Racism and Life Experiences Scales (RaLES): self-administration version*. Unpublished manuscript.

Harrell, J.P., Hall, S. and Taliaferro, J. (2003) 'Physiological responses to racism and discrim-ination: an assessment of the evidence', *American Journal of Public Health*, 93: 243–428.

Herrnstein, R.J. and Murray, C. (1994) *The Bell Curve: intelligence and class structure in American life*, New York: The Free Press.

Hickman, M.J. and Walter, B. (1997) *Discrimination and the Irish Community in Britain*, London: Commission for Racial Equality.

Home Office Research, Development and Statistical Directorate (2004) *2003 Home Office Citizenship Survey: people, families and communities. Home Office Research Study 289*, London: Home Office.

Huffman, M.L. (2004) 'More pay, more inequality? The influence of average wage levels and the racial composition of jobs on the Black-White wage gap', *Social Science Research*, 33: 498–520.

Hutnik, N. (1991) *Ethnic Minority Identity. A Social Psychological Perspective*, Oxford: Clarendon Press.

ISPO (1998) *1995 General Election Survey Belgium. Codebook and Questionnaire*, Leuven/Louvain La Neuve: ISPO/PIOP.

Jackson, J.J., Torres, M., Caldwell, C.H. *et al.* (2005) 'The national survey of American life: a study of racial, ethnic and cultural influences on mental disorders and mental health', *International Journal of Methods in Psychiatric Research*, 13(4): 196–207. See also http://rcgd.isr.umich.edu/prba/survey.htm

Jaffe, H.A. (1985) *History of Africa*, London: Zed Books.

Jordan, W.D. (1982) 'First impressions: initial English confrontations with Africans', in C. Husband (ed.) *Race in Britain*, London: Hutchinson.

Karlsen, S. (2004) 'Black like Beckham? Moving beyond definitions of ethnicity based on skin colour and ancestry', *Ethnicity and Health*, 9: 107–137.

Karlsen, S. and Nazroo, J.Y. (2002) 'Agency and structure: the impact of ethnic identity and racism in the health of ethnic minority people', *Sociology of Health and Illness*, 24: 1–20.

Karlsen, S. and Nazroo, J.Y. (2004) 'Fear of racism and health', *Journal of Epidemiology and Community Health*, 58: 1017–1018.

Kaufman, J.S., Cooper, R.S. and McGee, D.L. (1997) 'Socioeconomic status and health in blacks and whites: the problem of residual confounding and the resiliency of race', *Epidemiology*, 8: 621–628.

Kaufman, J.S., Long, A.E., Liao, Y. *et al.* (1998) 'The relation between income and mortality in U.S. Blacks and Whites', *Epidemiology*, 9: 147–155.

Krieger, N. (1990) 'Racial and gender discrimination: risk factors for high blood pressure?', *Social Science and Medicine*, 30: 1273–1281.

Krieger, N. (2000) 'Discrimination and health', in L. Berkman and I. Kawachi (eds) *Social Epidemiology*, Oxford: Oxford University Press, pp. 36–75.

Krieger, N. (2003) 'Does racism harm health? Did child abuse exist before 1962? On explicit questions, critical science and current controversies: an ecosocial perspective', *American Journal of Public Health*, 93: 194–199.

Krieger, N. and Sidney, S. (1996) 'Racial discrimination and blood pressure: the CARDIA study of young black and white adults', *American Journal of Public Health*, 86: 1370–1378.

Kuhn, M.H. and McPartland, T.S. (1954) 'An empirical investigation of self-attitudes', *American Sociological Review*, 19: 68–76.

Kundnani, A. (2000) '"Stumbling on": race, class and England', *Race and Class*, 41(4): 1–18.

Lillie-Blanton, M. and Laveist, T. (1996) 'Race/ethnicity, the social environment, and health', *Social Science and Medicine*, 43: 83–91.

McKenzie, K. and Crowcroft, N. (1994) 'Race, ethnicity, culture, and science', *British Medical Journal*, 309: 286–287.

McKenzie, K. and Crowcroft, N. (1996) 'Describing race, ethnicity, and culture in medical research', *British Medical Research*, 312: 1054.

Macpherson, W. (1999) *The Stephen Lawrence Inquiry: report of an inquiry by Sir William Macpherson of Cluny Cmnd 4262–1*, London: The Stationery Office.

Marmot, M.G., Adelstein, A.M. and Bulusu, L. (1984) OPCS *Immigrant Mortality in England and Wales 1970–78: causes of death by country of birth*, London: HMSO.

Massey, D.S. and Denton, N.A. (1989) 'Hypersegregation in US metropolitan areas: black and Hispanic segregation along five dimensions', *Demography*, 26: 373–391.

Miles, R. (1989) *Racism*, London: Routledge.

Miles, R. (1994) 'Explaining racism in contemporary Europe', in A. Rattansi and S. Westwood (eds) *Racism, Modernity and Identity: on the western front*, Oxford: Polity Press, pp. 189–221.

Ministry of Health (2004) *A Portrait of Health: key results of the 2002/03 New Zealand health survey*, Wellington: Ministry of Health. Available from: www.moh.govt.nz/PHI/Publications.

Modood, T. (1988) '"Black", racial equality and Asian identity', *New Community*, 14: 397–404.

Modood, T. (1997) 'Employment', in T. Modood, R. Berthoud, J. Lakey *et al.*, *Ethnic Minorities in Britain: diversity and disadvantage*, PSI Report 843, London: Policy Studies Institute.

Modood, T., Berthoud, R., Lakey J. *et al.* (1997) *Ethnic Minorities in Britain: diversity and disadvantage*, London: Policy Studies Institute.

Mosse, G.L. (1978) *Toward the Final Solution: a history of European racism*, London: Dent & Sons.

Murphy, R., Wedlock, E. and King, J. (2005) *Early findings from the 2005 Home Office Citizenship Survey 2005. On-line report 49/05*, London: Home Office.

Navarro, V. (1990) 'Race or class versus race and class: mortality differentials in the United States', *The Lancet*, 336: 1238–1240.

Nazroo, J.Y. (1998) 'Genetic, cultural or socioeconomic vulnerability? Expanding ethnic inequalities in health', *Sociology of Health and Illness*, 20: 714–734.

Nazroo, J.Y. (2001) *Ethnicity, Class and Health*, London: Policy Studies Institute.

Nazroo, J.Y. (2003) 'The structuring of ethnic inequalities in health: economic position, racial discrimination and racism', *American Journal of Public Health*, 93: 277–284.

Nazroo, J.Y. and Karlsen, S. (2003) 'Patterns of identity among ethnic minority people: diversity and commonality', *Ethnic and Racial Studies*, 26: 902–930.

Noh, S. and Kaspar, V. (2003) 'Perceived discrimination and depression: moderating effects of coping, acculturation and ethnic support', *American Journal of Public Health*, 93: 232–238.

Oakley, R. (1992) *Racial Violence and Harassment in Europe*, Strasbourg: Council of Europe.

Omi, W. and Winant, H. (1994) *Racial Formation in the United States: from the 1960s to the 1990s*, New York: Routledge.

Phinney, J.S. (1992) 'The multigroup ethnic identity measure: a new scale for use with diverse groups', *Journal of Adolescent Research*, 7: 156–176.

Rothon, C. and Heath, A. (2003) 'Trends in racial prejudice', in A. Park, J. Curtice, K. Thomson *et al.* (eds), *British Social Attitudes: the 20th report – continuity and change over two decades*, London: Sage.

Ruggiero, K.M. and Taylor, D.M. (1995) 'Coping with discrimination: how disadvantaged group members perceive the discrimination that confronts them', *Journal of Personality and Social Psychology*, 68: 826–838.

Saeed, A., Blain, N. and Forbes, D. (1999) 'New ethnic and national questions in Scotland: post-British identities among Glasgow Pakistani teenagers', *Ethnic and Racial Studies*, 22: 821–844.

Scott Jr, L.D. (2003) 'The relation of racial identity and racial socialization to coping with discrimination among African American adolescents', *Journal of Black Studies*, 33: 520–538.

Senior, P. and Bhopal, R. (1994) 'Ethnicity as a variable in epidemiological research', *British Medical Journal*, 309: 327–330.

Sibbitt, R. (1997) 'The perpetrators of racial harassment and racial violence', *Home Office Research Study 176*, London: Home Office and Statistics Directorate.

Smaje, C. (1996) 'The ethnic patterning of health: new directions for theory and research', *Sociology of Health and Illness*, 18: 139–171.

Smith, A.D. (1986) *The Ethnic Origins of Nations*, Oxford and New York: Blackwell.

United Nations (2000) *Report of the Committee on the Elimination of Racial Discrimination*, New York: United Nations.

Virdee, S. (1995) *Racial Violence and Harassment*, London: Policy Studies Institute.

Virdee, S. (1997) 'Racial harassment', in T. Modood, R. Berthoud, J. Lakey *et al.*, *Ethnic Minorities in Britain: diversity and disadvantage*, London: Policy Studies Institute.

Weber, M. (1922) *Wirtschaft und Gesellschaft*, Mohr: Tubingen.

Williams, D.R. (1997) 'Race and health: basic questions, emerging directions', *Annals of Epidemiology*, 7: 322–333.

Williams, D.R. and Collins, C. (2001) 'Racial residential segregation: a fundamental cause of racial disparities in health', *Public Health Reports*, September–October, 116: 404–416.

Williams, D.R., Neighbors, H.W. and Jackson, J.S. (2003) 'Racial/ethnic discrimination and health: findings from community studies', *American Journal of Public Health*, 93: 200–208.

Chapter 3

Doing research

Politics, policy and practice

Graham Scambler and James Y. Nazroo

Introduction

A central concern for the social sciences has been how far research can be, and should be, considered partisan or value-neutral. Hammersley (2000) identifies a number of ways in which social research can become partisan: the explicit alignment of the researcher with a political project (as in much feminist research); the conduct of research that serves the interests of professionals working in particular areas (as can happen in education research, for example); or research that is required to meet putative national interests (witness the declared aims of research commissioned by research councils in the UK and the National Institutes of Health in the US). Partisanship can influence research to varying degrees and at varying stages: how the research 'problem' is identified, how the research is carried out, strategies for analyses, the reporting of findings, and so on.

Hammersley argues that the description of value-neutral research as research that is free from the influence of all values glosses over a number of ambiguities. It obscures, in particular, how far a claim for value-neutrality is a principle guiding research rather than an attainable reality (can biases truly be eliminated?), the influence of practical concerns on how research questions are selected for investigation, and the evaluation of research findings for policy development. Nevertheless, it seems that a distinction can be drawn between the position of value-neutrality and partisanship.

It is not surprising that concerns of partisanship are present for research focusing on ethnicity. As Chapters 1 and 2 of this volume illustrate, ethnicity is a product of social relationships, relationships that often coincide with social inequalities. Ethnicity is inherently social and ethnicity research is typically concerned with explaining, redressing or justifying inequality. This makes it difficult to separate ethnic research from advocacy and taking sides; the concern with inequality that is embedded in much research around ethnicity, health and social care is, perhaps, inevitable. Indeed, Hammersley himself identifies anti-racist researchers as partisan in so far as they: 'see their task as to participate in the struggle against white racism' (2000: 16); but perhaps this, per se, should not worry us.

Beyond positivism and interpretivism

It has been a basic premise of that family of philosophies of science traceable to Hume, Comte and Mill, and going under the umbrella term of 'positivism', that scientists must take 'methodical' pains to exclude all intrusions of matters of value, whether moral or political, and remain strictly neutral when doing research. Central to this view is, of course, the assumption that the analysis of the social could be modelled on approaches used in the natural sciences, with the privileging of know-ledge gained from observation as opposed to theoretical analysis, thereby requiring observer objectivity. Such objectively produced knowledge can then lead to the iden-tification of rules that determine how societies operate, that can be tested and that allow for the explanation of, and prediction of, outcomes. What politicians and policy makers do with the results of scientific enquiry, the argument runs, takes us outside and beyond science. The investigation of an issue is a scientific matter. The devel-opment of policy in the light of scientific evidence engages moral and political values, warranting wider public engagement and debate.

Such approaches have, not surprisingly, faced fundamental challenges from those who have emphasised the significance of individual action in interpreting, assigning meaning to, and transforming social structures; so called interpretivism. The impli-cation is that society cannot be understood in terms of universal rules; instead, how individuals attach meaning to their activities and make sense of the world around them will influence the choices they make and govern outcomes. Perhaps paradoxic-ally, much funded social research remains broadly positivistic, with lip service still given to its neutrality premise long after this and other of its core premises have been debunked. It is as if there is reluctance, even in high and respectable places, to let it die and allow its memory to fade away.

Weber is often held to have attempted a synthesis of positivism and interpretivism, the latter allowing for due account to be paid to the ways in which people define their own situations. Like the positivists, he aimed at a philosophy of science that would deliver an empirical scientific sociology, or social science, whose propositions held independently of judgements of value. Unlike the positivists, however, he openly acknowledged that people's subjective perceptions were important constituents of objective explanations of social phenomena. Importantly, he also recognised that the topics and problems chosen for scientific investigation necessarily reflected the personal values of the social scientist and/or the collective values prevailing in the wider community (nowadays, perhaps, refracted through the micro-politics of fund-ing bodies). Thus, Weber distinguished usefully between value judgements of the researcher, which must not be permitted to contaminate scientific social research, and value reference, the context within which research topics are identified, which is an unavoidable precondition of all research programmes or studies. If all scientific research arises out of specifiable personal and/or collective values, however, it follows that these values are contestable. If scientific social research is, by definition, value-neutral for positivists, for Weber it never occurs in a socio-cultural vacuum and, therefore, values may insinuate themselves into the very framing of research proto-cols. In fact, it seems reasonable to contend that judgements of value are most worrying in social research when they go unrecognised as such. Where they are recog-nised, their influence can be analysed and countered.

To illustrate this, consider the high rates of admission to hospital for schizophrenia among Black Caribbean men in the UK. A study setting out to uncover explanations for this in *'pathological' individual behaviour*, such as drug abuse, or indeed in the *'pathology' of the Black Caribbean community*, such as lone-parenthood, will afford a very different profile of the causal linkages between ethnicity and health from a study established to discern the explanation for the same phenomenon in the *systematic stereotyping and racism of those who mediate hospital admission and apply the pertinent diagnostic label*. Moreover, both studies may be conducted in a manner that secures reasonable freedom from value judgements, although they clearly have value reference.

Weber goes on to distinguish also between the social scientist as scholar and the social scientist as intellectual or activist. However commendable the latter role, in his view it must be scrupulously separated from the research process. Recalling Hume, scholarship tells us what *is*; it cannot tell us what *ought* to be. To return to the example of the last paragraph, while both approaches to the study of high rates of admission to hospital for schizophrenia among Black Caribbean men might usefully inform health and social policy formation, their data cannot – logically – permit any direct inference to what these policies ought to be. And, although subsequent research might evaluate the 'effectiveness' of policy, this can only be done within the moral and political values that framed the aims of the policy.

While some contemporary social researchers may need reminding of Weber's early sophistication, much more needs to be said about the interface between moral and/or political values and the research process than this. In the next few paragraphs we shall reflect briefly and critically on seminal contributions from the American sociologists, C. Wright Mills, Howard Becker and Alvin Gouldner, prior to reaching what we believe is a philosophically viable and yet pragmatic stance. We shall then draw on these early paragraphs to consider the sensitive and often highly charged debates currently taking place among and between politicians, policy makers, funding bodies, researchers and researched in the domain of ethnicity and health.

Seminal positions

C. Wright Mills is usually recognised as the intellectual progeny of Marx and Weber, although commentators vary on how much he owed to each. Reacting against both the grand theory of Parsonian structural-functionalism and the neo-positivism or abstracted empiricism of Lazarsfeld in the US, he advocated a flexible and imaginative sociology oriented towards social problems identified as politically significant by sociologists acting as independent, but politically committed, intellectuals (Mills 1959). His was not a sociology geared to governments and policy formation, but rather a more radical and democratic project. Distancing himself from Weber, he had little sympathy with sociologists who entered politics, but saw sociology itself as fulfilling a progressive political role. According to the less than sympathetic Horowitz (1963), Mills felt sociologists might 'cure' social ills as well as explain them. Hammersley (2000) concludes that, unlike Weber, Mills fell foul of the 'is/ought' dichotomy, recommending that social science should move beyond providing accounts of what is in order to identify what ought to be and how to achieve it:

> what he appears to offer is a model that combines the traditional virtues of science as a specialized craft with the role of the intellectual as supplier of a comprehensive worldview, one that tells us what is right and wrong with the world and what needs to be done to remedy it.
>
> Hammersley (2000: 59)

This model, he continues, approximates more closely to that of Marx, while remaining: 'untarnished by the autocratic, indeed anti-intellectual, record of Marxism in power'.

Becker developed this position further. In his influential paper, 'Whose side are we on?' (1967), he argued that sociologists are inevitably partisan and should wherever possible make this partisanship explicit. Becker's statement needs to be understood against the background of both the 'Chicago School' and the decade of the 1960s. Hammersley discerns in what is undoubtedly a radical – if epistemologically ambiguous – paper, the durable Enlightenment view shared by many of sociology's pioneers, namely, that the production of social scientific knowledge is *by its nature* politically progressive (and maybe, too, that this is *desirable*). Becker seemed to maintain, further, that a condition of an ineluctably partisan, but progressive, sociology is sound empirical scholarship satisfying traditional methodological requirements (Becker and Horowitz 1972).

Gouldner appeared even more fiercely oppositional than either Mills or Becker. His most cited pieces carried the compelling rubrics of 'Anti-minotaur: the myth of a value-free sociology' (Gouldner 1962) and 'The sociologist as partisan' (Gouldner 1968). Central to his position was the contention that for all their overt professions of faith in value-neutrality, American social scientists *in fact* routinely produced work that was *not* value-neutral. For them, value-neutrality constituted a 'group myth'. While Weber's insistence on a scientific social science free of value judgements was vital in securing the autonomy of German sociology from political control, Gouldner (1973) claimed that a latent function of value-neutrality for postwar American sociologists was its role in building or furthering their careers. These careerists lived 'off' rather than 'for' sociology, retailing their skills to the highest bidder. Instead, the social scientist should be an intellectual no less than a professional, the former being someone who engages in social criticism and the latter someone who accommodates to 'the powers that be'. He announced his separation from Weber in the following terms:

> in the end, of course, we cannot disprove the existence of minotaurs who, after all, are thought to be sacred precisely because, being half man and half bull, they are so unlikely. The thing to see is that a belief in them is not so much untrue as it is absurd. Like Berkeley's argument for solipsism, Weber's brief for a value-free social science is a tight one and, some say, logically unassailable. Yet it is also absurd. For both arguments appeal to reason but ignore experience.
>
> Gouldner (1973: 12)

Hammersley has little time for this sloppy or casual abandonment of logic. Rather, he maintains that the only defence against Gouldner's 'powers that be' is an unyielding *and logical* insistence on the principle of value-neutrality, to free the researcher from undue influence.

This triad (Mills, Becker and Gouldner) of influential, if time-bound, offerings from talented and independent-minded American sociologists still carry weight. The durability of the problems they addressed and their subtly differentiated solutions retain their relevance despite an unhappy post-1970s, or 'postmodern', propensity to neglect positions staked out so long ago. They will serve as important resources in what follows.

Social research as a social science

The postmodern era has witnessed a bold attempt to re-define social sciences as post-Enlightenment or relativised disciplines, advancing one view among a plurality of competing views of the social world. Central to this is an emphasis on the importance of language in the construction of social life and the meaning it contains. It is a position favoured neither by the authors of this chapter, nor, less surprisingly, by the 'modernist' sociologists whose understandings of the sociological enterprise have just been briefly revisited. But the defence of sociology as a social *science*, that is, as a discipline that retains the potential to deliver a rationally compelling, because empirically accountable, 'overall picture' of the *hows* and *whys* at the interface of ethnic relations and health, requires a credible philosophical framework (Scambler 2002).

Critical realism offers such a framework, one that provides an alternative to positivism, interpretivism and postmodernism, and one that also helps develop our orientation towards value-neutrality and partisanship. Its advocates have defended a trinity of modernist positions: *ontological realism*, *epistemological relativism* and *judgmental rationality* (Archer *et al.* 1998). These three tenets underpin and inform our assessment of the interface between scientific social research on ethnicity and health and questions of value, both moral and political, that are intrinsic to policy formation and implementation.

Ontological realism states that there exist *real* objects of social scientific enquiry, *generative mechanisms* that govern and explain the *events* and *experiences* we observe in the social world, such as relations of class, command, status, gender and ethnicity. However, generative mechanisms are unperceivable and therefore theoretical, and the social world is an *open system*, rather than a closed system such as studied in experimental or natural science. This means that events are: 'conjointly determined by various, perhaps countervailing influences so that the governing causes, though necessarily appearing through, or in, events can rarely be read straight off' (Lawson 1997: 22). Generative mechanisms, therefore, result in *tendencies* in open systems rather than easily predictable relationships and outcomes. Further, because the social world is so dynamic and complex, events are typically 'unsynchronised with the mechanisms that govern them' (Lawson 1997: 22). This means that it is not possible to test generative mechanisms in the social world experimentally, rather we need to build up evidence by observing (demi-) regularities in the outcomes and relationships we observe. Although the underlying reasoning is complex, this seems unobjectionable enough, even if it raises awkward questions regarding evidence for those operating within a strictly positivistic tradition.

Epistemological relativism can be defined as the view that the social world can only be known in terms of available descriptions or discourses (Sayer 2000). Although the term carries with it a postmodern connotation, within critical realism it is associated with a rejection of judgemental relativism and acceptance of judgemental rationality. Judgemental relativism asserts that one cannot judge between different descriptions or discourses, that there is no rational and decisive way of determining that one is a better representation of the 'truth' than another. Judgemental rationality insists, to the contrary, that just because all knowledge is transitive and fallible, it does not follow that all knowledge is *equally* fallible; and just because all facts are theory-*dependent*, it does not follow that they are theory-*determined* (Danemark *et al.* 2002).

Having identified ontological realism, epistemological relativism and judgemental rationality as tenets that can underlie the important elements of the research process, we can now return to the issue of value-neutral or value-free research.

Towards pragmatic solutions

Enough has been said already to expose the traditional positivistic neglect of value as untenable. Weber's refinement, epitomised in the distinction between value judgement in the research process and value reference, the context of research, is of immense significance. The concept of value reference is especially pertinent. Good social science, however, is more than being up-front about one's partisanship, after the fashion of Becker. We also need to be aware of how social structures influence the nature of the research we conduct. Gouldner was right to point out the propensity of ambitious or careerist social scientists to accommodate to the powers that be.

This is a position explored in a way more germane to contemporary academic practice by Ritzer (2001), who refers disparagingly to the 'McDonaldisation' (the transformation towards the routine production of a uniform product) of social sciences. Key elements that have allowed this process are: the ubiquitous displacement of permanent by short-term contractual appointments in UK universities; the introduction of reward/punishment models of career advancement hingeing on appointees' potential to bring in – often commissioned – research funding; the kudos given to quantitative research, more easily done with large pre-established data sets; and the onus on publishing peer-reviewed papers conforming to set formats and lengths. All of these restrain the imagination of social researchers. But this (hyper-)rationalisation of academic work can also be read, and charitably at that, as a socially structured and non-arbitrary constriction of the field of value reference, as implied above. As in other fields, many, although not all, ethnicity researchers interested in health issues are under institutional pressure to seek funding for research the government or other appropriate 'clients' deem worthwhile using data sets that necessarily permit the asking and answering of a finite number of questions. Such processes represent an increasingly intense taming or colonisation of social research (Scambler 1996).

It needs to be acknowledged, beyond Weber's notion of value reference, that social research judged salient by radical or oppositional social scientists, in the mould of Becker and Mills, *should* not be sidelined by a profession overly eager to have its expertise sanctioned, underwritten and even commended by the powers that be. Social analysis should amount to more than an accommodation to the wealthy and powerful, lest its practitioners become mere handmaidens. One of us has contended, in fact, that there is a necessary rational *and moral* contiguity between the practice of socio-logy and resistance to 'colonisation' of the lifeworld by class and state interests, via the steering media of money and power (respectively), and the extension of deliber-ative democracy. There is a case to be made that the project of sociology necessarily commits its practitioners to the principles of justice and solidarity (Scambler 1996, 2002). Those who undertake scientific social research, in other words, are, like it or not, engaged in a moral enterprise; and one, paradoxically, that becomes most con-spicuously moral precisely when most constrained, McDonaldised or marginalised by

Mills' powers that be. Social scientists who deny this moral dimension to their work are faced with the difficulty of distinguishing their work from ideology.

What implications does this have for research on forms of association between ethnicity and health? Consider, for example, the 'problem' of the putative linkage between consanguinity (the marriage of first cousins) and birth defects within the Pakistani community in the UK. It is a problem made manifest both through consultations with general practitioners, during which parents are commonly 'blamed' for their offspring's condition (Ahmad *et al.* 2000), and through public health interventions designed to reduce consanguinity, or at least to increase the uptake of screening for the principal genetic disorders and birth defects. It is not enough merely to point out that the social construction of consanguinity as a problem is one of a number of possible by-products of value reference. This may be true, but it needs also to be recorded that it is a construction pre-structured by relations of ethnicity and command, reflective of generative mechanisms. Indeed, the discernment of consanguinity as a problem reflects relations of ethnicity, and its casting as an avoidable – and therefore potentially culpable – health risk, justifying health service interventions, reflects relations of command. In fact, considering the context of economic inequality and threats to security, a plausible case can be made that first cousin marriage carries social and economic benefits, particularly in post-migration communities. Consanguinity can be constructed as an opportunity as well as a hazard. In other words, the selection of areas or topics for empirical investigation tends to conform to dominant patterns of social relations. This is most explicit when research is commissioned to investigate an uncritically accepted 'problem' attached to marginalised or less powerful groups in society, as can often be the case in ethnicity research.

Conclusions

Acknowledgement of what amounts to a social structuring of value reference need not inhibit social researchers. One constant theme in the writings of anti- or postpositivists, such as Weber, Mills, Becker and even Gouldner, is the importance of maintaining standards in the process of conducting research, a theme that has guided the authors of this volume. There are, of course, difficulties concerning what passes as 'maintaining standards', not least because of the pressures on researchers to rationalise system-driven or McDonalidised projects as science (Scambler 1996). But, to recall the terminology of the critical realists, it remains possible to combine and reconcile ontological realism, epistemological relativism and judgemental rationality. Social scientists, like natural and life scientists, attend to real – although theoretical and unperceivable – objects, that is, social structures or relations acting as the generative mechanisms producing the events and experiences we observe. And although they necessarily take off from the *socially structured* descriptions and discourses available to them, making the rational judgement of rival theories difficult, it does not make this impossible. Indeed, what Weber refers to as value reference is, itself, a legitimate object of study. Why are consanguineous relationships a focus of health research? We suggest there exists a moral imperative to be reflexive, an imperative it is near-scandalous to resist in an era that has been dubbed one of 'reflexive modernization' (Beck *et al.* 1994). Value judgements should not, but can, and often do, intrude into the design and conduct of empirical studies. In just such micro-phenomena are macro-phenomena such as post-colonial ethnic relations acted out, making the study of such micro-phenomena worthwhile.

So no social research is conducted independently of value reference, and the values most likely to inform personal and collective research interests at any given time are those broadly compatible with the vested interests of the wealthy and powerful. The wealthy and powerful are, of course, overwhelmingly White males. Incompatible, or 'free', choices are unlikely to be funded or otherwise rewarded. Failure on the part of researchers to recognise this, that is, a lapse of reflexivity, is odd enough in contemporary society to demand investigation in its own right. If much social research at the interface between ethnicity and health stands to enhance our social scientific understanding, regardless of the values to which it 'refers', a not unreasonable hypothesis is that we *should* (also) examine, and as a matter of priority, precisely those phenomena most unlikely to be prioritised by those funding bodies with vested interests in lifeworld colonisation, namely, those resourced via the subsystems of the economy and the state. It is *always* too easy for social scientists to be sanguine about the status quo.

The type of social science emphasised here has been a reflexive critical sociology, and one oriented to public deliberation. It is important to appreciate that this is not to be dismissive of other varieties of sociological practice. The degree to which different forms of practice overlap and inform each other has been well made by Burawoy (2005), who delineates a division of sociological labour yielding four categories of knowledge: *professional*, *critical*, *policy* and *public*. Professional sociology here is characterised as instrumental knowledge aimed at an academic audience; critical sociology as reflexive knowledge aimed at an academic audience; policy sociology as instrumental knowledge aimed at an extra-academic audience; and public sociology as reflexive knowledge aimed at an extra-academic audience. The concept of a reflexive critical sociology that we have deployed cuts across Burawoy's categories of critical and public. One of the theses used to support the urgent need for the type of public sociology he defends insists that 'the standpoint of sociology is civil society and the defence of the social'. He adds: 'In times of market tyranny and state destruction, sociology – and in particular its public face – defends the interests of humanity' (Burawoy 2005: 24). While his view of sociology is consistent with ours, he rightly remarks that his four types of sociology display an interdependence. A successful public sociology can only be sustained alongside healthy professional, critical and policy sociologies.

References

Ahmad, W.I.U., Atkin, K. and Chamba, R. (2000) '"Causing havoc among their children": parental and professional perspectives on consanguinity and childhood disability', in W.I.U. Ahmad (ed.) *Ethnicity, Disability and Chronic Illness*, Buckingham: Open University Press, pp. 28–44.

Archer, M., Bhasker, R., Collier, A. *et al.* (eds) (1998) *Critical Realism: essential readings*, London: Routledge.

Beck, U., Giddens, A. and Lash, S. (1994) *Reflexive Modernization: politics, tradition and aesthetics in the modern world*, Cambridge: Polity Press.

Becker, H. (1967) 'Whose side are we on?', *Social Problems*, 14: 239–247.

Becker, H. and Horowitz, I. (1972) 'Radical politics and sociological research: observations on methodology and ideology', *American Journal of Sociology*, 78: 48–66.

Burawoy, M. (2005) 'For public sociology', *American Sociological Review*, 70(4): 28.

Danemark, B., Ekstrom, M., Jacobsen, K. and Karlsson, J. (2002) *Explaining Society: critical realism in the social sciences*, London: Routledge.

Giddens, A. (1991) *Modernity and Self Identity: self and society in late modern age*, Cambridge: Polity Press.

Gouldner, A. (1962) 'Anti-minotaur: the myth of a value-free sociology', *Social Problems*, 9: 199–213.

Gouldner, A. (1968) 'The sociologist as partisan', *American Sociologist*, May 103–116.

Gouldner, A. (1973) *For Sociology*, Harmondsworth: Penguin.

Habermas, J. (1987) *The Philosophical Discourse of Modernity*, Cambridge: Polity Press.

Hammersley, M. (2000) *Taking Sides in Social Research: essays on partisanship and bias*, London: Routledge.

Horowitz, I. (1963) *C. Wright Mills: an American utopian*, New York: Free Press.

Lawson, T. (1997) *Economics and Reality*, London: Routledge.

Mills, C. (1959) *The Sociological Imagination*, New York: Oxford University Press.

Ritzer, G. (2001) 'The McDonaldization of American sociology: a metasociological analysis', in G. Ritzer *Explorations in Social Theory: from metatheorizing to rationalization*, London: Sage.

Sayer, A. (2000) *Realism and Social Science*, London: Sage.

Scambler, G. (1996) 'The "project of modernity" and the parameters for a critical sociology: an argument with illustrations from medical sociology', *Sociology*, 30: 567–581.

Scambler, G. (2002) *Health and Social Change: a critical theory*, Buckingham: Open University Press.

Chapter 4

Engaging communities and users

Health and social care research with ethnic minority communities

Mark R.D. Johnson

Introduction

Central to the usefulness of research is the question of validity. Much attention may be paid, especially in health-related research, to questions of research quality assurance and the allocation of any research and guidance to a point on the accepted hierarchy. This is frequently achieved by the application of standards such as those delineated in the Cochrane (and now, Campbell) Collaborations and used to assess the entry of evidence into 'systematic reviews' (see also the guidance from the York Centre for Reviews and Dissemination: 'Undertaking Systematic Reviews of Research on Effectiveness' http://www.york.ac.uk/inst/crd/report4.htm). This approach has been particularly evident in relation to 'quantitative' research which measures or counts things and people – and their actions. Quality criteria here usually relate to the size of the sample, the accuracy of measurement, and sometimes the validation of the measurement instrument, be it a blood-pressure meter or a questionnaire. There are, however, few 'standardised' psychometric or quality-of-life (patient reported outcome) measures that have been validated for use with ethnic minority groups (Bhui *et al.* 2003). Another debate centres about the 'authenticity' of knowledge, which is more notable in the field of 'qualitative' research, but revolves around the same concepts of accuracy, applicability and measurement or understanding of reality. There are well-regarded systems for the assessment of research quality in the fields of qualitative research (Murphy *et al.* 1998). In both traditions, a critical issue is the question of accessing and selecting a legitimate, representative 'sample' of a population to inform the research. These points are universally important to social science, and other forms of research, but they fail to address the specific and central question asked in this volume. That is, what are the issues in conducting research in a society of diversity where a common set of values and ideas cannot be assumed, and the population is segmented along lines of 'race', culture or ethnicity. All research is only an approximation to the 'real world' (assuming that such an ideal exists), and all scientific research seeks to avoid systematic bias. Should the perceptions and values of a significant minority of the population be omitted, however, through what we may loosely term 'cultural discrimination', then that bias becomes inbuilt to the research, and its conclusions fatally flawed. That is to say, if a specific sub-group or 'type' of population is excluded (and this is not recognised and reported on), then the findings and conclusions of the study are flawed or biased. Some of these issues are explored elsewhere in this volume. In this chapter, the perceptions of 'minority' users, and the value of including them as partners in research, are more directly addressed.

However, from the outset it must be noted that from the perspective of minority populations there may be both 'too much' research – insofar as their particular ('peculiar') specific characteristics may attract research attention that is unwelcome or serves to stigmatise their community – or 'too little', insofar as they may be excluded from research that has measurable benefits or informs policy and practice shaping the provision of services they want or need. Following 'urban disturbances' in Britain in the 1970s and 1980s, ethnic minority groups felt that they were the focus of much research into their grievances, and the 'causes of riots', with little or no payoff for them, and seldom any sense of ownership of the results (Singh and Johnson 1998). Similarly, it has been observed that the discovery of genetic influences on health since the 1960s has 'turned the Pacific into a laboratory for exotic researchers' (Pearce *et al.* 2004), a comment that echoes Bhopal's comment over ten years ago that research had not yet delivered any 'health dividend' to ethnic minority groups in Britain (Bhopal 1990). The conclusion that 'there must be a strong community base for health research that is of community relevance, with a sustained community involvement in research planning and implementation' (Pearce *et al.* 2004: 1072) is hard to argue against, and one that finds resonances across minority and excluded communities everywhere.

Finally, there is another reason for researchers to wish to facilitate development in this direction, beyond the moral imperative of respecting human rights and entitlement to privacy and identity. Instrumentally, the researcher gains by entering a relationship with the minority communities, as thus we may obtain better, easier (or indeed, any) access to them as research subjects. Intellectually, science gains by making it easier to ensure that the tools we use are validated and produce more 'authentic' results. Further, politically, we need to recognise that, increasingly, those who fund research and those governing the conduct of research insist on ethical scrutiny and shared ownership of research processes. The move towards 'user involvement' in research has now become an unavoidable reality, even if sometimes the selection and the ethnic or social composition of those users, of the users who 'count', may itself be biased.

Research Governance

Research in Britain is increasingly subject to a number of forms of quality assurance and ethical scrutiny. In the health sector especially there have been significant recent developments in Research Governance, in addition to the traditional expectation that research should not do harm to patients and health and that certain accepted standards of scientific procedure be adhered to. In particular, it is important to note that a Research Governance Framework sanctioned by a UK Government Department has been promulgated and is widely accepted, especially in the field of health and social care (DH 2002, DH 2005 – see Box 4.1). This lays out for explicit consideration a number of ethical questions and means of protecting the public and other researchers. A key consideration is the inclusion of 'user' perspectives, following the activity, of INVOLVE (formerly Consumers in NHS Research) (Hanley 1999, Hanley *et al.* 2003). Over the last few years this group has produced extensive guidance and developed good practice relating to the inclusion of 'users' (now referred to more simply as 'the

---

Box 4.1 Research Governance and diversity

Research and those pursuing it should respect the diversity of human culture and conditions and take full account of ethnicity, disability, age and sexual orientation in its design, undertaking and reporting. Researchers should take account of the multicultural nature of society. It is particularly important that the body of research evidence available to policy makers reflects the diversity of the population.

Source: Originally published as: DoH 2002 *Research Governance Framework for Health & Social Care*, London: Department of Health – para 2.2.7– http://www.doh.gov.uk/research/rd3/nhsrandd/ researchgovernance.htm. Second edition now available at http://www.dh.gov.uk/PolicyAnd Guidance/ResearchAndDevelopment/ResearchAndDevelopmentAZ/ResearchGovernance/fs/en

---

public' or 'people who use services', rather than 'consumers' or 'lay people'). The change in terminology and the name of INVOLVE was deliberate, to reflect an extension of its concerns to a wider field of health and social care research as well as changes in the social use of terms such as 'patient' or 'consumer'. The publications of INVOLVE continue to demonstrate not only that it is possible to include 'user' perspectives at all stages of research from initiation to dissemination, but also that various benefits flow from this (Hanley 2005). The new DH guidelines also state quite clearly that it is no longer acceptable to design research that ignores the issue of diversity or continues explicitly to exclude members of minority groups and their needs (Box 4.1). In this, they are following a lead set in the US ten years earlier, when the National Institutes of Health (NIH) introduced mandatory guidelines for all health research supported by the US Government through the NIH, insisting on the appropriate inclusion of minority groups, including groups such as African Americans, and Hispanics, and also women (Hohmann and Parron 1996).

The same guidance, published by the Department of Health, lays out a number of 'Key Elements of a Quality Research Culture' that should be followed by researchers in designing and conducting their studies. These include:

- respect for participants' dignity, rights, safety and well being;
- valuing the diversity within society;
- personal and scientific integrity;
- leadership, honesty, accountability and openness.

It has to be admitted that there may be at present a different picture in practice. Few research papers give full details of the ways in which they seek to comply with these ideals, and even fewer discuss the ethical implications of this or their strategy to ensure maximal inclusivity. Indeed, most research is 'colour blind' and fails to take account of ethnic diversity. Further, significant numbers of studies explicitly exclude 'Non-English Speakers' – or even 'Minorities', as part of their research design. This has led to a number of problems – not the least is the fact that, for many purposes, the published research data available for designing guidelines on clinical practice and for social care are seriously flawed (Hussain-Gambles *et al.* 2004). In terms of the testing of clinical procedures and pharmaceutical products, further questions arise about 'product safety'.

A number of other issues arise in the governance of research in a diverse society. For example, the Department of Health guidelines state that 'Participants or their representatives should be involved wherever possible in the design, conduct and reporting of research' (DH 2002, see also DH 2005 and as published on the DH website http://www.dh.gov.uk/PolicyAndGuidance/ResearchAndDevelopment/Research AndDevelopmentAZ/ResearchGovernance/fs/en para 2.2.6), and it is generally accepted that all research should be undertaken against a background of 'informed consent'. This cannot always be assured if there is no proper translation of discussions into a common language, using a shared value base. Further, while most researchers would claim to work to some set of ethical standards, and most academic researchers now have to undergo scrutiny by an internal or external panel and subscribe to a set of standards such as the 'Helsinki Declaration' (World Medical Association 1964 *Declaration of Helsinki* WMA (South Africa): www.wma.net/e/policy/17-c_e.html), the DH places an additional suggestion for consideration: 'Research which duplicates other work unnecessarily or which is not of sufficient quality to contribute something useful ... is in itself unethical' (DH 2002, DH 2005, para. 3.4.2). It is not always clear that researchers do check this – and certainly, from the perspective of many members of ethnic minority groups, there is too much 'research' conducted on their communities that never gets published or used – and leads to repeated visits by further researchers seeking a natural social laboratory, supposedly available because of ethnic 'diversity', for their studies!

Who are users?

The inclusion of users in research governance is believed to have very important benefits, although it must be admitted that it is difficult to uncover good empirical research evidence for this, beyond the moral case, which is similar to that outlined above, in that inclusion goes some way towards assuring validity and public support for the research process. Nevertheless, 'INVOLVE' has concluded from its own work that involving members of the public leads to the production of research that is:

- more relevant to people's needs and concerns;
- more reliable;
- more likely to be used.

They note that: 'If research reflects the needs and views of the public it is more likely to produce results that can be used to improve health and social care services' (Hanley *et al.* 2003). They have, however, moved from their earlier terminology of 'consumers' or 'users' towards a more inclusive concept of 'the public'. This we may take to mean including not only patients or potential users of health and social care services, and informal carers, but also more generally members of the public who may be targeted by health promotion campaigns, and we might also include representative organisations and also groups who may get together to seek research because they fear that they have been exposed to potential hazards. All of these are, or might be, users, and all have a vested interest in being included in, and represented by, research.

Further, all of these categories occur among the BME population (or 'minority communities') as much as among the majority 'White' groups.

The definition of a 'user', then, must be wider than those who are already in contact with, or have taken up, the services of a health or social care provider. One of the most important groups, for example, will be those who are not using the service, perhaps because they have not heard of it, because it is not appropriate for their specific needs, or because those responsible have not thought about the need to widen the use of those services (Johnson 2000, Johnson *et al.* 2001). It is also true that researchers themselves, although clearly not 'lay people', may be users, or closely linked to someone who is themselves a 'user' – this may, indeed, be the spur to the research or the source of some of the research ideas. Indeed, as one major commissioner of research stated in interview, 'Everyone is a potential user, including me' (Johnson 2002). It is not that there is a particular 'right' or wrong definition, but that it is necessary to open up the debate and to clarify the descriptions used in discussions of 'user' involvement. An awareness of these issues is an essential part of the reflexive activity that should accompany any report of research, and might usefully be included in any 'declarations of interest' that are given (for example, when submitting articles for publication). For the purposes of this paper, we shall continue to use an inclusive definition.

Benefits and costs

Although the INVOLVE guidance (Hanley *et al.* 2003) does not give great consideration to this particular issue, many examples can be found that illustrate the specific usefulness of involving members of ethnic minority groups in research, and some of the issues that are intrinsic to this (e.g. Katbamna 1997, Culley *et al.* 2004, Dyson 1995, Dyson and Harrison 1997, Fleming and Ward 2004, Orford *et al.* 2004, Kelleher and Hillier 1996, Kai and Hedges 1999). Clearly, there are also costs or other disadvantages, some of which are considered below alongside the benefits (see also Hussain-Gambles 2003, Morjaria-Keval and Johnson 2005).

We may suggest a sort of taxonomy of significant issues as the key outcomes, or reasons for involvement, of people from ethnic minority groups in research and development activity. These are all, in general, of benefit to researchers and the quality of the research, but may also raise certain other implications. Increasingly, academic and practitioner research suggests that 'consumer involvement' and the development of collaboration or partnership, in what is now termed the 'empowerment' model, is of itself health-promoting, as well as ensuring better outcomes from the research and facilitating implementation of change arising from research (Fawcett *et al.* 1995). This is, in fact, a principal tenet of the 'Social Action' approach (Fleming and Ward 2004, Morjaria-Keval and Johnson 2005). The main factors benefiting the research itself, and the researchers, can be summarised as: diversity, sensitivity, access, language, expectation, profile and sustainability.

Diversity is, perhaps, one of the most useful (if obvious) outcomes from the involvement of minority users in research. As the reports from the Policy Studies Institute 'Fourth National Study' (Modood *et al.* 1997) demonstrate, and as shown in Chapter 1 of this volume, the more traditional sociological focus on 'race', or construction of categories such as 'Asian', commonly repeated by research reported in medical journals, overwrites and conceals significant variation within these categories. Sensitivity to issues of religion and language enables greater clinical relevance and precision to be obtained from research results, and also may show that combining two or more groups produces results that 'cancel out'. A simple example might be that while certain South Asian religio-cultural groups have very high levels of smoking, others abhor tobacco. Overall, 'South Asian' rates are close to the national average, but disease rates and appropriate health promotion action require that each individual group is considered separately (Johnson et al. 2000). Of course, such distinctions may be observed without the involvement of researchers or users from the groups concerned, but it appears that such differentials are more likely to be noted with the active involvement of 'users'.

Sensitivity, which includes an awareness of the multiple strands of diversity that may be acting in a community (language, religion, history, family allegiances etc.), is another significant part of the involvement of minority consumers. This goes beyond the kind of diversity awareness mentioned above, to ensure that researchers do not overlook other possible competing explanations for their findings. Working in partnership with communities also means that any recommendations arising from research will be sensitive to – and supported by – their concerns, such as a desire to see their cultural identity respected. Thus, Dyson's (1998) work on blood disorders is informed by close collaboration with community groups and includes a careful discussion about the use of appropriate terminology and the salience of this for treatment and professional awareness of client needs.

Another aspect of sensitivity, or of preventing a backlash following the reporting of 'sensationalised' research, can be drawn from examining the history of research into sexual health and HIV/AIDS. There are good examples of research by, and in partnership with, members of ethnic minority communities, including those with AIDS (Bhatt 1992), but many research articles have led to stereotyping and dramatic headlines in newspapers (Fenton et al. 1997: 'VD Epidemic revealed: Gonorrhea highest among Black people say top docs', front-page headline, *Voice* newspaper 16 June 1997). Such events lead to barriers for further research, while the collaborative approach tends to lead to more sensitive and accurate reporting, and may also have greater impact on behaviour because of a greater tendency to value and accept the message if it is delivered by those respected within the community.

While it is worth considering the importance of the sponsorship of research by organisations rooted in, and run by members of, ethnic minority communities, or the involvement of ethnic minority researchers, in facilitating acceptance of the results, this may raise other issues. It may sometimes be necessary to ignore or over-ride sensitivities about the discussion and investigation of problems that are denied, or seen as 'shameful', by communities. For example, there are increasingly members of minority culture community groups who are recognising the problems of drug abuse, although earlier non-acceptance of this was reported to be a barrier to engagement (Johnson and Carroll 1995). In such cases, it is particularly important to ensure that projects are seen to be sponsored or supported by consumers within the community concerned.

Access is the issue most often cited as provoking inclusion of community-based sponsorship or the use of fieldworkers drawn from the community, and the determination
of researchers to ensure community involvement in their work. Clearly, in many cases
the recruitment issue relates to questions of language, but other issues may also be
significant, including acceptability of interviewers to the community being researched,
and willingness of interviewers to work in certain areas such as the 'inner city'
(Luchterhand and Weller 1979). Community leaders and groups are sometimes
unwilling to become involved in research activity unless there is significant input
from minority workers or other direct benefit for the community. This is particularly
the case for over-researched or marginalised groups who feel under threat from state
interference, such as members of refugee and asylum groups (Hynes 2003, Temple
and Moran 2006). A very significant trend is the increasing use of 'lay interviewers'
drawn from the community and provided with basic training in social research methods
before being paid to conduct interviews for the study (see Fleming and Ward 2004).

Language remains an 'access issue' and is often the principal reason for employing
community ('consumer') workers on projects, but it is also clear that this is not simply
about translation and interpreting. The language of research includes many concepts
and technical terms that do not translate easily, and may have no direct equivalent
in the language and culture of certain minorities (Bhopal *et al.* 2004). Working with
'lay' colleagues enhances the researchers' awareness of differing concepts and
priorities. Indeed, much social science research is based on models of decision
making and logic deriving from western science and society which do not facilitate
understanding of minority cultural explanations. An American report describes how
researchers were denied access to work in a 'reservation' area among native Americans
until they had explained their objectives more clearly (Red Horse *et al.* 1989), and
in New Zealand the Maori community has used the principles of the Treaty of
Waitangi and the concept of 'cultural safety' to ensure that no research intrudes
on their community without first being agreed by a 'community' sponsor (McPherson
et al. 2003, www.newhealth.govt.nz/toolkits/tow.htm).

Expectation is an important issue, since conducting research with the involvement of
consumers inevitably raises expectations, both of action and of feedback. A common
theme of health services needs-assessment exercises is the low level of knowledge
and of expectation among potential consumers. This actually makes it difficult to ask
about the use of services that have not been heard of. Their involvement in research
and development activity may be seen as a means of raising both expectation and
knowledge. However, if these expectations are not met (for example, if there is no
reporting back or no change is seen by the communities 'on the ground'), resentment
will be generated and future research made more difficult (Singh and Johnson 1998).
'Action' research approaches, however, are often designed with change built into
them, and the common recognition of the so-called 'Hawthorn' effect suggests that
there is now no real expectation among researchers that they are, in social research
at least, operating invisibly and without changing the thing (society) that they are
studying.

The *Profile* of agencies involving consumers and communities may also be an
important benefit (or, if as above unsuccessful, hazard) of the process. Many agencies,

particularly those paying attention to Equal Opportunity policies and their obligations under the Race Relations (Amendment) Act 2000, seek actively to be seen as 'good partners'. This is particularly important for Local Authorities who need to be seen to address local minority concerns, but also has implications for higher education establishments and others who wish to be seen as 'good neighbours'. A desire to be seen as ethical actors, meeting Good Practice targets, is increasingly a common feature of organisational mission statements.

Sustainability is important because 'short-termism' has been frequently identified as one of the main barriers to change and to improving the services and the situation experienced by members of ethnic minority groups. Many initiatives designed to overcome social exclusion or racialised inequalities are funded out of 'project' budgets, and never make it into the mainstream. When the initial funding ceases, the intervention, and the organisational development and learning associated with it, are lost. Too often, 'ethnic minority' needs are not regarded as proper charges upon mainstream funding, and are therefore met by 'special' funds. Quite apart from the perceptions of the communities concerned, staff in such settings also feel marginalised and are unable to develop proper career patterns: they therefore cannot be expected to commit to a project and may leave half-way through it, leading to inefficiency and wastage. If the community and 'users' are more involved in the research, there will be a wider constituency and higher level of commitment to the implementation of changes based on the research, and the maintenance of some form of 'institutional memory'.

Levels of involvement

There are, obviously, different levels at which 'users' may be involved in the design, conduct and reporting of research. Arnstein's (1969) 'ladder of participation' is commonly cited as an illustration of involvement in decision making, and provides a basis for a similar ladder or hierarchy of involvement in research (see Box 4.2). This also raises questions of power relationships in research, an issue that has been much debated in the field of 'feminist' research but is implicit in the hierarchy proposed here, and has important implications for the publication and dissemination (and use) of research results. The inclusion of 'user' representatives in research governance – almost as much as the commissioning of research by bodies drawn from 'user' communities, begins to subvert the traditional relationships and create new ones.

It can be seen that often the population or the service user is seen as an 'object' of research, and participates only as a research subject, undergoing interviews and tests. At best, for many projects, they may be 'consulted' about the study, perhaps before it takes place, and may be given an opportunity of having a copy of a report from the project – if one is ever produced. Dissemination of results usually follows a strict hierarchy, with the project sponsor having the first sight of the results, and sometimes (it is alleged) preventing further spread of them. Inclusion of representatives of the target population(s) on steering groups may form a higher level of 'consultation', but may also be subject to tokenism and exclude them, as 'non-experts' (*sic*) from real decision making, despite their expertise in (or on) their own community.

Box 4.2 A hierarchy of involvement

Project originators and sponsors
⇑
Partnership
⇑
Professional investigators
⇑
Fieldworkers and research assistants
⇑
Steering groups
⇑
Consultation and dissemination
⇑
'Research subjects'

Apart from this, as we have seen above, the only real involvement of lay members of (ethnic minority) user groups is often as fieldworkers or research staff, employed because of their ability to speak a particular language, or to gain access to certain groups, or perhaps because gender is an issue and male researchers cannot easily speak with females of a specific group. This, of course, may be necessary even if the principal investigator, the person who has designed and run the research, is a member of an ethnic minority group him (or her) self.

Consequently (and, by inversion, to protect the autonomy of both investigators and the researched), it is important that members of all ethnic or otherwise-defined groups should be able, free and willing to conduct and take part in research in a partnership with members and organisations representing minority interests – and, especially, that those minority groups should be regarded as legitimate and capable of designing, commissioning and managing research, with a researcher of good quality, to follow up their own interests. There are examples of such research, but they seem to be few, and they are rarely cited or highly regarded in academic and scientific literature. This is greatly to be regretted, since these are frequently found to be the best at getting to grips with the specific questions relevant to the access to, and efficacy of, services – and to have the most accurate and insightful definitions of the relevant character-istics of the minority community groups with which they are concerned (see Szczepura *et al.* 2005, Szczepura *et al.* 2004). (Further examples can be found at the website of the Centre for Evidence in Ethnicity Health and Diversity: www.ethnic-health. org.uk). However, there may be a debate as to whether, when the user becomes the commissioner of research themselves, they remain 'users'.

Users may be involved at a number of points in the research process, and at different levels. These all have their part to play, and are associated with different types of impact on the research: they also have consequences for the whole process of the research. In reviewing a number of research projects which had been funded specifically to look into the health care needs of ethnic minority groups (Johnson 2002), the following types of involvement emerged.

Investigator

While it may be unusual to consider the researcher as being (him- or herself) a 'user', it must be recognised that, especially for many professionals of ethnic minority origin, their ethnic origin is a significant influence in their life, both personal and professional. Similarly, of course, the researcher needs to be reflexive about other aspects of their identity and the effect that this has on their agenda – including, for example, religious orientation, physical impairments or disability, and gender. It needs to be clearly stated that the processes, or the professionalism, of researchers from 'minority' backgrounds are no different, from those of White researchers. More fundamentally, it can be seen that some research questions are more likely to be asked by those who have personal experiences or insights to draw upon. The growth of 'reflective' approaches to science and learning in health, however, suggests that there is growing recognition of this fact (Dooher and Byrt 2003).

Research assistant/fieldworker

The largest single category where there is a strong involvement of users from ethnic minority groups is the growing trend for research projects to adopt a 'community development' or 'action research' approach, and work with community members, perhaps recruiting interviewing staff or fieldworkers to projects directly from within the community being researched. This, too, is not a new or exclusively 'ethnic minority' phenomenon, having been used, for example, by (the late) Professor Mark Abrams in a pioneering study in Sunderland in the late 1950s. However, there are particular advantages for researchers working with communities whose first language is not English, or who live in inner city areas where conventional field-force workers may be reluctant to work. Equally, it may be said that there are also benefits for the communities (consumers), both in terms of training and employment, and in their ability to affect the research agenda, particularly in the development of survey instruments and the dissemination of the results. These issues have been discussed by some researchers, notably Dyson:

> Learning points to emerge include the importance of . . . debriefing workshops . . . and reflexive data in reports; the importance of devolving organisational aspects of the research to community members . . . the pros and cons of monetary reward for community researchers . . . the nature of the required commitments to feedback and the limits to further pressurising clients who live in challenging social circumstances.
>
> (Dyson and Harrison 1997: 203)

There is, further, a well established body of evidence that, while White researchers can interview in Black (and other minority ethnic) communities and obtain similar results, levels of participation (response rates) are generally lower than when ethnic minority interviewers are used (McIver 1994) – see Chapter 9 for further discussion of this.

Steering group

A smaller level of involvement, but one that may be significant, is the inclusion of 'lay' or consumer representatives on the steering or management groups of research projects. There are clearly difficulties with the approach, not the least of which is, as for the 'majority' community, the difficulty of finding someone with the ability to contribute articulately to the management of research while being a 'lay' person. In most cases, 'representatives' seem to be drawn either from the professional 'elite' of the minority community, or be community workers and officers of social or religious organisations. Other issues more specific to ethnic minority groups, which have been also raised in connection with Trade Union and similar 'participative democracy' activities, include the timing of meetings, their location, and the question of payment for attendance to make it possible for unemployed people, or those working in less flexible occupations and on low wages, to attend without financial hardship. We might also include this point under our earlier discussion of 'costs and benefits'.

'Consultation'/dissemination

The lowest level of involvement of consumers in research and development may be the organisation of public meetings or provision of other opportunities to comment on reports and plans. It is clear that even this is regarded by ethnic minority people as being absent from the practice of many researchers. Examples of good practice could be found, which may require some departure from customary practice, such as arranging meetings in minority organisations' buildings, separately for men and women, with interpreter support, and perhaps with some other 'social' incentive, or at times that were less convenient for officers and professionals.

Sponsorship and origination

It is important to note that ethnic minority communities and their community organisations are also frequently the sponsors and managers of research projects. As with the charitable agencies of the majority community, there are 'ethnic minority' groups that have raised funds, proposed projects and employed researchers. The question of the dynamics of such projects has yet to be researched, even if the author has experienced it and observed the difference that it makes (Tomlins *et al.* 2000).

Conflicting needs and expectations of stakeholders

Evidently, from consideration of the types of stakeholder and roles examined above, there will from time to time be problems of conflict. These may stem from religious or cultural beliefs or matters of 'honour' and community image, but they are also sometimes associated with expectations relating to the end-use and outcome of research. From the point of view of socially excluded or deprived communities, the very activity of research and of documenting their everyday lives and experiences is a luxury and a form of exploitation – they, individually or collectively, 'know' their situation and can at least intuitively assert the solution to social needs and problems. The need for 'evidence' (especially when a community has experienced repeated bouts of external scrutiny or research) may be a contested priority.

Solutions to these sorts of conflict can be found, but rely on the good faith and commitment of the researcher to ensuring that users really are equal partners. This means maximising inputs from user representatives and viewpoints at all stages of the research, from the initial formulation of the 'research question' to the dissemination and implementation process. This will determine the relevance and acceptability of the research agenda, its methods and techniques, and the questions actually asked. It may be a matter of style and presentation, or a fundamental structural concern, to ensure that the 'user' input is not seen as tokenistic, reliant on the presence or influence of a single individual, or an 'inconvenience': ideally, such inputs should permeate the whole research structure, and the 'user' be seen as a partner rather than as a subject. Clearly, this is hard to avoid when they are the funder/commissioner of the research. It does, however, mean that they must have a significant role in any priority setting exercises, and in managing the project, including not only shaping and steering the research instruments (questionnaires etc.) but also in determining what might be left out, added, or when a project should be halted. Users will also then have legitimate expectations that the dissemination process will include presentations in languages or formats and locations that are accessible to their communities.

Finally, affirmation of user views before the final draft of the report is produced, is desirable to ensure that the researcher has not misunderstood or ignored key elements, although we should not ignore the possibility that there may be unresolved conflict and that the researcher may be right, or at least more 'honest', at times, too. The above is not an argument for 'politically correct' research: a partnership must be established in which the researcher brings skills and knowledge – and sometimes authority or the ability to legitimate the demands of the community by reference to prior evidence from other places. Acting as a 'critical friend', the researcher gains by the collaboration, but so does the community.

A model of good practice

A model of research that seeks to overcome some of the difficulties expressed in this chapter, is the 'social action research model' (Fleming and Ward 2004), which attempts to bring together the discipline and approach of traditional scientific research with the accessibility and insight (and ethical stance) idealised in the above discussion (see Box 4.3). In this model, qualified academic or professional researchers will follow the normal processes of searching the literature – but will pay especial attention to the so-called 'grey' (or 'fugitive') literature that does not appear in databases of scientific, peer-reviewed publications, but may be reports, administrative or internal documents, and studies conducted by members or organisations of minority communities that have not been submitted to the scientific review process.

Following this, the researchers need to recruit and work with partners from within the minority community(ies), to establish common ground and shared understandings about the principles of the research, and to test understanding of the conclusions of

---

Box 4.3 The social action research model – working with and through communities

- Literature review, incorporating grey literature
- Collaborative eliciting of key factors
- Community involvement in design of data collection
- Training of community-based interviewers
- Community-based data capture
- Academic rigour in analysis and collation of data
- Validation by community feedback
- Presentation and publication
- Submission of selected material for peer review
- Publication in accessible formats

---

the literature reviewed, giving higher priority to the expressed views of community members if they feel that these studies have misrepresented their community culture. From this, the team may design a more appropriate research instrument (such as a questionnaire, etc.) with more sensitive and effective questions, and train members of the community in the core skills of interviewing, active listening and report writing (Johnson and Verma 1998, Morjaria-Keval and Johnson 2005). Those peer field-workers, who have been active partners in the design of the study, can then be employed to collect, and even partially to analyse, the data required. They will often provide a translated transcript in English from discussions conducted in a minority language. The analysis process, however, should not abandon the normally accepted rules and processes for quality assurance (as may be appropriate for the technique – whether grounded theory, narrative analysis, or statistical review of survey data) in the field or discipline of the researchers. However, an additional stage of quality assurance is imposed – of 'feedback' and validation by presenting the initial results to the fieldwork partner team and other members of their communities, to ensure that what the researchers have 'heard' and reported, reflects what the researcher subjects and fieldworkers thought they were saying. Only then should the report be presented for the sponsor, publication and wider dissemination. That latter process should include ensuring that copies are made available in accessible formats (taking language, style and medium into account) to ensure that the communities 'researched' are also able to access and use the knowledge produced.

It has to be accepted that this approach is not without its problems. There are real costs involved, including the costs of translation, and supporting and training people from the communities, some of whom (but not all) may not have experienced such research and scientifically rigorous approaches before. There is also the cost of publication and dissemination, particularly in the growing 'open access' era, where some forms of publication will have to be paid for. That said, most researchers who adopt this route discover unsuspected sources of expertise and well-qualified individuals working and living within the communities that have been designated as under-researched, hard-to-reach or disadvantaged. At the same time, the research may have to bear the real costs of participation by those communities, including the costs of attending interviews, travel, and child care which may be absorbed in other research among more affluent groups. There may also be, at times, a degree of manipulation and management by some members of the community of interest, seeking to use their position to obstruct or obtain advantage from gatekeeper roles, and even, where several projects are seeking to access a particular group of interest, a form of price war and bidding-up of the costs of participation.

These, however, are not problems specific or peculiar to ethnic minority groups. What may be more problematic, especially for 'outsider' researchers, is the question of how much people are prepared to reveal about discreditable aspects of their own community. This may or may not be easier when using insider informants and peer research interviewers, when it is difficult for people to reveal to their fellow community member, for fear of exposure or because they know (or expect) that the interviewer from their own background will be more aware of how shameful an action, such as drinking alcohol or smoking tobacco, may be. There are also problems if peer fieldworkers are chosen who themselves represent a 'biased sample' and only access a particular substrate of the population that they know or approve of. Again, these are issues common to all research, and are discussed further in the next chapter of this volume.

Solutions can be found to most of the problems outlined. In general, it is true that the greater the degree of partnership, and the legitimacy obtained by working in an open and equal way with organisations that exists within, and are trusted by, the members of the community, the less these difficulties will arise. Proper planning and consideration of the likely real costs needs to be discussed with sponsors – and if done well, may mean that waste of resources on ineffective research or planning that fails to take into account the real needs and responses of key minority groups, is avoided. A longer-term relationship, and proper follow-up (including better dissemination) will also reduce 'research fatigue' and raise the willingness of the group to be involved in future research. Similarly, some provision of training and feedback empowers the community and 'puts something back' as well as ensuring higher quality and acceptability (and maybe implementation) of the findings. This benefits all participants, including the researchers and the wider general population.

Conclusions

The so-called 'colour-blind' approach, where no 'special' or specific attention is paid to the needs and concerns of ethnic minority groups, cannot be said effectively to reflect national or local population and consumer priorities. There are many issues that may comprise a distinctive set of priorities and concerns, but people of ethnic minority origin also have the right and need to be allowed to express their concerns on any issues that affect the 'general public' and community. However, most research in which ethnic minority groups have been explicitly involved has been short-term in its nature, funded by specific project money, and frequently qualitative rather than quantitative in its approach. Furthermore, inclusion of a minority consumer perspective tends to widen the focus of attention to include issues of discrimination and racial harassment.

The composition of research teams, and the origins of those proposing research, are matters of significance in the design of research. This is not to suggest that 'White/ majority' researchers cannot investigate 'ethnic minority' issues. Nor do researchers of minority origin necessarily, or in any sense exclusively, have an affinity with, or need to concern themselves with, minority community matters. However, there are clearly pressures, advantages and problems in all possible combinations, which need to be considered explicitly and reflectively as part of the research process. In a sense, this is only a subset of the wider question, since all researchers are part of social groups (families, among others) which use services, as well as themselves sometimes being users, and this will necessarily affect their insight and approach.

There are some risks involved in ensuring that ethnic minority user perspectives are adequately incorporated in research and development activity. It is necessary to ensure that such involvement is neither tokenistic, nor individualised – that is, dependent upon the input of particular individuals. Such research can also take longer than planned, partly at least due to the need to develop trust between the partners. It is also necessary to avoid the perception that minority cultures and practices are themselves 'unusual' and potentially problematic or pathogenic. There is a fine balance between 'care' and 'control' when research investigates culturally or ethnically specific questions. Taking advice and guidance from community members could easily become a form of censorship, just as the expertise of the researcher could become paternalism.

Significant benefits arise from the involvement of ethnic minority users and consumers in research. These include a greater awareness of the extent of diversity in the population, and its implications for practice; a greater sensitivity to such diversity (which enhances the applicability of the research for the whole population); better access to specific groups and communities; the ability to overcome barriers such as those of language and comprehension; a wider awareness of the holistic approach, including other factors affecting people's health and health behaviours; and an improvement in the 'equal opportunity' profile of the research sponsors or practitioners, potentially opening up new areas or populations. It should also be noted that there are significant resources of expertise within minority communities, and that research informed by an 'ethnic minority' perspective does not necessarily exclude or prove irrelevant to, the needs of the majority 'White' populations. Good research is good research; we are all members of the same human family and society – so what is learned in one community must have resonances for all societies. Bad research, which ignores diversity, is, equally, bad research and may lack transferability.

References

Arnstein, S. (1969) 'Eight rungs on the ladder of citizen participation', *Journal of the American Institute of Planners*, 35: 216–224.

Bhatt, C. (1992) *Aids and the Black Communities*, London: Black HIV/AIDS Network.

Bhopal, R.S. (1990) 'Future research on the health of ethnic minorities: back to basics', *Ethnic Minorities Health: A Current Awareness Bulletin*, 1(3): 1–3.

Bhopal, R. (1992) 'Future research on the health of ethnic minorities', in W.I.U. Ahmad (ed.) *The Politics of 'Race' and Health*, Bradford: Bradford University Race Relations Research Unit, 51–54.

Bhopal, R., Vettini, A., Hunt, S. *et al.* (2004) 'Review of prevalence data in, and evaluation of methods for cross cultural adaptation of, UK surveys on tobacco and alcohol in ethnic minority groups', *British Medical Journal*, 328(7431): 76.

Bhui, K., Mohamud, S., Warfa, N. *et al.* (2003) 'Cultural adaptation of mental health measures: improving the quality of clinical practice and research', *British Journal of Psychiatry*, 183(3): 184–186.

Culley, L., Johnson, M., Hudson, N. *et al.* (2004) 'A study of the provision of infertility services to South Asian communities', *Report to NHS Executive (Trent)*, Leicester: De Montfort University.

Dooher, J. and Byrt, R. (eds) (2003) *Empowerment and the Health Service User*, vol. 2, Quay Books (Mark Allen).

Dyson, S. (1995) 'Clients as researchers: issues in haemoglobinopathy research', *Social Action*, 2: 4–10.

Dyson, S. (1998) 'Race, ethnicity and haemoglobin disorders', *Social Science and Medicine*, 37: 121–131.

Dyson, S. and Harrison, M. (1997) 'Black community members-as-researchers: working with community groups in the research process', *Groupwork*, 9: 203–220.

Fawcett, S.B., Paine-Andrews, A., Francisco, V.T. *et al.* (1995) 'Using empowerment theory in collaborative partnerships for community health and development', *American Journal of Community Psychology*, 23: 677–697.

Fenton, K., Johnson, A.M. and Nicoll, A. (1997) 'Race, ethnicity and sexual health: can sexual health programmes be directed without stereotyping?', *British Medical Journal*, 314: 1703–1704.

Fleming, J. and Ward, D. (2004) 'Methodology and practical application of the social action research model', in F. Maggs-Rapport (ed.) *New Qualitative Research Methodologies in Health and Social Care: putting ideas into practice*, London: Routledge.

Hanley, B. (1999) *Involvement Works: second report of the standing group on consumers in NHS research*, London: Department of Health.

Hanley, B. (2005) *Research as Empowerment*, York: Joseph Rowntree Foundation.

Hanley, B., Bradburn, J., Barnes, M. *et al.* (2003) *Involving the Public in NHS, Public Health, and Social Care Research: briefing notes for researchers*, Eastleigh, Hants: INVOLVE (2nd edn).

Hohmann, A.A. and Parron, D.L. (1996) 'How the new NIH Guidelines on inclusion of women and minorities apply: efficacy trials, effectiveness trials, and validity', *Journal of Consulting and Clinical Psychology*, 64: 851–855.

Hussain-Gambles, M. 2003 'Ethnic minority under-representation in clinical trials: whose responsibility is it anyway?', *Journal of Health Organisation and Management*, 17: 138–143.

Hussain-Gambles, M., Atkin, K. and Leese, B. (2004) 'Why ethnic minority groups are under-represented in clinical trials: a review of the literature', *Health and Social Care in the Community*, 12(5): 382–388.

Hynes, T. (2003) 'The issue of "trust" or "mistrust" in research with refugees: choices, caveats and considerations for researchers', *Working Paper 98 – New Issues in Refugee Research*, Geneva: United National High Commission for Refugees (Evaluation and Policy Analysis Unit) www.unhcr.ch.

Johnson, M.R.D. (2000) 'Perceptions of barriers to healthy physical activity among Asian communities', *Sport Education and Society*, 5: 51–70.

Johnson, M.R.D. (2002) 'Involvement of Black and minority ethnic groups in health research', *Seacole Working Paper 3*, Leicester: Mary Seacole Research Centre.

Johnson, M.R.D. and Carroll, M. (1995) *Dealing with Diversity*, London: Home Office Drugs Prevention Initiative.

Johnson, M.R.D. and Verma, C. (1998) *It's Our Health Too: Asian men's health perspectives*, Southern Birmingham Community Health NHS Trust and NHS Ethnic Health Unit, University of Warwick CRER Research Paper 26.

Johnson, M.R.D., Bains, J., Chauhan, J. *et al.* (2001) 'Improving palliative care for minority ethnic communities in Birmingham', A Report for Birmingham Specialist Community Health NHS Trust and Macmillan Cancer Relief (Seacole Working Paper 5) Leicester: Mary Seacole Research Centre.

Johnson, M.R.D., Owen, D., Blackburn, C. *et al.* (2000) *Black and Minority Ethnic Groups in England: the second health and lifestyles survey*, London: Health Education Authority.

Kai, J. and Hedges, C. (1999) 'Minority ethnic community participation in needs assessment and service development in primary care', *Health Expectations*, 2: 7–20.

Katbamna, S. (1997) *Experiences and Needs of Carers from South Asian Communities*, Leicester: Nuffield Community Care Studies Group.

Kelleher, D. and Hillier, S. (eds) (1996) *Researching Cultural Differences in Health*, London: Routledge.

Luchterhand, E. and Weller, L. (1979) 'On reaching out-of-school, hard-to-reach youth: notes on data gathering', *Adolescence*, 14: 747–753.

McIver, S. (1994) *Obtaining the Views of Black Users of Health Services*, London: King's Fund.

McPherson, K., Harwood, M. and McNaughton, H.K. (2003) 'Ethnicity, equity and quality: lessons from New Zealand', *British Medical Journal*, 327: 443–444.

Morjaria-Keval, A. and Johnson, M.R.D. (2005) 'Our vision too: improving the access of ethnic minority visually impaired people to appropriate services', *Seacole Research Paper 4*, Leicester: MSRC with Housing Corporation and Thomas Pocklington Trust.

Modood, T., Berthoud, R., Lakey, J. *et al.* (1997) *Ethnic Minorities in Britain: diversity and disadvantage*, PSI Report 843, London: Policy Studies Institute.

Murphy, E., Dingwall, R., Greatbatch, D. *et al.* (1998) 'Qualitative research methods in health technology assessment: a review of the literature', *Health Technology Assessment*, 2: 16.

Orford, J., Johnson, M.R.D. and Purser, B. (2004) 'Drinking in second generation Black and Asian communities in the English Midlands', *Addiction Research & Theory*, 12: 11–30.

Pearce, N.B., Foliaki, S., Sporle, A. *et al.* (2004) 'Genetics, race, ethnicity and health', *British Medical Journal*, 328: 1070–1072.

Red Horse, J., Johnson, T. and Weiner, D. (1989) 'Cultural perspectives on research among American Indians', *American Indian Culture and Research Journal*, 13 (3/4): 267–271.

Singh, G. and Johnson, M.R.D. (1998) 'Research with ethnic minority groups in health and social welfare', in C. Williams, H. Soydan and M.R.D. Johnson (eds) *Social Work and Minorities: European perspectives*, London: Routledge.

Szczepura, A., Johnson, M.R.D., Gumber, A. *et al.* (2004) 'RR221 – Review of the occupational health and safety of Britain's ethnic minorities', London: Health & Safety Executive (on-line report) (www.hse.gov.uk/research/rrpdf/rr221.pdf).

Szczepura, A., Johnson, M.R.D., Gumber, A. *et al.* (2005) *An Overview of the Research Evidence on Ethnicity and Communication in Healthcare*, Report to the Department of Health Coventry: Warwick Medical School (CEEHD) (ISBN 0 9535430 4 8).

Temple, B. and Moran, R. (eds) (2006) *Doing Research with Refugees: issues and guidelines*, Bristol: Policy Press.

Tomlins, R., Johnson, M.R.D., Line, B. *et al.* (2000) *Building Futures – meeting the needs of our Vietnamese communities*, London: An Viet Housing Association.

Ethnic and language matching of the researcher and the research group during design, fieldwork and analysis

Ini Grewal and Jane Ritchie

Introduction

There is a widely held opinion in social research that the answers given may depend on who asked the questions. In other words, the identity of the interviewer[1] can shape the input to the research and hence its outcome. Like any individual, interviewers get their sense of identity from many sources: culture; religion; colour of skin; age; gender; ethnicity; nationality; social class; sexuality; educational qualifications; language; employment; health status; and so on. With reference to the theme of this chapter, this raises a fundamental question: when so many factors are at play, is it possible to identify the influence of ethnic and language matching? We shall return to this question later in the chapter, but let us begin by taking a step back and considering why we want to ethnic and language match in the first place.

The case for ethnic and language matching may be considered axiomatic. But the question must be addressed as to whether this is based simply on wisdom (in other words, that common sense and logic would seem to suggest that 'it is a good thing') or whether it is evidence-based (for example, from practical experience, through observation or experiments).

In relation to language matching, common sense would suggest that a shared language (or, better, a shared dialect) would facilitate communication. In addition there is a body of work reporting that language matching does influence data collection or the nature of the data collected. Some research indicates that it does this in a positive way by enabling the respondent to ensure that their views have been fully communicated and understood (Hughes *et al.* 1995, Marshall and While 1994, Bradby 2001, 2002, Fallon and Brown 2002). The conclusions of other studies are less clear cut, suggesting that while there is a language-of-interview effect (Lee 2001), its impact is not presumed always to be a positive one. For example, the interviewer may judge the status and performance of a respondent who is conversing in a language other than English in a particular way. Similarly, the respondent may consider the status, motivation and legitimacy of an interviewer putting questions in a language other than English differently from that of an English-speaking interviewer. But fundamentally, the need to communicate the questions and understand the answers means that a shared vocabulary, which language matching brings, is paramount.

Common sense would also suggest that a shared ethnicity might foster a sense of mutual experience and trust that can facilitate rapport, an ingredient that is felt to be critical in obtaining sound and reflective information from respondents. The crux of the case to support ethnic matching is similar to that advocated for any form of peer matching, which is, put simply, that 'a respondent is more likely to say how they really feel to someone they can relate to and who they think can relate to them'. Some feminist researchers employed this line of reasoning to promote gender matching, arguing that women were willing to share the depth of information about their lives because they expected a female interviewer 'to understand what they meant simply because . . . [they were] another woman' (Finch 1984: 76). They also argued that the shared experience of being a woman helped to redress a power imbalance.

More recently, the call for, and the practice of, other forms of peer matching has increased. Examples include age matching for both older people (Warren *et al.* 2000) and children/young people (Fast Forward Positive Lifestyles 1996, Kirby 1999) and disability matching (Faulkner and Layzell 2000, Barnes 2003). The grounds remain the same, that peer matching reduces the power imbalance between the interviewer and the interviewee thereby encouraging a willingness on the part of the respondent to give fuller information in interviews. So, for example, young people may welcome talking to people closer in age because they are presumed to have shared references and meanings, especially if the young people are deferential to those who are older (which may vary across cultures) and thus offer views that they perceive are expected of them. However, the 'peer' status enjoyed by the young interviewer can be weakened simply by the very act of setting up an interview situation whereby their status shifts from 'peer' to 'interviewer'. Another reason for the rise of peer matching is that it is championed as a way of empowering the individuals (for example, older people, children, and people with disabilities) to carry out the research. Of course, this is only really possible if these same groups are setting the research agenda rather than merely following it, a point that we will return to later in the chapter, but which is also discussed in Chapter 4.

As with language matching there is research-based evidence that indicates that ethnic matching can influence the data collected. Although this chapter focuses on the *ethnicity*-of-interviewer effects, we can draw on the body of work regarding the race-of-interviewer effects (RIE)[2] in surveys to consider the pros and cons of ethnic matching. The evidence suggests that the influence of the ethnicity of the interviewer can be productive or obstructive. There are findings from studies showing that a shared ethnicity can give the interviewer 'insider' status (Zinn 1979, Reese *et al.* 1986, May 1993, Phoenix 1994, Egharevba 2001) that facilitates rapport and yields rich data. However, there are also findings (Merton 1972) implying a shared ethnicity can lead to incorrect assumptions whereby interviewers presume they know the answers and do not explore issues fully, or the 'insider' status of the interviewer makes the respondent reluctant to share their views for fear of being judged. Added to this difference of opinion about whether ethnic matching helps or hinders rapport, there are two key reasons why it is difficult for any evidence-based research to be conclusive. The first is the range of definitions of ethnicity that are used in studies, and the second is the difficulty of separating the impact of the individual's ethnicity from all the other factors at play. Both these issues will be explored later in the chapter.

Before further assessing the evidence (rather than the wisdom) for ethnic matching and language matching, it is critical to make very clear one point that will shape the rest of the discussion. The literature on the subject of ethnic and language matching is concentrated around the fieldwork stage of the research process (in other words how the interviewer's ethnicity/language affect fieldwork) and much less consideration has been given to the activities that come before and after it (namely, design and analysis). For this reason, our discussion of the role of ethnic and language matching will start with fieldwork and then move on to examining similar arguments and issues as they relate to the design and the analysis stages of the research process.

We shall be drawing on the following studies[3] to illustrate issues and points:

* Ethnic inequalities in the quality of life of older people (Quality of life study).
* Ethnic minority psychiatric illness rates in the community (EMPIRIC).
* Exploring ethnicity and sexual health (ExES).
* Health Survey for England: the health of minority ethnic groups 1999 (HSE).
* Fourth National Survey of Ethnic minorities (FNS).

As will be explained, all of these studies employed some form of researcher matching but none were carried out with the primary aim of exploring the role of ethnic and language matching. In other words, the studies were not designed in a way that allows any conclusions to be drawn about the effects of ethnicity and language on the integrity and nature of the data collected – or on the research findings. Instead, the studies are used to help to describe and debate the issues arising when some attempt at ethnic and language matching has been made.

Our consideration of the role of ethnic and language matching will cover both quantitative and qualitative research methodologies. Most crucially, we shall be examining ethnic matching and language matching separately because, as is evident from the discussion above, they raise very different issues and are based on quite different assumptions.

Ethnic matching

We start by considering what is actually meant by 'ethnic matching', and whether there is a shared understanding of this concept within the research community. A trawl through research suggests that the debate is still going strong. Some researchers appear reluctant to operate within a fixed definition, instead arguing that 'ethnicity is a fluid concept and depends on context' (Bhopal 1997: 1753). Those who have attempted to construct a classification, include one or more of the following factors in their definition: shared history, homeland/land of origin (place of birth/place of birth of parents), cultural values (reflected in, for example, family structures, dress, diet), common language and religion. While some aspect of ethnicity of the researched (usually place of birth, language or religion) is described, the ethnic makeup of the interviewer is rarely defined at all. The description commonly takes the form of 'interviewers were ethnically matched'. From this the reader must assume that the interviewer and the interviewee have the same ethnicity *but only* based on whatever definition of 'shared ethnicity' (common history, homeland/land of origin – place of birth/place of birth of parents, cultural values, language or religion) that the study is applying.

Let us take just one of the possible bases of ethnic matching, say shared cultural values between the interviewer and interviewee, and see the strength of the assumption. If we consider this from the perspective of a second-generation interviewer, who was born in England but whose parents were, say, born in India; how likely are they to have a shared history or cultural values with an interviewee who is first-generation Indian? Less likely, perhaps, than a first-generation interviewer. Certainly less likely than a first-generation Indian with the same religious and regional background as the respondent. But more likely, perhaps, than a White interviewer. So perhaps we should be thinking of matching on a scale that runs from not matched to perfect match. To put it in another way, and quite crudely, how many points would an interviewer have to score to be technically described as matched with the interviewee? Is there a point when an 'insider' becomes an 'outsider'? In the quality of life study, data were collected through Indian Punjabi Sikhs interviewing Pakistani Punjabi Muslims, mixed ethnicity people interviewing non-mixed people, and all were second-generation individuals interviewing first-generation respondents. Do these qualify as ethnically matched interviews? Did these interviews offer any of the advantages that ethnic matching claims to provide? In order to address these issues let us consider how ethnic matching can influence research.

Influence of ethnic matching

The literature identifies the influence of ethnic matching at each stage of the research process, from study design and data collection, to analysis, interpretation and impact of the research. Ethnic matching is believed to:

1   have impact on the relationship between the interviewer and interviewee;
2   shape the study design (including data collection tools);
3   affect the process of accessing participants;
4   influence data analysis and interpretation; and
5   have some bearing on the credibility of the research.

Interviewer and interviewee relationship

Much of the debate about ethnic matching has been concentrated on data collection, with strong cases being made for and against its benefits. In both camps, the argument hinges on the relationship between the interviewer and the interviewee which is seen as being critical to the success (or failure) of the data collection. This is because everything about the interviewer – their appearance, their manner, the way they ask the questions, the way they respond to the answers – can influence how the respondent feels about the interview and, consequently, how they engage with the research. A research interview (even an unstructured in-depth qualitative interview) is not a conventional conversation. It does not play by the usual rules of social dialogue since both parties do not engage in asking questions, or share details of personal experiences. There are two different but equally important roles in a research interview – the interviewer is there to ask the questions, the interviewee to answer them – and one of the factors that can influence how willingly the interviewee accepts that role is the quality of the rapport between the two parties. Rapport can be created by a feeling of trust, familiarity and a sense of shared experience. And the argument is that a shared ethnicity can be used by both parties as a 'quick start' to building rapport – with the interviewer implying, and the interviewee assuming, a shared understanding.

The above is equally applicable to both qualitative and quantitative methodologies of data collection. With the former the case may be more obvious in that the interviews are unstructured leaving the interviewer with more scope for shaping the interview, which may influence the relationship with the interviewee. With the latter, even though the standardisation of questioning leaves less opportunity for variations, there is evidence that the impact of the person, administering a questionnaire, on the respondent can be just as critical. As noted earlier, much has been written about the 'race-of-interviewer-effect' in surveys. A recent example of this was a survey that sought views from the Asian community about the 11 September attacks and subsequent military action (Worcester and Kaur-Ballagan 2002). It found that British Asians were more likely to express a view that was less in keeping with the perceived national mood when speaking to an interviewer with a shared ethnic background.

In the quality of life study, the depth of information collected would suggest that there was good rapport between the interviewers and the respondents. If this rapport is to be attributed to a shared ethnicity then two points need to be highlighted. First, the study could not (and does not) claim to have attained ethnic matching. It involved qualitative interviews with older people of White English, of Punjabi Pakistani, of Indian Gujarati and of Black Jamaican backgrounds. Only the interviews with Indian Gujarati older people could be described as ethnically matched – interviews were undertaken by an Indian Gujarati first-generation interviewer. As noted earlier, the others involved data collected through Indian Punjabi Sikhs interviewing Pakistani Punjabi Muslims, mixed ethnicity people interviewing non-mixed people, and there were second-generation individuals interviewing first-generation respondents. But before we surmise that maybe even low level ethnic matching (for example, interviewers of broadly similar ethnicity) might have aided rapport, we need to consider that there was also evidence of strong and instant rapport between the minority ethnic interviewers and White English respondents. This may be explained by the fact that the interviews were conducted by second-generation interviewers who may have had sufficient shared cultural values to build rapport with White English older people as with those from minority ethnic backgrounds. This may be a peculiarity of second-generation immigrants whose sense of history does capture points both in their parents' place of birth and that of their own. This interpretation is given further weight by the fact that 'you know how it is' type responses arose in both 'matched' (at some ethnic level) and 'unmatched' interviews. And equally in both, interviewers countered this by nevertheless probing and asking for clarification (with the justification that they wanted to make sure that they had understood the respondent's point).

The experience of conducting this qualitative study is not unique since 'perfect' ethnic matching rarely takes place. The same is true in quantitative research. For example, the 1999 HSE did not involve ethnic matching. The justification for this was based on weighing up the possible benefits of ethnic matching (which were considered to be limited given the standardised nature of the survey) and the practicalities of ethnically matching large numbers (both in terms of the number of individual minority ethnic groups included and the overall number of respondents involved). This is not to conclude that 'perfect' ethnic matching is never proactively pursued. Researchers involved in the Fourth National Survey of Ethnic Minorities engaged in similar debates before deciding that recruiting an ethnically matched fieldforce would increase their opportunities to obtain the data they required to answer the research questions.

However, the practice of ethnic matching is not without its detractors. One counter argument is that the notion of the interviewer and respondent making assumptions about each other is actually detrimental to the data collection. Whereas the pro-matching argument is that it encourages respondents to 'tell more' because of the trust and rapport that it brings, there are equal concerns that for precisely the same reason the respondent may 'tell less'. The line of reasoning is that with a non-ethnically matched interviewer, the interviewee may feel the need to offer a fuller explanation of their answers believing that the interviewer is not familiar with their way of life (Atkinson *et al.* 1994, Rhodes 1994). But with an ethnically matched interviewer the respondent may not make explicit the information as they may assume the interviewer already knows. Indeed, the argument continues that the interviewer themselves may more readily accept answers without requesting explanation or clarification, instead assuming that they have a shared understanding.

The above points demonstrate how the ethnicity of the interviewer could adversely affect the standard of a qualitative interview because of insufficient probing and inadequate rapport (both essential to qualitative research). However, this is not to dismiss the negative impact of shared ethnicity in quantitative research. While the standardised nature of a survey does not require the same level of probing, nor, some would argue, the same degree of rapport, the negative influence of a shared ethnicity can nevertheless be at play. In other words, deference to the interviewer with a shared ethnicity could make the respondent give acceptable answers.

Literature also suggests that the nature of the research topic can influence the effect that the ethnicity of the interviewer has on the respondent (Elam *et al.* 1999). These topics are described as 'sensitive' and include issues such as 'race', 'racism', sexuality, and drug taking. An illustration of this point arose in the quality of life study when respondents were asked to describe their ethnicity. Individuals within all the groups selected an ethnic identity – whether it be in terms of colour (e.g. black or white), geographical area (e.g. Indian, English), religion (e.g. Christian, Muslim) or nationality (e.g. British). However, it was the minority ethnic interviewer interviewing the older White English people who received responses of the 'well you'll know better than me' ilk, followed by much effort to assure the interviewer that they were 'not a racist'. It is possible to attribute these reactions to the ethnicity of the interviewer.

Furthermore, there is evidence that with certain research topics, individuals actually prefer to be interviewed by an 'outsider' (Phoenix 1994). This may be because they are concerned about either confidentiality or sensitivity and do not want to risk being interviewed by someone who may be from their community. Where the interviewer and the interviewee are from a relatively small population in this country, these concerns about confidentiality may be reasonable, since both the interviewer and interviewee may be known to each other's community. The anxiety about sensitivity is based on the fear of the adverse impact of shared knowledge that is derived from experience. For example, if the interviewee is going to be discussing their support for an issue that is considered a taboo within their community, being interviewed by someone from the same community may make them assume (possibly incorrectly) that the interviewer is coming with 'all the community baggage' about that subject, and will therefore judge them. This could perhaps be described as the reverse of 'ethnicity-of-interviewer effect' noted earlier, in that a shared ethnicity could actually damage data integrity. An example, albeit untested, comes from the ExES study which explored people's sexual attitudes, practices and behaviours. There were some concerns that respondents might be reluctant to reveal sexual practices that were discouraged or disapproved of in their home culture (such as homosexuality, casual sex or sexual partnerships outside of marriage) to another person from their own community.

Informed study design

Our discussion started at the fieldwork stage because that is the focus of much of the research on the subject of ethnic matching. However, as many have noted (Gunaratnam 2003) the relevance of a shared ethnicity is not limited to interview interactions. The influence of involving ethnically matched researchers (at whatever level of matching) can in fact begin at the study design stage.

Subject expertise is often used as a valuable guide to assembling a high quality research team. For example, there would seem to be obvious merit in involving someone who has worked extensively on family relationships and childcare in a study looking at 'changes in parenting roles', or someone whose research experience covers employment, working conditions and pensions, in a study exploring 'influences on industrial relations'. Indeed, it is common practice for non-subject focused research organisations (or those venturing into new territory) to illustrate in research tenders how they propose to build subject expertise into their work. An example of this is the inclusion of disability awareness training for researchers working on a disability-related study.

With ethnic matching, a shared ethnicity can be viewed as one of the expertises needed. In such cases the ethnically matched researcher is believed to be in a position to be able to contribute 'insider' information. The argument is that having a 'lived', rather than an academic, understanding of an ethnic group, brings with it an inherent awareness of culture and customs, and an instinctive sensitivity to subtleties and nuances in behaviour and conduct. Having such knowledge of a particular subject, and in this case of an ethnic group, should help to develop an informed study design by identifying pertinent issues and designing appropriate data collection tools.

Let us consider the latter point – designing appropriate data collection tools – a little further. An 'insider' researcher may be able to draw on their expertise to determine an appropriate method of data collection, for example, whether the primary consideration to build rapport, to address a particular research question using focus groups, should be age or gender. Their expertise may also feed into the design of appropriate questions and this is particularly important for the development of surveys. While there is the opportunity during a qualitative interview to adapt or adjust the line of questioning, using respondents' language and terms, a survey does not offer a similar degree of flexibility. It is critical, therefore, that the questions 'fit' the lives and circumstances of the research population.

All the studies included here involved a team of researchers from a range of ethnic backgrounds (some of whom share an ethnicity with the research population) in the study design. But the influence of ethnic matching is not an easy path to trace.

For example, in the ExES study people 'matched' with each of the studied communities, participated in the design of the interviews and provided what were felt to be thoughtful contributions to its coverage. Equally, advice was taken from experts in the field of sexual health but precisely who contributed what in terms of final coverage is hard to say since the history of an idea was not traced or documented, and probably never could be. Similarly, the quality of life study drew on knowledge gained vicariously through academic study and on knowledge gained directly through personal experience. The former came from members of the research team who had a wealth of experience in the field of ethnic research. And the latter came from both research team members and freelance interviewers (not team members) who shared an ethnicity with the research population. The combination provided for a lively discussion and identification of the pertinent issues and how they should be addressed.

Access to study participants

Accessing participants is a key part of the fieldwork stage and could have been included in the discussion about the interviewer–interviewee relationship. Indeed, many of the issues are similar. However, we have chosen to discuss it separately, partly because ensuring access to the target population is a key aspect of study design, but also because it receives very limited coverage in other literature on ethnic matching.

Minority ethnic communities are often included in the list of research populations that are described as 'hard-to-reach'. The case made for ethnic matching at this stage is that being approached to take part in a study by someone who 'looks like you' is likely to be successful because it brings with it a sense of familiarity and trust. Where the population is to be approached through gatekeepers (for example, places of worship, community centres) a shared ethnicity can sometimes act as a facilitator. However, it is important to be aware that issues not necessarily related to ethnicity, such as protectiveness of members, or group leaders having a different agenda to its membership, could also be influencing negotiations with gatekeepers.

Bearing this in mind, one feature that is believed to have contributed to engaging some Gujarati participants in the quality of life study, was the involvement of an ethnically matched interviewer who was able to use her identity to comfortably recruit (the term often used for such initial approach stages) participants. With the same proviso, it is also believed that the EMPIRIC study was able to involve individuals who may not have taken part in the study if the recruitment had not been carried out by ethnically matched interviewers. In contrast, the 1999 HSE did not report significant difficulties in recruiting its sample using non-matched interviewers. The recruitment was carried out in English, with the offer of the interview to be conducted in the language that the respondent specified. It could be that the relatively short encounter between the respondent and the person recruiting meant that the need for ethnic matching was not so critical. As with data collection, it may be that the level of rapport that a person recruiting needs to convince an individual to take part in an unstructured interview is greater than that required to ask individuals to take part in a survey. For this reason the criticality of the ethnicity of the person recruiting may depend on what the respondent is being asked to do.

Informed analysis

The ethnicity of a researcher is also relevant when considering analysis. But little is written about the role of ethnic matching in the analysis of data. Some would argue that this only has relevance for qualitative analysis since the nature of quantitative data leaves it less open to alternative interpretations. However, this is debatable and certainly others would claim that no part of the research process, including the analysis of quantitative data, is value free. In other words, the quantitative researcher is deciding how the data are analysed and how particular statistics are described.

If we follow the pro ethnic matching argument through – that it can help to facilitate informed study design – then it may also enable informed analysis. In other words a shared ethnicity may make the analyst sensitive to details, illustrations, descriptions and explanations in the data that can help them to answer the research question. One of the findings of the quality of life study was that 'control' was uniformly seen as a contributor of quality to peoples' lives, but that concepts of 'control' appeared to be shaped by ethnicity. It could be claimed that having an intimate knowledge of a culture or community makes such discovery more likely. But, again, the sources of such insights are difficult to trace and certainly no comparative studies that might test such influence have been undertaken.

Language matching

The case for language matching is perhaps easier to defend than ethnic matching, since all social research requires some form of communication. In both qualitative and quantitative research, respondents need to be able to tell their stories and the researcher needs to be able to hear and respond to those accounts. This can best be achieved if both parties are able to (literally) understand each other. Therefore, unlike ethnic matching there does not appear the same need to go to great lengths to make a case for language matching in fieldwork, and definitely no need to present a case against the approach. Again, our discussion will start with the role of language matching in the data collection stage and then move on to address other aspects of the research process.

Language matching in fieldwork

With qualitative research, where the emphasis is on hearing the respondent's story in their own words, the need for a shared vocabulary is paramount. Qualitative interviews aim to elicit opinions, explanations and descriptions. This requires the respondent to discuss their feelings, thoughts and emotions in considerable depth. For interviews conducted in English, limited use of the language would not allow the respondent to fully engage in such a discussion. This problem would occur equally in interviews conducted through an interpreter where the complexity of issues raised would be almost impossible to capture in a three-way exchange. For example, the quality of life study wanted to look at post-retirement activity. The study wanted to go further than establishing *how* the older people spent their time. It also wanted to understand, for example, why the individual did the things that they did, how they felt about doing these things, their history with such activities, what else they might have liked to do, and so on. A shared language was central to achieving the study's aim.

A shared language can be equally critical to a quantitative survey reaching its objectives. There is evidence that answers given by survey respondents differ depending on whether an interview is conducted in a matched language or in English, even when sample characteristics have been taken into account (Lee 2001). One explanation offered is that an interview conducted in a respondent's first language may evoke in them a sense of identity of what it means to be a member of a minority ethnic community.

In terms of enabling the respondents to tell their stories, the criticality of language matching appears to be more serious in qualitative research. There are examples (the quality of life of older people study and EMPIRIC) where respondents, who had completed a questionnaire in English, found that their fluency in English was insufficient to fully take part in a follow-up qualitative in-depth interview. Nevertheless, unlike ethnic matching, language matching is usually actively pursued in both quantitative and qualitative research.

Role of language matching in other parts of the research process

The advantages of language matching in collecting data are to a large degree obvious. However, it is the value of a shared language in other parts of the research process, namely, design and analysis, that appears to be less considered or debated. As we will see there are similar kinds of requirements for shared language at both the design and analysis stages.

Role of language matching in design

Language matching is vital in the design of the data collection tool, be it a topic guide for a qualitative interview or a questionnaire for a quantitative study. Furthermore, language matching is not achieved by a straightforward translation of the data collection instrument. Rather, it entails the 'translation' of the *concepts* used in the instruments so that there is a shared understanding between the interviewer and the interviewee.

Steps need to be taken to ensure that the specific areas of questioning are appropriately adapted for people whose first language is not the same as the language in which the data collection tool was created. Check lists for this have been developed, an example of which is Herdman *et al.*'s (1998) model of assessing cross-cultural equivalence in adaptation of HRQoL (health related quality of life) instruments. They note six types of equivalence – conceptual, item, semantic, operational, measurement and functional (see Box 5.1) – that need to be addressed when deciding whether and how to adapt an instrument.

Although the work in this area has focused on questionnaires, much can also be broadly applied to qualitative topic guides. A data collection tool, then, is only language matched if the concepts within it are adapted to, rather than simply translated into, another language. Checks need to be made that the concepts have the same meaning in all the languages to be used to collect the data (Hunt and Bhopal 2004). An illustration can be taken from the quality of life study. One of its aims was to explore how people spoke about old age (the study involved people aged above

---

Box 5.1 Types of equivalence

Conceptual equivalence between questionnaires is achieved when the questionnaire has the same relationship to the underlying concept in all the cultures under investigation.

Item equivalence exists when items estimate the same parameters on the latent trait being measured and when they are equally relevant and acceptable in all cultures under investigation.

Semantic equivalence is concerned with transfer of meaning across languages, and with achieving a similar effect on respondents in different languages.

Operational equivalence refers to the possibility of using a similar questionnaire format, instructions, mode of administration and measurement methods. Equivalence is attained when these elements do not affect the results.

The aim of investigating *measurement equivalence* is to ensure that different language versions of the same instrument achieve acceptable levels in terms of their psychometric properties, primarily in terms of their reliability, responsiveness and construct validity (including an instrument's discriminant, evaluative and predictive properties). The degree of measurement equivalence is therefore defined as the extent to which the psychometric properties of different language versions of the same instrument are similar, though not all of these properties will be expected to be the same.

Functional equivalence can be defined as the extent to which an instrument does what it is supposed to do equally well in all the cultures under investigation.

(Herdman *et al.* 1998: 324–331)

---

pensionable age). At the design stage the concepts 'old age' and 'older people', which in Punjabi can carry connotations of 'wisdom' or of 'frailty', was one example of a concept that needed further thought in conceptual translation. Further illustrations of how concepts need to be adapted to achieve equivalence in another language can be found in the 1999 HSE. One such case was the need to develop a descriptive sentence rather than a single word to adapt the term 'wheezing'. Another involved discussion about red and white meat consumption. In the English version the question about eating red meat was asked before that for white meat. However, in communities that made no distinction between red meat and white meat (all meat was described as red), these questions were confusing if consumption of red meat was raised first. This situation was resolved by reordering the questions.

The nature of surveys, which requires standardisation in terms of how and in what order questions are asked, as well as what responses are offered, means that *all* of the groundwork to ensure that concepts are transferable across languages has to be completed before going into the field. While such advance thinking is equally important in qualitative research, an unstructured interview allows the opportunity to discuss, explain, correct, and even adopt the word, phrase or style used by the respondent to ensure understanding of a concept. Furthermore, a translated concept may not mean much without some explanation, which is possible to accommodate in a qualitative interview but is a little more difficult in a questionnaire.

Whatever the stage at which the issue of adaptability of concepts is considered, it is usual for the design of, and musing about, the data collection tool to be done in English. Unless the study is being carried out by language matched researchers, this is a reality of research. What is important then is that the same space and opportunity is provided for producing a 'translated' version of the tool, and that it is a two-way process. For example, if the discussion of a concept in Punjabi reveals a better way of approaching a topic, the idea should be returned to the English questionnaire to see whether it could improve questioning in that context too.

Also worth noting is that in terms of accessing respondents, the same argument made earlier about the influence of ethnic matching applies to language matching.

Role of language matching in analysis

The influence of language extends to analysis but, as noted earlier, the requirement here appears to be greater for qualitative than quantitative data. Once qualitative data have been collected, the next stage is to translate it into English, in order for it to be analysed. The analysis then requires data management, of some kind, before moving on to descriptive, explanatory and interpretative analyses. Dealing with translated data has an equally critical impact at each of the stages. However, with statistical enquiries, the numerical data is ready to analyse from responses to the pre-structured questioning. This is another reason why it is so critical that the concepts used in a questionnaire are meticulously 'translated' and adapted before going into the field.

The data management stage involves generating a set of themes and concepts and applying them to the raw data. 'These themes and concepts should remain close to the participants' own language and understandings' (Ritchie and Lewis 2003: 214). However, the analyst will be working from transcripts that have been translated into English, which will not therefore strictly contain 'raw' data in that they no longer comprise the literal words of the respondents. A degree of interpretation by the person transcribing and translating the taped interview has already taken place. The translator has to deliver a translation that not only remains true to the words of the respondent but also has to ensure that its meaning is understood by the analyst. This demands a degree of judgement and reasoning by the translator. This is not usually seen as part of the analysis process, but given its pivotal role in interpreting the data, perhaps it should be. Using the quality of life study as an example of the different ways of defining 'older people', if the translator interprets it in a different way to that intended by the respondent then that will be the 'raw' data that the analysts will be working with.

This raises the issue of how the responses are translated for analysis. A common practice with qualitative studies is to use the person who carried out the interview to transcribe and translate the taped interview, because they will be as close as possible to the meaning intended by the respondent. Sometimes a further stage is involved where the translated transcription is then translated back into the original language by another person to check its integrity and relation to the original words.

A second task in analysis is to prepare descriptive accounts. Here the 'analyst makes use of the ordered data to identify key dimensions, map the range and diversity of each phenomenon and develop classifications and typologies' (Ritchie and Lewis 2003: 217). One of the two features that Ritchie and Lewis (2003) state as being central to descriptive analysis is 'language – the *actual* words used by the study participants' (Ritchie and Lewis 2003: 214, their emphasis). This, they maintain, portrays the 'richness or "colour"' that a given phenomenon holds for them (Ritchie and Lewis 2003: 214). Again as noted above, translated transcripts are not made up of the original words of the respondent but, rather, the interpretations of those words by the translator.

In some studies translators make every effort to add notes in brackets to clarify meanings in transcripts which help retain the 'colour'. With a study such as EMPIRIC, which set out not only to explore the substance of what individuals said about a particular phenomenon but also the idioms they used to discuss mental health, this meant that these had to be captured and retained through translation.

Later stages of analysis involve developing explanatory accounts, which is done by finding patterns and associations as well as contradictions and exceptions in the data and explaining why those patterns and outcomes have occurred. Because analysis of qualitative data is an iterative process with the analyst continuously moving between the raw data, assigned categories and classifications, and more abstracted and explanatory accounts – and often in the process refining the way the evidence is put together – the importance of a shared language continues throughout the process.

The way forward

In order to move the debate further we need to take note of two very important points. First, discussions of 'ethnic matching' and 'language matching' need to be separated since each is based on different assumptions and raises very different issues for the design and conduct of research. Second, 'ethnic matching' and 'language matching' should be considered with reference to the whole research process and not just limited to the data collection stage.

Conventional wisdom dictates that both ethnic matching and language matching are 'good things'. It is believed that a common language will facilitate communication, which is critical for individuals to be *able* to tell their stories. And the notion of ethnic matching is based on the belief that shared experiences will facilitate rapport, which is important for an individual to *want* to tell their story. It is when we move on to assess the evidence to support the wisdom that the strength of argument for ethnic matching becomes more blurred.

Language matching is something that is actively pursued at the data collection stage, as a matter of course for qualitative interviews, but also as good practice in surveys, whereas ethnic matching can sometimes be a by-product of language matching. In other words, the primary criterion for using an interviewer may be that they speak the same language as the respondent, for example, Punjabi, but they may also coincidentally share the same ethnicity, for example, be Pakistani. However, an Indian Punjabi speaker might be just as readily employed.

Regardless of whether the matching (of either type) is sought, it is an approach that is usually applied to the data collection stage. We would suggest that the data collection stage is probably the part of the research process where it is especially difficult to disentangle the impact of a single factor from all the others that are at play. This is particularly the case for assessing the impact of ethnic matching. While we can turn to research-based evidence and map out the role that language matching has played in data collection, the contribution of ethnic matching is a less proven one, as we have discussed.

Therefore, we would propose that rather than being discouraged by the complexity of the task of extricating the influence of ethnic matching in data collection, we should widen our consideration of ethnic (and language) matching to other parts of the research process. We would argue that the strengths that matching brings to data collection are equally applicable to research design and data analysis. In other words, setting parameters of a research question, selecting an approach and methodology, and analysing and interpreting data, would also benefit from insights, understanding and sensitivity that ethnic matching can bring. Similarly, conceiving and developing ideas at the design stage or staying close to the actual words used for as long as possible during qualitative analysis, offers a role for language matching that is wider than just fieldwork. Furthermore, we would suggest that the design and analysis stages lend themselves to a more systematic assessment of the impact of ethnic matching (and language matching) than has hitherto taken place.

One way of applying this learning to real world social policy research is to adopt the idea of 'culturally competent' researchers suggested by Papadopoulos (2002). This approach recognises that resources and logistics will not allow ethnic matching to be achieved in all circumstances. It advocates that all researchers need to be culturally aware (conscious of how the cultural backgrounds of the researcher and the respondent interrelate); culturally knowledgeable (understanding of similarities and differences in order to avoid essentialism); and culturally sensitive (this may involve language matching and ethnic matching alongside the awareness that there are other factors such as gender and socio-economic status at play). Papadopoulos claims that by synthesising and applying these, a culturally competent researcher will be 'aware of their own background and how this might affect their perceptions of other groups' (Papadopoulos 2002: 263). However, in aiming for a culturally competent team we should not overlook the importance of research competence. An example of this is the practice of recruiting freelancers predominantly for their language and/or ethnic matching without paying due consideration to their research skills, which can then compromise the quality of the research and the individual's career development (Nazroo and Grewal 2002).

All research endeavours to achieve credibility so that findings are more likely to be accepted and acted upon. A key way of strengthening the integrity and credibility of research is to employ robust methods. If this is understood as asking the right questions, in the right way, of the right people, and not misinterpreting their answers, then recognising the full breadth of the role of language matching and ethnic matching may go some way to meeting that requirement (see also the discussion of culturally competent research in Chapter 6). This will strengthen credibility not only among commissioners and researchers, but also within the communities that are researched.

Notes

1   For qualitative research 'interviewers' and 'researchers' are sometimes synonymous but this is not the case for quantitative research. This is because in a qualitative study the same people usually collect the data as well as designing the study and analysing the data, and they are referred to as 'researchers'. However, in a quantitative study, those who collect the data are a different set of people to those who design the questionnaire or analyse the data. The data collectors are described as 'interviewers' and the designers and analysts as 'researchers'. In order to avoid confusion, we shall refer to the person who carries out in-depth qualitative interviews or administers questionnaires as 'the interviewer'. For all other circumstances we shall use the term 'the researcher'.

2   In research into survey methodology, the examination of interracial interviewing in the United States in the 1950s and 1960s that focused mainly on ethnic minority participants, led to the concept of 'race-of-interviewer effects' (RIE). This concept has been employed to refer to the 'response bias' and 'measurement error' that has been recorded in the 'adjustment' that people make to their opinions and attitudes when questioned by an interviewer from another ethnic group, e.g. White respondents are more likely to express a willingness to vote for an African American candidate in the presence of an African American interviewer than in the presence of a White interviewer (Finkel *et al.* 1999).

3   **Summary of studies**

Ethnic inequalities of quality of life of older people (quality of life study)

The study investigated inequalities in the circumstances of older people from minority ethnic groups. It was conducted in two phases: the first used qualitative methods and the second, quantitative. This chapter draws only on the qualitative phase, which involved in-depth interviews with respondents from four ethnically 'homogeneous' groups (Jamaican Caribbean, Gujarati Indian Hindu, Punjabi Pakistani and White English). The sample was drawn from the Fourth National Survey of Ethnic Minorities. The study explored ethnic differences in influences on and levels of quality of life, relating this to the circumstances and biographies of respondents. (Qualitative findings reported in Grewal *et al.* 2004.)

Ethnic minority psychiatric illness rates in the community (EMPIRIC)

This consisted of both a quantitative survey and a qualitative study. Again, this chapter draws only on the qualitative part of the study, which involved in-depth interviews with a sample drawn from the quantitative survey of people from six ethnic groups (Bangladeshi, Caribbean, Indian, Irish, Pakistani and White). The study aimed to conduct a detailed examination of ethnic differences in the way in which people both experience and express mental distress. (Qualitative findings reported in O'Conner and Nazroo 2002.)

Exploring ethnicity and sexual health (ExES)

This study involved in-depth qualitative interviews with Indian, Bangladeshi, Jamaican, Nigerian and Ugandan people. It aimed to inform both sexual health promotion and future research in this area by providing detailed information on the factors that might influence sexual lifestyles and how these might vary across different ethnic groups. (Elam *et al.* 1999.)

Health Survey for England: the health of minority ethnic groups 1999 (HSE)

The Health Survey for England comprises a series of annual surveys, of which the 1999 survey is the ninth. The 1999 survey was the first to increase the representation of minority ethnic adults and children from Black Caribbean, Indian, Pakistani, Bangladeshi, Chinese and Irish communities. The 1999 Health Survey was designed to augment existing research on the health of minority ethnic groups by interviewing a representative sample of minority ethnic, and by covering an extensive range of health issues in an interview associated with objective physical measurements and the taking of blood samples. (Erens *et al.* 2001.)

Fourth National Survey of Ethnic Minorities (FNS)

The FNS was a large representative survey of ethnic minority and White people living in England and Wales. The ethnic groups included: Caribbean; Indian (including East African Asians); Pakistani; Bangladeshi; Chinese; and White. The aim of the survey was to describe and explain the experiences of ethnic minority people living in England and Wales. In order to do this the following topics were covered in detail: household and family structure; socio-economic position, including economic activity, sources of income and size of income; perceptions of the quality of the neighbourhood; education; dimensions of ethnic identity; experience of crime and harassment, including 'low-level' racial harassment; social networks and participation; both general and specific health outcomes; and use of health and social services. (Modood *et al.* 1997, Nazroo 1997.)

References

Atkinson, P., Batchelor, C., Bloor, M. and Owens, D. (1994) *The Advantages and Disadvantages of Qualitative Methods for Studying Health Beliefs and Barriers in South Asian Communities*, Cardiff: University of Wales.

Barnes, C. (2003) 'What a difference a decade makes: reflections on doing "emancipatory" disability research', *Disability and Society*, 18: 3–17.

Bhopal, R. (1997) 'Is research into ethnicity and health racist, unsound, or important science?', *British Medical Journal*, 314: 1751–1763.

Bradby, H. (2001) 'Communication, interpretation and translation', in L. Culley and S. Dyson (eds) *Ethnicity and Nursing Practice*, Basingstoke: Palgrave.

Bradby, H. (2002) 'Translating culture and language: a research note on multilingual settings', *Sociology of Health & Illness*, 24: 842–855.

Ecob, R. and William, R. (1991) 'Sampling Asian minorities to assess health and welfare', *Journal of Epidemiology and Community Health*, 45: 93–101.

Egharevba, I. (2001) 'Researching an-"other" minority ethnic community: reflections of a black female researcher on the intersections of race, gender and other power positions on the research process', *International Journal of Social Research Methodology*, 4: 225–241.

Elam, G., Fenton, K., Johnson, A. *et al.* (1999) *Exploring Ethnicity and Sexual Health (ExES)*, London: Social and Community Planning Research.

Erens, B., Primatesta, P. and Prior, G. (eds) (2001) *Health Survey for England: the health of minority ethnic groups 1999, (Volume 1: Findings, Volume 2: Methodology and Documentation)*, London: The Stationery Office for the Department of Health.

Fallon, G. and Brown, R.B. (2002) 'Focussing on focus groups: lessons from a research project involving a Bangladeshi community', *Qualitative Research*, 2: 195–208.

Fast Forward Positive Lifestyles (1996*) Scottish Schools Drugs Survey*, Glasgow: Scotland Against Drugs.

Faulkner, A. and Layzell, S. (2000) *Strategies for Living: a report of user-led research into people's strategies for living with mental distress*, London: The Mental Health Foundation.

Finch, J. (1984) '"It's great to have someone to talk to": the ethics and politics of interviewing women', in C. Bell and H. Roberts (eds) *Social Researching: politics, problems, practice*, London: Routledge & Kegan Paul, pp. 70–87.

Finkel, S.E., Guterbock, T.M. and Borg, M.J. (1999) 'Race-of-interviewer effects in a pre-election poll: Virginia 1989', *Public Opinion Quarterly*, 55: 313–330.

Grewal, I., Nazroo, J., Bajekal, M. *et al.* (2004) 'Influences on quality of life: a qualitative investigation of ethnic differences among older people in England', *Journal of Ethnic and Migration Studies*, 30: 737–761.

Gunaratnam, Y. (2003) *Researching 'Race' and Ethnicity: methods, knowledge and power*, London: SAGE.

Herdman, M., Fox-Rushby, J. and Badia, X. (1998) 'A model of equivalence in the cultural adaptation of the HRQoL instruments: the universalist approach', *Quality of Life Research*, 7: 323–335.

Hughes, A.O., Fenton, S. and Hine, C.E. (1995) 'Strategies for sampling black and ethnic minority populations', *Journal of Public Health Medicine*, 17: 187–192.

Hunt, S.M. and Bhopal, R. (2004) 'Self report in clinical and epidemiological studies with non-English speakers: the challenge of language and culture', *Journal of Epidemiology and Community Health*, 58: 618–622.

Kirby, P. (1999) *Involving Young Researchers: how to enable young people to design and conduct research*, York: York Publishing Services.

Lee, T. (2001) *Language-of-interview Effects and Latino Mass Opinion*, Harvard University: John F. Kennedy School of Government.

Marshall, S. and While, A. (1994) 'Interviewing respondents who have English as a second language: challenges encountered and suggestions for other researchers', *Journal of Advanced Nursing*, 19: 566–571.

May, T. (1993) *Social Research: issues, methods and process*, Buckingham: Open University Press.

Merton, R.K. (1972) 'Insiders and outsiders: a chapter in the sociology of knowledge', *American Journal of Sociology*, 78: 9–48.

Modood, T., Berthoud, R., Lakey, J. *et al.* (1997) *Ethnic Minorities in Britain: diversity and disadvantage*, PSI Report 843, London: Policy Studies Institute.

Nazroo, J.Y. (1997) *The Health of Britain's Ethnic Minorities Findings from a National Survey*, London: Policy Studies Institute.

Nazroo, J. and Grewal, I. (2002) 'Qualitative methods for investigating ethnic inequalities: lessons from a study of quality of life among older people', *ESRC Growing Older Programme Newsletter*, Issue 4, Spring.

O'Connor, W. and Nazroo, J. (eds) (2002) *Ethnic Differences in the Context and Experience of Psychiatric Illness: a qualitative study*, Norwich: The Stationery Office.

Papadopoulos, I. and Lees, S. (2001) 'Developing culturally competent researchers', *Journal of Advanced Nursing*, 37: 258–264.

Phoenix, A. (1994) 'Practising feminist research: the intersection of gender and "race" in the research process', in M. Maynard and J. Purvis *Researching Women's Lives from a Feminist Perspective*, London: Taylor & Francis, pp. 49–71.

Reese, S.D., Danielson, W.A., Shoemaker, P.J. *et al.* (1986) 'Ethnicity-of-interviewer effects among Mexican-Americans and Anglos', *Public Opinion Quarterly*, 50: 563–572.

Rhodes, P.J. (1994) 'Race-of-interviewer effects: a brief comment', *Sociology*, 28: 547–558.

Ritchie, J. and Lewis, J. (eds) (2003) *Qualitative Research Practice: a guide for social science students and researchers*, London: SAGE.

Smith, P. and Prior, G. (1996) *The Fourth National Survey of Ethnic Minorities: technical Report*, Social and Community Planning Research.

Warren, L., Maltby, T. and Cook, J. (2000) 'Older women's lives and voices: participation and policy in Sheffield', *Generations Review*, 10: 15–16.

Worcester, R.M. and Kaur-Ballagan, K. (2002) 'Who's asking? Answers may depend on it', *Public Perspective*, 42–43.

Zinn, M.B. (1979) 'Field research in minority communities: ethical, methodological and political observations by an insider', *Social Problems*, 27: 209–219.

Chapter 6

Culturally competent research

A model for its development

Irena Papadopoulos

Introduction

A number of factors have been identified that point to the difficulties in doing culturally competent research, which is here defined as research that both utilises and develops knowledge and skills that promote the delivery of health care that is sensitive and appropriate to individuals' needs, whatever their cultural background.

Despite the cultural diversity of most societies in today's world, Porter and Villarruel (1993) argue that a unicultural perspective in research prevails, which assumes that concepts and explanations of relationships between concepts are universally applicable across different cultures. Research continues to exclude 'culture', and its related concept of 'ethnicity', as essential variables even though in the last 25 years there has been a growing realisation that our understanding of health and illness has to be considered not only in terms of biological factors, but also in terms of social and cultural determinants (Dahlgren and Whitehead 1991). One reason for this, is the historical domination of the health research agenda by positivistic approaches with a focus on objective measurement, emphasis on facts, prediction, and production of value free, universal truths. Further, most of the research in the UK (and other developed countries) continues to be focused on the majority culture and is undertaken by researchers who belong to the majority culture. This inevitably has affected the way research priorities and research problems are conceptualised, defined and funded. However, the research agenda is very slowly becoming more balanced, primarily due to the persisting health inequalities worldwide, which are forcing governments to invest in research that aims to understand the impact of the socio-economic and cultural factors on health. In addition, the pluralistic nature of our society has heightened awareness for the need for research paradigms that can deal with the needs of culturally and ethnically diverse populations, in more effective and sensitive ways. The need for new paradigms is also becoming more evident and compelling in a global world. Health problems in one country quickly become problems of all countries. The recent outbreak of SARS in China amply demonstrated the importance of generating knowledge across national and cultural divides. Irrespective of the scale of the research projects – international, national or local – researchers need to understand the world views of their collaborators and target populations, otherwise the chances of generating invalid results are high.

New research paradigms cannot be achieved overnight. In order to move towards more effective paradigms, researchers need to overcome the existing indifference and superficiality of treatment of ethnicity and culture, and must at least be convinced of the centrality of culture when developing their research programmes. Current WHO and UK health policy, is making an impact and we are beginning to see a more serious consideration being given to culture and ethnicity. However, Senior and Bhopal (1994) in discussing the use of 'culture' and 'ethnicity' as variables in research, high-light the problems that may arise due to the lack of precise definitions of these terms. They argued that the lack of agreed definitions leads to difficulties of measurement, as well as to an inability to represent the heterogeneity of the populations being studied; further they are concerned that a focus on culture may result in essentialist research designs. McKenzie and Crowcroft (1996: 1054) suggested, however, that: 'Given our diversity, the fact that ethnicity is now most often self-classified, and that both ethnicity and culture are dynamic it seems unlikely that an agreed taxonomy can be achieved.' Until a consensus is reached on how culturally or ethnically to demarcate the people of the world, they advise that researchers collect a range of information that will help to describe the groups being researched. Papadopoulos and Lees (2001) reported that another major factor impeding the development of culturally competent research designs is the absence of appropriate training to help researchers become culturally competent practitioners. They undertook a review of a number of key research textbooks that were recommended in the curricula of various postgraduate courses that included a research component; they found that the majority of textbooks did not address concepts such as culture, ethnicity, language, culturally knowledge-able or sensitive research methods, cultural comparisons, racism, ethnocentricity, etc.

It is important to clarify at this point that we are all cultural beings. Therefore, a culturally competent research approach is not aimed only at researching the health needs and problems of minority ethnic groups. It is also important to realise that such an approach does not only apply to qualitative research, but it equally applies to quan-titative research designs. Henderson (1992) states that culturally sensitive research is not research about another culture, but research done with a raised consciousness concerning the impact of culture on the persons and/or phenomena being studied, on the research process itself, and on the researcher.

There is considerable evidence that suggests that the absence of the cultural per-spective in health research results in the failure to produce, for example, knowledge about the values, health needs, disease patterns, health behaviours, religious practices, and other problems such as socio-economic inequality, racism, etc., of people from different cultural and ethnic groups. This lack of information impedes the under-standing of service providers, resulting in inappropriate provision that is either ineffective or not utilised. It could be argued that the hitherto neglect by health researchers to undertake culturally competent research has contributed to the persist-ence of health inequalities. Therefore, the need for research training that reflects the diversity of cultures and the plurality of needs, is both urgent and the key to the future development of policy.

A model for the development of culturally competent researchers

Papadopoulos et al. (1998) first proposed a model for developing culturally com-petent health practitioners, which consisted of the four constructs: cultural awareness,

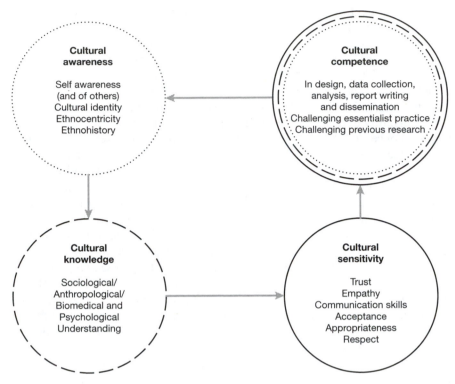

Figure 6.1 Concepts of cultural competence of research.

Adapted from Papadopoulos *et al.* (1998).

cultural knowledge, cultural sensitivity and cultural competence. Papadopoulos and Lees (2001) have adapted these constructs to address culturally competent research as they believe that a framework, rather than a 'pot-pourri', approach to training is far more preferable and effective (Figure 6.1).

Cultural awareness

This begins with the researchers examining and challenging their own personal value base and understanding how these values are socially constructed. This culminates in the process of being reflexive whereby researchers reflect on how their own values, perceptions, behaviour, or presence, and those of the respondents, can affect the data they collect (Parahoo 1997). Reflexive researchers should be conscious of the need to be explicit about their position in the research process and how their cultural backgrounds and those of respondents interrelate. Leininger (1995) points out that without cultural awareness researchers tend to impose their beliefs, values and patterns of behaviour upon cultures other than their own. She suggests that this leads to invalid research data. In relation to researching minority ethnic cultures, Hunt and Bhopal (2003) state that researchers should be cognisant of the customs, values and beliefs of the target group(s) before designing any project. Becoming aware of the ethnohistory of the group or groups to be studied will raise the researchers' awareness around important issues such as politics, historical events, religion, language, family structures, gender issues, and so on, all of which are affected by, and affect, the group's culture. Furthering cultural awareness can be achieved through the collaboration between researchers and/or consumers from the cultures one intends on studying, as discussed in Chapter 4 of this volume. However, simply having a multicultural team does not protect against ethnocentric views and cultural bias, which every individual of the research team needs to become aware of and try to minimise during all stages of the research. As this is not necessarily a straightforward or a quick process, leadership is required to facilitate the development of cultural awareness. But it should be viewed as an investment for the team members some of whom will have to learn new ways of researching. Ovretveit (1998) suggests that culturally competent trained researchers develop tolerance, patience and persuasive diplomacy; skills that are important qualities for leading projects in multicultural societies or across cultures.

Bennett's (1986) useful heuristic model suggests that in order to move from our ethnocentric positions to more ethnorelative ones, we must move through a number of stages, which require skilful facilitation. These stages are: denial, defence, minimisation, acceptance, adaptation and integration. Although this is primarily a linear process, Bennett states that the boundaries of each stage are blurred and that it is possible to skip a stage or, in some cases, go backwards a stage. In the stage of 'denial', one's own culture is seen as the only culture, thus cultural differences are not recognised. In extreme cases of denial the humanity of members of other cultures is suppressed. One example of denial in research is the infamous Tuskegee syphilis study of the US Public Health Service, when, in order to observe the effects of untreated syphilis, almost 400 Black men with syphilis were told they were being treated for 'bad blood', never told they had syphilis and never given penicillin. Many of them died from the disease or its complications. During the stage of 'defence', cultural differences are recognised, but are defended against by the belief that one's own culture is superior. In the 'minimisation' stage cultural differences may be recognised, but the magnitude of their impact is still minimised. An example of this is the frequent use of research instruments that have been standardised within the dominant White culture to study populations of other cultures. In the 'acceptance' stage, differences are acknowledged and seen as valid and part of a dynamic process; individuals begin to understand their own culture more deeply and realise that it is also dynamic and changeable. It is at this stage, which I call cultural awareness, that culturally sensitive research can begin to take place. In the 'adaptation' stage, an individual is able to adapt to a different culture. This is what happens to migrant researchers (and migrants in general) who successfully adapt to the culture of their host country. Finally, 'integration' occurs when an individual is able to move comfortably among cultures and simultaneously take into account the various elements of different cultures. This is what I would call a culturally competent person.

Cultural knowledge

Although cultural knowledge is drawn from many disciplines, such as anthropology, sociology, history, psychology and biomedicine, contact with people from different cultural groups is highly desirable. Knowledge derived from these disciplines is required in order to understand the similarities and differences of cultural groups. For example, sociologists have provided explanations about the structural forces in society, such as the power of health care professionals and the role of medicine in social control. Such forces are profoundly influential in the creation or perpetuation of health inequalities within and between groups. Another example of the application of cultural knowledge is the avoidance of essentialism, which assumes that there are essential cultural differences between people that always override other aspects of their being. Douglas (1998) suggested that a common essentialist practice in research is the assignment of health problems to the culture of an individual to the exclusion of other important influences, such as country of origin, area of residence, socio-economic status and gender. Essentialising knowledge that derives from culturally incompetent research is dangerous, and may lead to stereotyping, prejudice and discrimination. Cultural knowledge should be reflected in the conceptualisation of the research project, its design, data collection methods, analysis and presentation of findings.

Cultural sensitivity

Considering research participants as true partners is an essential component of cultural sensitivity and a crucial element in anti-oppressive practice (Dalrymple and Burke 1995). Partnership demands that power relationships are challenged and that real choices are offered. These outcomes involve a process of facilitation, advocacy and negotiation, which can only be achieved on a foundation of trust, respect and empathy. Telford *et al.* (2003) undertook a study to find out the successful ways of involving consumers in research. Even though the investigation did not declare a cultural stance, the principles derived from the study can be applied to achieve cultural sensitivity in the research design and process. The principles include the importance of costing the consumer involvement, the provision of training and support to consumers involved in research, the desirability of involving consumers in decisions about how research participants are both recruited and kept informed about the progress of the research, and the reporting of their involvement in research reports. Patel (1999) provides a set of guidelines to be used to improve sensitivity when researching health issues related to minority ethnic groups. She recommends that researchers should always consult members of the community or group to be studied while being aware that minority ethnic communities are not homogeneous nor can their members be entirely representative of all those belonging to their community. She goes on to state that the power differentials between the researcher and those being researched should be considered throughout the research process.

Interviews are a common method of data collection in research. An example of culturally sensitive research is the notion of content equivalence. This requires the researcher to ensure that the questions asked are relevant to the target culture and that they do not include concepts that are offensive, as for instance asking a devout Muslim to state how much alcohol he consumes per week, or an orthodox Jew if his newborn son will be circumcised. Naturally, if there is a strong rationale for conducting research on such culturally sensitive topics, this must be done following an extensive immersion into the particular culture and in collaboration with appropriate people from that culture, in order to prepare the data collection phase in as sensitive a way as possible.

Another example of culturally sensitive research is the matching of the ethnicity and culture of the interviewer and participant whenever possible (see the discussion in Chapter 5). This approach should not be applied lightly as there are numerous and complex reasons as to why this may, in fact, be undesirable. Notwithstanding the fact that cultural or ethnic groups can be very heterogeneous, this approach when used appropriately encourages a more equal context for interviewing which allows more sensitive and accurate information to be collected. A researcher with the same ethnic and cultural background as the participant will possess 'a rich fore understanding' (Ashworth 1986), an insider/emic view (Leininger 1991, Kaufman 1994), will have more favourable access conditions leading to the co-operation of a large number of people (Hanson 1994), and a genuine interest in the health and welfare of their community (Hillier and Rachman 1996). Care should be taken to counteract the disadvantages of ethnic/cultural matching. As far back as 1978, Kratz suggested that researchers who share the target community's culture and ethnic background may take some of what the research participant is saying for granted; s/he is less likely to ask those naive questions that could yield useful explanations. Hammersley and Atkinson (1995) advise that in order to avoid over-identification and over-rapport with the population being studied, the researcher should aim to adopt a marginal position of simultaneous insider/outsider, and be intellectually poised between familiarity and strangeness. Although they acknowledge that this is very difficult to achieve, it is not impossible. Burman (1996), on the other hand, suggested that having easy access and co-operation may result in exploitation of the group. For this reason, culturally competent research should be underpinned by both professional ethics and internationally agreed codes of ethics and human rights.

Cultural competence

This requires the synthesis and application of previously gained awareness, knowledge and sensitivity. An important component of this stage is the ability to recognise and challenge forms of racialised/discriminatory thinking such as essentialism, ethnocentricity, and racism. Here I discuss how key stages of the research process can be made culturally competent, illustrating my points with examples from the EMBRACE[1] UK Project (Papadopoulos and Gebrehiwot 2002), which investigated the beliefs, migration and adaptation processes, and the experiences with the health care system of Ethiopian refugees.

Study design

As discussed above, the involvement of consumers is crucial at the study design stage. Such involvement will ensure that the research problem is firmly responding to the realities and perceptions of the target groups, and is sensitively articulated and presented. The challenge here is to decide who to involve and how? If the researcher is approached by a particular cultural group to become involved in investigating an issue they are concerned about, then clearly issues around involvement become easier to address. However, if the researcher wishes to respond to a call for proposals by a funder, then the issues of involvement need serious consideration. For example, the EMBRACE UK Project was initiated by myself. I contacted an Ethiopian organisation in London and discussed with them my intentions to develop a research proposal. The leader of the organisation was enthusiastic about my proposal and became committed to working with me. I obtained information about the organisation in order to familiarise myself with the work they did, their size and complexity, the extent of services they provided and the credibility they had within their community. Having satisfied myself that this was an organisation that would make a good partner, I questioned whether other similar organisations should also be invited to participate. I was convinced by them and my investigation that this was not necessary as the organisation had extensive links with its community and was widely used by members of the community UK-wide. At a very early stage, the roles of each partner were clarified and agreed ensuring that equal involvement was achieved. A steering committee chaired by an eminent member of the Ethiopian community was established with representation of all key stakeholders assured.

It was important for me to learn as much as I could about the Ethiopian culture, the numerous sub-cultures that it consists of, the history, politics and recent conflicts of its people, the reasons why many fled Ethiopia, the health systems they were used to in Ethiopia and their self-care practices. My readings were augmented and grounded in reality by my Ethiopian partners. I soon discovered that not all Ethiopian migrants were of the same tribe, religion or political affiliation. Knowing this enabled me to avoid making mistakes in the research design and its operationalisation.

Research participants

It is essential that clear and detailed inclusion and exclusion criteria for research participants are developed in consultation with the collaborating organisation/s or the community representatives involved in the research design. It is important not to exclude sections of the target group/s because they are difficult to reach, reluctant to participate, or even discouraged to participate, as in the case of women in some cultural groups. Nevertheless, numerous ethical dilemmas may arise so broad ethical principles, such as avoidance of actions that may violate the moral standards of the cultures involved, or avoidance of causing harm, should be upheld. Guidance and advice from the community representatives is also crucial and the research team may have to modify their commonly used techniques of sampling to more unconventional ones. For example, it may be more realistic to opt for a purposive sample for a survey, as a random sample would be impossible to achieve. If data are needed from various age groups, the research team must ensure that the age bands used are meaningful to the communities being studied. For example, in the EMBRACE UK project, we used three age groups based on the advice given by our partners: 12–25 (adolescents and young adults), 25–59 (mid-life), and 60+ (elders). We opted for a combination of snowball and quota sampling. Having a community organisation as partner partly addressed the access issues.

Data collection

Culturally competent researchers realise that data collection raises numerous language issues. What language do the targeted research participants speak? Should information material and data collection tools be produced in different languages or will this be ineffective because large numbers of the target group/s are illiterate in their own language, or even do not have a written form of the language they speak? If interviews are to be used for collecting data, should the use of an interpreter be preferred over the use of a bi-lingual researcher? If data are collected in a language other than English how is the translation handled to assure quality and accuracy?

Birbili (2003), reports that collecting data in one language and presenting the findings in another is now increasingly common among social researchers. The factors that affect the quality of translation include the linguistic competence of the translator and the translator's knowledge of the culture of people under study. Temple (1997) points out that the use of translators and interpreters is not merely a technical matter that has little bearing on the outcome, it has epistemological consequences as it influences what is found. Temple (1997) argues that researchers who use translators need to acknowledge their dependence on them, not just for words, but to a certain extent for perspective. In doing so, researchers need to constantly discuss and debate conceptual issues with their translators in order to ensure that conceptual equivalence has been achieved. Similarly, readers of the research report need to be informed about who those people were and what kind of role they played at all stages of the research endeavour.

In the EMBRACE UK project, the advice given by our partners was that most interviews would have to be conducted in an Ethiopian language; it was anticipated that most participants would speak the official Ethiopian language, which is the Amhara. The decision was also taken that it would be desirable to recruit bi-lingual researchers to match the characteristics of the participants. Part of the role of those conducting the interviews was to recruit participants with the help of the community organisation. Further, we saw the recruitment of a number of Ethiopians for the data collection and first level analysis as capacity building for the Ethiopian community. Eight Ethiopian research assistants were recruited to work on the project on a part time basis. They all attended a structured training programme to familiarise themselves with the aims of the project, develop and/or refine their interview skills and become fully cognisant of their role. This included: recruiting research participants, gaining consent, arranging a venue for the interview, conducting the interview in the participant's preferred language, tape recording the interview, keeping field notes, attending supervision sessions, transcribing the interviews verbatim, translating the interviews if needed, and identifying what in their views were the main issues of each interview. During their training the research assistants helped to test the interview schedule. A verbal agreement was reached regarding the comparability of meaning of the concepts to be explored, which were written in English, and those to be used in Amharic. In order to test the accuracy of the translated concepts, the first interview of each research assistant was considered as a pilot. Conceptual comparability or equivalence needs to be taken very seriously as often concepts in one language do not exist in another. For example, Hunt and Bhopal (2003) reported that the term 'feeling blue' has different connotations in different languages, whereas the terms 'check up' and 'Pap smear' have no conceptual equivalence in any Chinese language. Helping the research assistants to adopt the marginal position of simultaneous insider/outsider was another topic focused on during training. Particular attention was given to ensure that researchers could follow the lead questions with relevant probing, thus avoiding taking what was said for granted. The research assistants were encouraged to become reflexive and were required during the study to record in their field notes the effect they may have had on research participants and the communication process, as well as how they dealt with a difficult situation, such as being asked to offer help or advice by the research participants during the interview, or when talking about a very sensitive topic such as depression or despair when they may have had much to identify with that particular situation. The supervision process enabled them to discuss any problems they had encountered and to explore solutions or alternative ways. In fact, the research assistants provided useful insights and made practical suggestions, which improved the data collection process.

Translating and back-translating interview transcripts

In qualitative research, data may be collected through a variety of methods such as one-to-one interviews, focus group interviews, observation, self-completed questionnaires and so on. If data are not in English, written translation to English is a must, even if the research team are fluent in the language used to collect the data. Skipping the translation and back-translation process must be avoided as crucial meanings will be missed. The practice of producing only a summary of the data into English should also be avoided. Unfortunately, this poor practice still goes on and is being excused as necessary due to lack of time and/or resources. However, a culturally competent researcher would ensure that these processes are adequately resourced within a realistic timetable.

Usunier (2003) reports that even basic concepts such as autonomy, leadership, friendliness, motivation, satisfaction, authority, well-being, shame and guilt, etc. are often used in research questionnaires as if they had universal meaning. However, words often express meaning shared only in the particular cultural and language group, especially when they relate to perceptions and interactions. If concepts are understood differently, there is a great chance that findings are, to a large extent, a reflection of differences in understanding.

Once the data are fully translated into English, back-translation should follow in order to assure the accuracy and quality of the translation and to eliminate any translation-related problems. Back-translation ensures that translation was not an exercise of mere lexical equivalence, but one of conceptual equivalence too. First, target language transcripts are translated into English and then the English transcripts are translated back to the target language by a second bi-lingual person (not involved with the original translation efforts). The two versions of the target language transcripts are then compared to determine how closely they match. A close match indicates that the translator is competent.

As discussed above, the bi-lingual interviewers of the EMBRACE UK project also transcribed and translated the interviews into English. The project employed three Ethiopian academics to act as back-translators. At the early stage of the data collection processes, a random translated transcript from each interviewer was selected and submitted for back-translation. The original Ethiopian transcript and the one produced by the back-translator were then read and carefully compared by the leader of the partner organisation who was also the co-director of the project. Differences in expression were identified but the reviewer was satisfied that the conceptual meaning remained true to the original transcript. This process assured the research team that the English translations were of good quality and none of the original meaning was lost or misrepresented. For, despite the training and supervision given to interviewers and the fact they are more likely to understand the meaning intended by the interviewees than an 'outsider' researcher, there is a danger of producing an edited English version of the original transcript for a number of reasons. For example, in another study conducted under my supervision, where the interview included questions on the sexual behaviour of Arab Muslim women, it was discovered through the back-translation process that the interviewer/translator had omitted or re-phrased small portions of the interview that, in her view, were portraying these women in a negative light.

Data analysis and validation

The methodological rigour described above prepares the way for a rigorous analysis. However, even this may not guard the researchers against unwitting ethnocentricity and cultural bias during the analysis process. This could result in the perpetuation of essentialist views and may lead to oppressive and racist attitudes among policy makers and service providers. It is therefore important that various approaches are adopted to ensure that this does not happen and that the analysis is accurate, fair and sensitively presented. Validating the analysis is an important process in qualitative research. Silverman (1993) suggests that there are two forms of validation particularly appropriate for qualitative research, that of triangulation and that of respondent validation. Triangulation is the process through which different kinds of data, or data derived from different methods, are compared to see whether they corroborate one another. Researcher triangulation has also been suggested as good practice. Respondent validation occurs when the findings are taken back to the subjects being studied in order to be verified.

The qualitative data of the EMBRACE UK project was analysed using a constant comparative process of defining and redefining any emerging themes in the light of new data. The emerging themes were elaborated conceptually using theoretical and empirical constructs from the literature. The initial first level analysis of the interview data was performed by those who conducted the interviews. Independent analysis of a random sample of transcripts was performed by three members of the research team who agreed on the final coding frame to be used in order to identify the major themes. Although the pure form of respondent validation was not undertaken, researcher and methodological triangulation were utilised. Further, the preliminary findings were presented at two peer review conferences, which provided an opportunity for discussion, reflection and validation. The findings were also presented to the steering committee, which was constituted by community representatives (proxy respondent validation) as well as other stakeholders. Given the methodological rigour of the project, and the advantages of a research team that included both 'insiders' (Ethiopians) providing the 'emic' perspective, and 'outsiders' (non-Ethiopians) providing the 'etic' perspective, the research team was confident that the findings were free from cultural bias (non-essentialist), had truth value (credibility), were dependable (reliability) and that they could be applicable to the rest of the Ethiopian UK community (generalisability).

Reporting and disseminating the findings

Reporting the findings should be done in sensitive and inclusive ways. First, it is crucial that community representatives are not excluded during this stage. Second, the voices of the participants must be allowed to be heard. Third, the report, or at the minimum its executive summary, must be translated into the community language/s of the participants, and if necessary into other formats such as audio tapes, to enable them easy access to the findings. Fourth, dissemination activities such as conferences should not be the exclusivity of the academics, but should involve members of the partner organisation/s. Fifth, community mass media should be used, as many cultural groups now have access to these media. Sixth, the reporting and dissemination of the findings must avoid essentialism for all the reasons given in the previous sections. Finally, the research report must include an action plan for change. This is an act of respect to the participants who gave up their time, and often much more, in order to contribute to a project which they believed would benefit their community.

The EMBRACE UK report was edited by myself and the Ethiopian project co-director. Its chapters have been co-authored by some of the Ethiopian members of the research team. Extensive direct quotations are used that allow the voices of the participants to be heard. The research report contains an extensive executive summary and, crucially, a detailed plan of action. The findings have been presented by the Ethiopian Radio. Numerous conferences and workshops have been presented jointly and two articles, written jointly, have been published in peer review journals.

Concluding considerations

It could be argued that a culturally competent approach to research is unrealistic as it may be perceived as long winded, time consuming, resource intensive and a needlessly politically correct approach. I would argue that culturally incompetent research is wasteful, dangerous and unethical. It is true that many of the skills I described as essential for culturally competent research need time to be developed, but then competencies of any kind take time to develop. Since most of us would not accept culturally incompetent health care (even though many of us have to for lack of an alternative), why should we find knowledge or evidence that was derived through culturally incompetent ways as acceptable? And if we believe that research should be rigorous and appropriate then we must factor into our proposals adequate funding and time, and funding bodies must support this. Culturally competent research promotes inclusivity and fairness. Further, I suggest that the principles I described above are applicable to all types of research. Within the global context of today's information flows, culturally competent research can facilitate high quality cross-cultural and comparative research at national and international levels.

Note

1   EMBRACE UK stands for Ethiopian Migrants, their Beliefs, Refugeedom, Adaptation, Calamities and Experiences in the United Kingdom.

References

Ashworth, P. (ed.) (1986) *Qualitative Research in Psychology*, Pennsylvania, PA: Duquesne University Press.

Bennett, M.J. (1986) 'A developmental approach to training for intercultural sensitivity', *International Journal of Intercultural Relations*, 10: 179–196.

Birbili, M. (2003) Publishing on the internet, *Translating from one language to another*, Social Research Update 31. University of Surrey. Available HTTP: http://www.soc.surrey.ac.uk/sru/SRU31.html (accessed 18 September 2003).

Burman, E. (1996) 'Interviewing', in P. Bannister, E. Burman, I. Parker and M. Taylor *Qualitative Methods in Psychology. A research guide*, Buckingham: Open University Press.

Dahlgren, G. and Whitehead, M. (1991) *Policies and Strategies to Promote Equity in Health*, Stockholm: Institute for Future Studies.

Dalrymple, J. and Burke, B. (1995) *Anti-Oppressive Practice. Social care and the law*, Buckingham: Open University Press.

Douglas, J. (1998) 'Developing appropriate research methodologies with black and minority ethnic communities. Part 1: reflections on the research process', *Health Education Journal*, 57: 329–338.

Hammersley, M. and Atkinson, P. (1995) *Ethnography Principles in Practice*, 2nd edn, London: Routledge.

Hanson, E.J. (1994) 'Issues concerning the familiarity of researchers with the research setting', *Journal of Advanced Nursing*, 20: 940–942.

Henderson, D.J. (1992) 'Toward culturally sensitive research in a multicultural society', *Health Care for Women International*, 13: 339–359.

Hillier, S. and Rachman, S. (1996) 'Childhood development and behavioural and emotional problems as perceived by Bangladeshi parents in East London', in D. Kelleher and S. Hillier (eds) *Researching Cultural Differences in Health*, London: Routledge.

Hunt, S. and Bhopal, R. (2003) 'Self reports in research with non-English speakers', *British Medical Journal*, 327: 352–353.

Kaufman, K.S. (1994) 'The insider/outsider dilemma: field experience of white researcher "getting in" a poor black community', *Nursing Research*, 43: 179–183.

Kratz, C.R. (1978) *Care of the Long-term Sick in the Community*, London: Churchill Livingstone.

Leininger, M.M. (ed.) (1991) *Culture Care, Diversity and Universality: a theory of nursing*, New York: NLN Press.

Leininger, M.M. (1995) *Transcultural Nursing. Concepts, theories, research and practices*, New York: McGraw-Hill.

McKenzie, K.J. and Crowcroft, N.S. (1996) 'Describing race, ethnicity, and culture in medical research', *British Medical Research*, 312: 1054.

Ovretveit, J. (1998) *Comparative and Cross-cultural Health Research. A practical guide*, Abingdon: Radcliffe Medical Press.

Papadopoulos, I. and Gebrehiwot, A. (eds) (2002) *The E.M.B.R.A.C.E. UK Project. The Ethiopian Migrants, their Beliefs, Refugeedom, Adaptation, Calamities, and Experiences in the United Kingdom*, London: Middlesex University.

Papadopoulos, I. and Lees, S. (2001) 'Developing culturally competent researchers', *Journal of Advanced Nursing*, 37: 258–264.

Papadopoulos, I., Tilki, M. and Taylor, G. (1998) *Transcultural Care: a guide for health care professionals*, Salisbury: Quay Books.

Parahoo, K. (1997) *Nursing Research: principles, process and issues*, Houndmills: Macmillan.

Patel, N. (1999) *Getting the Evidence. Guidelines for ethical mental health research involving issues of 'race', ethnicity and culture*, London: TCPS and Mind Publications.

Porter, C. and Villarruel, A. (1993) 'Nursing research with African American and Hispanic people: guidelines for action', *Nursing Outlook*, 41: 59–67.

Senior, P. and Bhopal, R. (1994) 'Ethnicity as a variable in epidemiological research', *British Medical Journal*, 309: 327–330.

Silverman, D. (1993) *Interpreting Qualitative Data: methods for analysing, talk, text and interaction*, London: Sage.

Telford, R., Boote, J. and Cooper, C. (Autumn 2003) 'Principles of successful consumer involvement in NHS research: results of a consensus study and national survey', *INVOLVE newsletter*, p. 6.

Temple, B. (1997) 'Watch your tongue: issues in translation and cross-cultural research', *Sociology*, 31: 607–618.

Usunier, J.C. (2003) *Publishing on the Internet*, Université Louis Pasteur, *The use of language in investigating conceptual equivalence in cross-cultural research*. Online. Available http://marketing.byu.edu/htmlpages/ccrs/proceedings99/usunier.htm (accessed 18 September 2003).

Chapter 7

Approaches to conducting qualitative research in ethnically diverse populations

Karl Atkin and Sangeeta Chattoo

The growing popularity of qualitative methodologies has been accompanied by an increasing interest in research into health and healthcare of ethnic minority populations living in the UK (see Ahmad 2000). Such research raises particular methodological challenges. Current debates, for example, struggle to engage with ethnicity, often reinforce essentialized notions of the "other" and fail to deal appropriately with ideas about equity and access (Atkin 2004). This, however, embodies a more fundamental tension. Research related to ethnic minority populations often finds itself marginalized and relegated to a sub-speciality of "ethnicity" subordinated to more "mainstream" concerns.[1] This is reflected, for instance, in how people representing these populations are conveniently excluded from an overwhelming majority of clinical trials (Hussain-Gambles *et al.* 2004), as well as qualitative studies (Ahmad *et al.* 2002). At a more mundane level, although equally worrying, is the appropriation of this "left-over," marginalized field by researchers from diverse professional backgrounds, without any particular theoretical orientation. This often results in descriptive and poorly contextualized studies that ignore the complexity and theoretical rigor of qualitative approaches. These studies not only undermine the value of qualitative methodologies but also fail to explain difference and diversity.

It is, therefore, useful to go back to first principles and explore the philosophical basis of qualitative methods and examine their value in researching health within an ethnically diverse society. This is the focus of the first section of this chapter, to be followed by a brief discussion of some of the practical aspects of research design. We will then broaden the discussion by looking at the process of doing qualitative research and explore the potential for adopting a research method that is rigorous and provides the opportunity for critical insight into the field of health and social care within a multiethnic society. We will specifically look at ways in which qualitative approaches can help us understand the experience of ethnic minority populations as part of the larger society, using examples from research done in the UK.

It is not our intention to offer a general introduction to qualitative approaches. There are many excellent books available on the subject and we do not wish to go over familiar ground (see, for example, Bryman and Burgess 1994, Creswell 1994, Denzin and Lincoln 1998, Mason 1996, Wengraf 2001). We are more concerned with the significance of qualitative strategies within the broader context of making 'meaningful' observations about the experiences of ethnic minority people (see Taylor 2004, for a broader discussion of these issues) and providing explanations that will add to our current understanding. With this in mind, we end by exploring how qualitative research methods might contribute towards positive change in policy and practice in terms of addressing issues of diversity, inequalities and discrimination at a collective level, and how the notion of reflexivity is central to this process.

The origins of qualitative research

We begin with a brief philosophical prologue on the origins of qualitative methodologies. Admittedly, in doing so, we run the risk of simplifying what are extremely complex and diverse debates.[2] Nonetheless, our aim is to get across some key ideas that provide an insight into the origins and developments of qualitative research, which will be of interest to a general reader.

In Western Europe, nineteenth-century social scientists, such as August Comte (1798–1857), Emile Durkheim (1858–1917) and Herbert Spencer (1820–1903), assumed that social reality was like any natural phenomena, and could be observed with comparable tools resulting in scientific explanations, predictions and probable laws of social behavior. This positivist or structural-functionalist mode of thought implied that society is *sui-generic*, existing independently of the individuals who make it up. This became the dominant thinking in the development of social science inquiry, but it left little room to explain conflict of interests, contradictions in perspectives and social change, which became the main focus of Karl Marx's (1818–1883) approach to dialectical materialism (following on from G.W.F. Hegel, 1770–1831 and George Feuerbach, 1804–1872). This perhaps explains why, towards the turn of the century, other philosophers such as Friedrich Nietzsche (1844–1900) were beginning to question an understanding of social reality that was premised on shared meaning and notions of truth derived from Christianity and to shift the focus to human agency, social action and meaning assigned by social actors, thereby providing the seeds for the future developments in reflexive social science and sociology.

Influential works of late nineteenth- and early twentieth-century writers, which questioned the value of using natural science methods to investigate the social world, for example, led to the development of hermeneutic analysis.[3] This applied the idea of looking beyond the 'here and now' and emphasized the importance of "interpretation" and "meaning" when making sense of the social world. This development followed on from the Kantian distinction between *phenomenon* (relating to the physical world) that can be *known* with the help of scientific methods and *noumena* (the abstract realm of feelings, experiences and emotions) that could be *understood* (see Immanuel Kant, 1724–1804). With this, came the possibility that human behavior, unlike that of the physical world, could be understood with reference to the meanings and purposes attached by human actors to their activities. Such views began to influence historical analysis. For William Dilthey (1833–1911) and Johann Gustav Droysen (1806–1884), 'understanding' or *verstehen* came to emphasize the value of looking at how people made sense of and interpreted the circumstances in which they found themselves (see Outhwaite 1986 for a broader discussion). Max Weber (1864–1920), writing at the turn of twentieth century and building on the work of Dilthey and Droyson, began to apply some of the principles of *verstehen*, as he attempted to establish a methodology for the social sciences that would enable "meaningful" empirical observations to take place.

Qualitative research, therefore, can trace its roots to the method of *verstehen*, which came to be associated with understanding social reality, by going beyond surface meaning – "the here and now" – and engaging with the process of "interpretation," "meaning" and "the construction (and representation) of meaning." There is an obvious tension here between the two epistemological stands of realism regarding the existence of social reality out there that can be interpreted with appropriate tools, and relativism arising from the constructivist perspective related to the idea that meaning is subjective and assigned by social actors. Hammersley (2002) suggests that adopting a framework of subtle realism and reflexivity can be one way of reconciling this tension. We will explore this further, as we discuss the value of qualitative methods and the particular importance of reflexive practice in addressing issues of access to health and social care.

The value of qualitative research

At the very outset, we have to acknowledge that our approaches to research have particular historical bearings (see Denzin and Lincoln 1998). The twin focus on ethnicity and the use of qualitative methods in investigating health and access to healthcare within sociology, for example, is located in wider post-1950s shift in epidemiology and better understanding of the role of social and economic factors influencing patterns of health and illness; and the steady increase in the incidence of chronic diseases alongside rises in life expectancy. The 1960s and 1970s saw the rise of new ideas and approaches, which moved away from Parsons' functionalist theory towards Marxism, conflict theory (Zola 1972) and issues of structured disadvantage (Taussig 1980), and inter-actionist perspectives (Gerhardt 1989). This involved a shift of focus towards the meaning of illness, and negotiations of ideas and relationships related to illness. More importantly, the rise of feminism, the social model of disability and anti-racist methodologies in the 1980s (Oakley 1980, Gilman 1985, Stacey 1988, Oliver 1990, Arber 1994, Arber and Ginn 1991) had a huge influence on how we look at pathology, difference and disadvantage related to gender, age, class, ethnicity, sexuality and disability. Finally, post-modern approaches (Bauman 1992, Giddens 1991) have reinforced the notion of the contingent nature of self and society, and shifted focus on how individuals negotiate different sources of information and authority, and notions of citizenship, related to illness and health-related behavior (for a review see Bury 1997).

We start with the basic assumption that methodologies cannot be true or false, only less or more useful in relation to the aims of research (see Silverman 2000). Debates that try to prove the superiority of one method over the other obscure the importance of choosing the most appropriate method for a particular research question (Creswell 1994). As suggested earlier, a certain degree of caution and methodological reflexivity (as explained below) is necessary when outlining the value of qualitative approaches. The twin fields of ethnicity and health, and qualitative approaches, are currently popular and often invoked together as a *mantra* for a safe and successful bid for funding. One of the common, methodologically unconvincing, justifications for using qualitative methods is that it is best suited for researching an area where not enough is known.

Much of qualitative research within the field, however, is synonymous with an uncritical following of Glaser and Strauss' grounded theory approach (1967) – rather than the intended intermeshing of data collection and theoretical reflection leading to "discovery of theory from data" (Bryman and Burgess 1994: 4–6). The grounded theory approach, itself a method rather than a theoretical perspective, is used as an "approving bumper sticker" (Richards and Richards 1991: 43) – a soft option for circumventing the need for any serious theoretical engagement with the research question. It is perhaps not surprising that within a fast track, multidisciplinary, policy oriented research culture, there is no acknowledgment of the discursive practices informing the research project and the influence of such practices on how the research is conducted, data analyzed and represented in a textual form.

Similarly, ethnographic research becomes disengaged from its interpretative underpinnings, and internal critique of realism, relativism and crisis of representation (see Clifford 1988, Clifford and Marcus 1986). It is used to give the illusion of gravitas within a largely post-positivist framework to what are little more than descriptive and poorly contextualized accounts. Ethnography has been misappropriated as a communal mode of sharing observations, interviews and analysis; defeating the underlying principles of holistic logic[4] – not to speak of the feminist, post-modern engagements with locating the subjectivity of the participant as well as the researcher within the text (see Denzin and Lincoln 1998, Hammersley 2002).

Most of us are guilty, in some measure, of contributing to this fragmentary and theoretically impoverished, multidisciplinary research culture. However, recognizing this is an important first step in developing *methodological* reflexivity that helps us engage with epistemological and ethical concerns arising from a particular piece of research. As suggested by Hammersley (2002: 75), this implies developing, "ways in which we monitor our assumptions and the inferences we make on the basis of them, and investigate those that we judge not to be beyond reasonable doubt." *Ideological* reflexivity, on the other hand, implies positioning the researcher within the intersecting representations of the field, and recognizing the partiality of a particular perspective rather than an "authentic" vision, more objective than others. Post-modern social theory has been criticized for embodying a pessimistic stance valorizing difference, relativism and endless forms of narrativization on self and society. However, ideological reflexivity remains central to critical research and social theory, informed by post-modern understandings, committed to change and restructuring of social relations of power and domination in society (Kincheloe and McLaren 1998: 279).

Following from above, we need to develop criteria that enable us to debate the quality of qualitative research within a shared framework, a practical step towards achieving methodological reflexivity. In some ways this is straightforward, and Box 7.1 provides an initial framework on which to base critical appraisal of qualitative methods (taken from criteria developed from Ryan *et al.* 2001, Waterman *et al.* 2001, Pope and Mays 1995, Mays and Pope 2000, Popay *et al.* 1998, Critical Appraisal Skills Programme 2002).

Such critical appraisal can introduce accountability and reflexivity into the research process and remind us that good qualitative research, just like good quantitative research, follows a logical and rigorous methodology; has a clear set of aims and objectives; follows a clear sampling strategy; justifies the method of data collection

---

Box 7.1 Critical appraisal of qualitative research

- Was the need for the research discussed?
- Was there a clear statement of research aims?
- Was the research method chosen appropriate to these aims?
- Was the connection with the existing body of knowledge made clear?
- Was the context of the research described so that a reader could relate the findings to other settings?
- Was the study design responsive and flexible?
- Was the sampling strategy made explicit, justified and related to the aims of the research?
- Was the method of data collection appropriate and relevant to the research questions?
- Was the approach to data analysis adequately explained and was it sufficiently rigorous and justified? How were themes and concepts identified from the research material? Was the relationship between evidence and interpretation transparent?
- Was there a clear statement of the findings?
- Were the findings appropriately contextualized in broader debates and a clear link made between data and commentary?
- Was the impact of the methods on the material obtained discussed?
- To what extent are the findings transferable?
- Does the research provide useful insights and contribute usefully to existing understanding?

---

and analysis; locates findings within the broader literature; and draws meaningful conclusions. Of course, qualitative techniques have a different emphasis to more quantitative strategies. There is, for example, less concern with hypothesis testing and establishing generalizable principles from large sample sizes, or demonstrating causal relationships between variables (Denzin and Lincoln 1998).

The ontological assumptions underlying qualitative methods help to capture a range of individual responses that reflect a diversity of attitudes and experiences related to various social variables or institutions, such as gender, age, socio-economic position, race, ethnicity, sexuality and disability (see Hammersley 1996). Further, the qualitative emphasis on *understanding* makes it an ideal strategy for gaining an insight into the complex nature of wider processes of "being" and "becoming," through which individuals engage with the broader relations of power, ideology, politics, economy and history (see Chamberlayne and King 2000).

Theoretically, at least, qualitative research by emphasizing the importance of understanding, interpretation and context, allows for *etic* (outsider) accounts to be challenged by local contexts, in which *emic* (insider) views can assume prominence and demonstrate the inappropriateness of certain dominant discourses in making sense of such experience (Denzin and Lincoln 1998). This, of course, is ideal for those exploring difference, diversity and inequalities related to health. This distinction also relates to another important feature of qualitative approaches – an ability to engage with bureaucratized, state and professional discourses on ethnicity that constitute the needs and experiences of ethnic minority communities through reified ideas of difference (also see Bhopal 1997).

Qualitative methods, for example, have successfully demonstrated how the assumptions of practitioners and policy makers deny ethnic minority populations the support they need from public organizations (see Mason 2000 for an overview and Bowler 1993, for a more specific example). In looking at how the needs of ethnic minority populations are interpreted and acted upon by those responsible for providing and managing the welfare state, we also have detailed accounts of the multi-faceted nature of institutional racism (Atkin 2004). In short, qualitative methods can address both the micro level of individual experience and the macro level of policy issues and, by doing so, suggest ways for bridging the gap between institutional policies protecting the rights of ethnic minority communities in principle and practice (see, for example, Gunaratnam 2001). This theme is further explored in our discussion of the more practical aspects of doing research.

Doing qualitative research

Up to now, our discussion has largely focused on the broader theoretical issues informing qualitative research. We now look at the actual process of conducting research in a multiethnic setting and the specific aspects that inform research design. In doing so, we will specifically relate our discussion to the criteria of critical appraisal outlined above and the broader context of reflexivity, which such appraisal implies. As we have mentioned, our intention is not to provide an introduction to all aspects of the research process but, rather, to ensure that qualitative research is appropriately grounded in broader debates about difference and diversity. Further, we would like to reiterate that critical qualitative research must recognize and address the gaps and issues related to equitable provision of health and social care within an ethnically diverse society.

As a starting point, it is perhaps important to mention that qualitative research does not have a distinct set of methods that it can claim for itself (Denzin and Lincoln 1998). Qualitative researchers can use a variety of techniques – such as face-to-face interviews, focus groups, observation, ethnography, reflective diaries and secondary sources to collect material – which can then be subject to a variety of different analytical strategies. Nonetheless, what underpins these different techniques and strategies is a concern with the systematic collection, organization and interpretation of data (Malterud 2001).

One of the important aspects of the research process is to clearly define the scope of the study. In practical terms, this implies making specific decisions about aims and objectives; sampling size and strategy; the method of data collection; the approach to analysis; and the purpose of the dissemination process: as well as ensuring these processes are linked and justified. The need to make such decisions is not, of course, peculiar to doing research with multiethnic populations, although the responses we adopt – as we shall see – have particular implications for the ways we frame and report our research. Further, the decisions we make in response to, say, sampling, for example, have implications for other aspects of the process, such as analysis. Consequently, ensuring a consistent theoretical approach, which facilitates and supports the generation of "meaningful" findings from the empirical material, addressing the objectives of research, is essential to a good research design and – more generally – the reflexive process.

Deciding the research focus

We begin by looking at how we decide the focus of the research and, in particular, establish the aims and objectives. Prior to this, however, is another important question: is the research really necessary? A critical approach is necessary to make sure that we are not reinventing the wheel in replicating previous research. This is of particular relevance when doing work in an area where a body of literature is already available. In formulating our research question, we might wish to consider, for example, whether primary research is really the answer. In a much researched area, would a review, using secondary resources, be more appropriate?

The relevance of a field of research shifts with time and new research must respond to the changing political and socio-economic scene. We may also have to accept that many local studies can sometimes be commissioned by statutory agencies as an excuse for inaction. We have, for example, accumulated a great deal of evidence outlining the process and outcomes of racism, disadvantage and discrimination in a wide variety of settings (Mason 2000). We need, therefore to think more creatively about situations, where we know little or where we can gain novel and fresh perspectives on previously researched areas.

Let us explain some of these issues further with the help of the following example of sickle cell disorders. Literature in the field of sickle cell disorders suggests that further research exploring the general difficulties faced by African-Caribbean people with sickle cell disorders in the UK, as they struggle to gain access to appropriate healthcare, may not be necessary (see Anionwu and Atkin 2001 for a detailed account of these problems). A more strategic approach to issues not explored or less understood is more appropriate. There is little work, for instance, exploring the broader social consequences of the condition. Looking at why service delivery fails to respond to the needs of those with hemoglobin disorders, for example, might prove equally productive as would specific evaluations of emerging service initiatives such as the introduction of neo-natal screening for those at risk of sickle cell disorders.

At a macro level, we might wish to reflect on why, despite our considerable evidence base explaining the process of discrimination, we struggle to translate these insights into improvements in service delivery. This would suggest a particular need for more research that explores how services can best meet the needs of ethnic minority populations. As part of this, it would be helpful to understand more about what constitutes good practice at a local level and how such practice can be sustained and replicated in other localities. Without addressing such questions, we are in danger of doing sterile research that wastes valuable public resources and people's time. More importantly, we are also in jeopardy of doing research that becomes little more than a token gesture, leading to increasing disillusionment and estrangement among ethnic minority populations.

Another fundamental problem concerns how the research question is framed and, more specifically, how it relates to current discursive practices about ethnic difference and diversity. Ironically, when research recognizes the importance of ethnicity to issues of health and social care, it often works to the disadvantage of ethnic minority populations. Sometimes this is the consequence of ill-informed views about the cause and epidemiology of diseases (see Bhopal 1997); at other times it is the use of inappropriate myths and stereotypes which, although purporting to explain the behavior and beliefs of ethnic minority populations, do little more than misrepresent their experience (see Parekh 2000 and Atkin 2004 for a discussion of these issues).

To begin with, research often identifies health and social care problems experienced by ethnic minority populations as arising from cultural practices (Ahmad 2000). This results in research often blaming ethnic minority communities for the problems they experience, because of their deviant, unsatisfactory and pathological lifestyles (Atkin 2004). The current obsession in research with the association between "poor birth outcome" and consanguineous marriages provides a good example of this (and how prior assumptions can corrupt the research process (Ahmad *et al.* 2000)).

Health professionals often relate low birth rate or childhood illness among Pakistani families to consanguineous marriages. This constructs congenital health problems within Pakistani communities as being self-inflicted, located within presumed cultural and biological deviance (Darr 1997). The relationship between consanguineous marriage and the incidence of childhood poor health is complex. In some cases, marrying a first cousin can increase a family's risk of giving birth to a disabled or chronically ill child, especially if there is a history of certain conditions in the extended family (Modell and Darr 2002). First cousin marriage, however, is not the only cause of disability or chronic illness in Pakistani families, and there is good evidence to suggest its influence has been over-emphasized (see Ahmad *et al.* 2000 for a review of the evidence). Such an approach not only carries with it an implicit (and misleading) criticism of "Asian" cultural practices; it also misrepresents the origins of ill health (Atkin *et al.* 1998). The pre-occupation with consanguineous marriage in explaining morbidity also means that other important explanations – such as poverty, poor maternal health, inappropriate housing, or inadequate service support – are rarely mentioned.

Low socio-economic status, for example, seems far more influential than ethnic origin or cultural difference in explaining ill-health among South Asian populations in general (Nazroo 1997). We also know that poor antenatal and postnatal care might be closely related to impairment and ill health among children in South Asian families, rather than any specific cultural practices (Mir and Tovey 2003). The process of service provision and continuity of care might, therefore, be a more legitimate and meaningful research focus rather than exotic beliefs and cultural practices. Clearly, a focus on culture, within such a context, draws our attention away from structural issues of inequality in access to services and forms of institutional cultures and racisms that reinforce these inequalities (see Gunaratnam 1997 and Ahmad 1996 for a review).

Sampling strategy

Once we have decided our research question and whether it is a legitimate focus for qualitative research, we have to develop a sampling strategy. In light of the above discussion, a theoretical definition of ethnicity is central to how the sample is selected (see Bradby 2003 and Karlsen and Nazroo 2002 for a broad discussion of these issues). The initial difficulty is how to define ethnicity and, more specifically, how to draw criteria of inclusion and exclusion for particular ethnic groups. Any definition of ethnicity then of course, needs to be related to the needs of the research question (Oakley *et al.* 2003). Collecting material on child feeding practices of "Indians" for a local Primary Care Trust, to help formulate local policy, would be of little use as it fails to take account of religious and regional differences and does not distinguish between people of Indian origin born in the UK and those born and brought up in India and Africa.

Ethnicity often refers to a shared sense of identity related to heritage, area of origin, religion, language and culture. At the same time, it also serves as a convenient surrogate term for attributes of race within the British context (see Anthias 1992, Ahmad 1996, Parekh 2000). Ethnicity is also increasingly seen as a political symbol, defining not just exclusion by a powerful majority but also a source of pride and belonging (Parekh 2000); a mobilizing resource that enables ethnic minority populations to celebrate their difference and make legitimate demands as citizens (Husband 1996).

Previous understandings that classify people according to their country of origin seem no longer sustainable, particularly since nearly 40 percent of those we regard as ethnic minority populations are born in the UK (Modood *et al.* 1997). Young people, for example, are beginning to redefine their identity and adopting such terms as British Muslim or British Caribbean (see Ahmad *et al.* 2002 for a discussion of these broad issues). In some ways, the multi-faceted nature in which we have come to understand "ethnicity" has the advantage of highlighting the context within which ethnicity, gender and socio-economic position intersect differently to shape individual and collective experiences of disadvantage and discrimination (see also Bhopal 2001).

To address the practical issues of sampling we must ask: does a research question require us to convey the experience of a wide range of ethnic minority groups or is it more appropriate to focus on just one? A common mistake is attempting to design a sample that includes too many different ethnic groups without a particular rationale. Those who fund research can be especially guilty of encouraging this since we have often been told that a research design representing the experiences of one defined ethnic group is too narrow in focus. Sometimes it is appropriate to focus on, for example, a sample of people of Pakistani origin. This might bring greater clarity and depth to the research findings, particularly if these are to be contextualized within the broader literature. In other instances, we may wish to broaden our sampling strategy to include a range of ethnic groups comprising South Asian populations. If a range of different ethnic groups is to be included, special attention must, however, be given to criteria of inclusion depending on how comparisons are to be drawn in analysis. The eventual decision ultimately depends on what the focus of the research is and the types of issues we wish to address.

A straightforward approach would be to use census categories as a guideline for sampling. This might be especially useful if we wish to draw comparisons between our findings and those of other researchers using these categories. Given the issues related to self-perception and fluid boundaries between ethnic groups, it is increasingly common to use a combination of ethnic origins as census categories with self-perception of participants about where they belong. Hence, for some purposes it is useful to have a sample representing broad categories of Pakistani Muslim, Indian Muslim or Bangladeshi Muslim. For other purposes, one might need a sampling strategy that distinguishes between Mirpuri-speaking Muslims and Pashto-speaking Pathan Muslims to draw out the significance of ethnic boundaries marked by region and language within the same religious and/or national group. Similarly, we might need a sampling frame that draws out differences and similarities between Gujarati-speaking Hindus who moved from Kenya and those who moved straight from Ahmedabad or Bombay to look at the specific features of different histories of migration within communities.

Once we have a workable definition of "ethnicity," it is important not to treat that ethnic group as homogeneous, but recognize that ethnic groups, whether minority or majority, are diverse in terms of social class, gender, age and history (Nazroo 1997, Smaje 1995). Sampling strategies need to reflect this diversity; otherwise they will risk the danger of presenting a skewed population, misrepresenting the experience of those who might be classified as belonging to that ethnic group. This has implications for appropriate sample size. As a rule of thumb, sample size must address both the diversity within an ethnic group and yet make theoretical generalizations for subgroups meaningful. However, there is no statistical logic of validity informing the right number of individuals/cases, and these issues are addressed theoretically in relation to the kind of data required as well as approach to analysis. Gareth Williams's essay (1993) is a classic example of robust analysis using one individual case study of a woman's experience of rheumatoid arthritis, located within wider social and cultural values related to the welfare state and disability at a collective level. We shall return to this issue when we discuss analysis.

Accounts that solely focus on the experience of various ethnic minority populations can be useful, although broader sampling strategies can provide a larger, structural context for understanding their experience. We have already discussed the possibility of including a range of different ethnic minority groups. It might also be appropriate to consider whether a sample of the majority/White population is necessary, given that ethnicity is not simply the preserve of (ethnic) minority populations. We also need to pay more attention to how we use White as a generic category, which is an equally difficult concept to define (Bradby 2003). Using a broad comparative framework, either from primary or secondary sources, is invaluable in avoiding the problem of attributing all differences in attitudes or experience to ethnicity.

The work of Chattoo and Ahmad (2003), for example, explored the meaning of end stage cancer for South Asian people and their families. They were able to contextualize the experience of South Asian people by also drawing a White sample. In doing so, they found that South Asian families shared many experiences with their White counterparts. More importantly, they were able to analyze how different people within the same ethnic group might attribute a similar experience, to different causes. Hence, for some Indian patients and carers a bad experience with nursing care at the hospital was experienced as yet another example of the racist attitudes of nursing professionals. For others, such experiences were perceived as reflecting problems within nursing care at a generic level within the NHS, and did not imply their own ethnicity in the equation since they had seen White patients receiving equally poor quality of care.

It is, however, important to add that contextualization might not always necessitate the inclusion of a White sample. In many areas, we have far more research that looks at the experience of a White or majority population. This research evidence can be used as a point of contextualization and comparison during analysis, instead of needing to include a White sample in the research design. The example of family care is an excellent case in point. We know, for example, that the experience of family caring has many generic features, which occur irrespective of ethnicity. Gender, for example, cuts across some of the variations in the experience of caring across ethnic groups (Atkin and Rollings 1996).

As with any other group, the experience of ethnic minority populations is interpreted, framed and acted upon within the context of service delivery and professional attitudes (Smaje 1995, Nazroo 1997, Atkin *et al.* 1998, Bhakta *et al.* 2000). There is research evidence to suggest that professional attitudes to care and patterns of referral to secondary services are informed by the gender, class and ethnicity of patients and carers (Smaje 1995). We know that, for example, referrals for community services are made less often for ethnic minority patients (Nazroo 1997). Further, health professionals may not always take the concerns of patients and carers of ethnic minority communities seriously (Atkin *et al.* 1998, Bhakta *et al.* 2000). To offer a meaningful account, it is sometimes necessary to engage with professional perspectives and the organizational culture within which these are located. This allows us to explore the ways in which legitimacy is sought for particular discursive practices related to notions of ethnicity and how this impacts on practice. Hence, inclusion of a sample of practitioners and managers of service provision might, at times, be useful in locating this broader context. Triangulation of data sources can also be important in analyzing and explaining similarities and differences in experiences of people from different ethnic backgrounds. This, in turn, can contribute to greater reflexivity in professional practice by shifting the focus on professional assumptions and cultures underlying particular health and social care practices (see Atkin *et al.* 1998).

This, however, raises a more philosophical point. Welfare provision, in principle, is premised on a collectively agreed notion of need. In practice it confronts difference and diversity of values related to ethnicity, gender and socio-economic position among other markers of stratification, within society. Consequently, welfare provision is, by its nature, complex, full of ambiguities, contradictions, inconsistencies and compromises, reflecting a mix of individual and collective solutions. Recognizing the subjectivity of individual citizens can only be addressed through bureaucratized notions of rights and justice (see Habermas 1986). Policy does not exist in a theoretical and moral void but embodies historically constructed, widely contested ideas and values regarding health, welfare, justice, social relationships and institutions, realized and given meaning through particular discursive practices (see Rojeck *et al.* 1988).

Such observations, though somewhat tangential to our discussion, are necessary to achieve a degree of ideological reflexivity, while also providing the opportunity to ground policy and practice recommendation in the everyday reality of organizational practice. Much policy and practice guidance, for example, seems to exist in a vacuum, often criticizing the essence of professional practice, without providing an alternative framework for action (see Hunter and Killoran 2004). Better understanding of the dynamics of professional practice can, therefore, help facilitate change. This is an issue we return to, when we discuss dissemination. More generally, framing research also needs to take into account broader power relationships and the context in which people's experiences are located and negotiated, as well as the political context within which research takes place.

Collecting material

As we have seen, there is no one method specifically appropriate to researching ethnic minority populations. Admittedly, there has been some debate about whether Euro-centric methods of data collection, such as the face-to-face interview, which are grounded in particular assumptions about individualism, adequately reflect the experience of other cultures, premised on alternate ways of constructing accounts of the self. This, however, is a complex debate to disentangle since our research methods – and underlying epistemological and ontological assumptions – are bound to be ethnocentric and rooted within a particular world view informing the discipline. It is difficult to transcend these assumptions without recourse to drawing simple polarities between East and West; the industrial and the non-industrial; the traditional and modern; and the modern and post-modern worldviews. It is possible, however, to take a skeptical position premised on reflexivity – where difference and diversity are recognized but not considered immutable within the context of research, given the broader principles of *verstehen* outlined in the introduction. As we have argued, methodological and ideological reflexivity in research design and analysis can begin to address these problems and debates and provide insights into received ideas and specific power relations that inform the process of doing research (see, for example, Willis 2000).

Tools for collecting qualitative material need to critically engage with these debates and also address the practical aspects of doing research with people for whom English may not be their first or second language (Marshall 1994). The importance of appropriately translated research material has been covered elsewhere in this book (see Chapters 6 and 9). What is, however, important to consider here is the use of translation and interpretation during the process of collecting research material. Informing people about the purpose of the research and the process of gaining consent should, of course, be produced in the relevant languages. It should be remembered, however, that some languages, such as Mirpuri or Pushto, spoken in the North-West frontier region of Pakistan, have no written script. While theoretically it is possible to use the Arabic/Urdu script for the vernacular, not everybody is necessarily literate in a language that they speak fluently (or use as a second language). Hence, in certain situations, the possibility of conveying such information on an audio cassette or other means might be more appropriate.

When collecting research material, a decision has to be taken about the types of questions one asks. At one level, this seems straightforward since what kind of data is collected depends on the kinds of questions the research is engaging with or trying to answer. However, this process needs to be made explicit, particularly since there is a tendency in qualitative research to obscure the process of generating questions or framework for observation. In other words, the data or material collected is informed by theoretical considerations and aims of research that inform the whole research process and analysis.

The difficulties of using interpreters in collecting information have been considered in Chapter 6 and, generally, we agree that their use does not produce sufficiently detailed or contextualized material on which to base qualitative analysis. It is preferable to use same-language interviewers rather than rely on interpreters. The use of certain qualitative methods, such as ethnography, specifically excludes the possibility of using interpreters since these methods rely on thick description and immersion in the field (Geertz 1973). In-depth interviews require a degree of understanding of the field as well as listening, probing and communicating skills that help build a rapport between the interviewer and interviewee that, we feel, is central to the qualitative research process as a whole.

Translation (and back-translation) is, indeed, necessary where interviews, focus groups or other forms of data have been collected in a language other than English. Ideally, it is sensible to rely on the person who collects the material to translate it, given the significance of the social context and non-verbal cues of communication within face-to-face interviews or focus group settings. This provides for a degree of consistency and immersion in the data set and helps locate the researcher in the text. However, given the pragmatic constraints of time, number of languages and typescripts one is working with, translating work is often commissioned to professional agencies. One of the basic rules of thumb is that, while translating, emphasis should be on providing conceptual rather than literal translations, attempting to preserve the use of local metaphor and the meaning intended by the person. Poor translation can have serious consequences for the quality of analysis and it is imperative to maintain quality control, especially when dealing with more than one regional language. It is, therefore, important to use skilled translators who can strike a balance between listening carefully without attributing their own meaning to the speech. Given the complex nature of translating from one language to another, it is also useful for a second person to cross-check the translated accounts to ensure quality and consistency for back-translation. This can help improve validity and meaning of the research findings in the same way as inter-reliability coding among members of the research team.

Finally, it is often believed that in engaging with ethnic minority populations, it is advisable to offer research participants a choice of who they speak to, in terms of say, gender, age and ethnic background (see Mclean and Campbell, 2003). Without going into the pros and cons of this rather complex 'insider-outsider' debate (see for example, Stanfield, 1998), which are discussed in more detail in Chapter 5, our experience suggests that the emphasis needs to be on appropriate language and communicative skills that facilitate a relationship of respect and trust, rather than matching ethnic background and gender of the participant and the researcher. Much, at times, depends on the nature of the topic under discussion and interpersonal skills of the researcher and to what extent s/he is comfortable with the topics being explored. To this extent fieldwork relationships are negotiated and not imposed or predefined (Burgess, 1984), and participants in any piece of research set boundaries of interaction that the researcher must respect.

Analysis

Clearly, our approach to analysis is mediated by other decisions taken at previous stages of the research design, especially sampling and the kind of questions probed.

There are several different strategies to qualitative analysis, although the basic principles remain the same. The purpose of analysis is to offer an explanation for a particular phenomenon, experience or institution rather than a mere description of a range of observations, responses or narrative accounts of subjective experiences. Most importantly, analysis explores concepts and establishes linkages between concepts implied in the research question and the data-set; and provides explanations for patterns or ranges of responses or observations from different sources (see Bryman and Burgess 1994 for a more detailed account).

Qualitative analysis often involves understanding the meaning of actions, beliefs, attitudes and relationships, from the range of participants' views on particular issues. This approach enables a comparative analysis of variations in experience, as well as the significance of an individual's background in making sense of this experience. Whether we are using the comparative method or a case study approach, it is possible to look at individual experience within the context of larger social institutions, and provide explanations for the individual as well as collective levels without reducing one to the other. Analysis must carefully look at the kind of data and nature of generalizations that can be made.

Analyzing material drawn from ethnic minority populations, however, raises several more specific issues. As discussed earlier, dominant discursive practices surrounding ethnicity, health and social care in the UK tend to present ethnic minority populations as the distant "other" and offer essentialized accounts of cultural practices, with little reflection on differences within, and similarities across, communities. As observed earlier, this focus on culture deflects attention away from structural issues of inequality in access to services and forms of institutional cultures and racisms that sustain these inequalities (see Gunaratnam 1997). Such essentialized accounts can also focus too much on potential ethnic differences, rather than considering ethnicity within a broader social context. As a starting point to addressing this issue, analysis needs to engage with the relationship between ethnicity, socio-economic status, age and gender and recognize these as generic markers of difference within any ethnic group (Smaje 1995, Nazroo 1997, Chattoo and Ahmad 2003, Atkin 2004). South Asian women, for example, sometimes struggle to convince doctors that their child is seriously ill and find themselves being dismissed as being "neurotic" or "overprotective" (Atkin *et al.* 1998). Lack of language support and assumptions about the passivity of South Asian women contribute to such views. Nonetheless, their treatment is not wholly a consequence of their ethnic background, but can be explained by doctors' more general sexist attitudes (Green and Murton 1996). Without contextualizing the experience of these women within broader literature, we would have mistakenly attributed the doctor's response to racism, when in fact sexism is the main explanatory factor.

Hence, at a theoretical level, as part of our concern with understanding diversity, we need to accept that in some ways ethnic minority populations may not be all that different from the general population (Mason 2000). Every significant finding from the data might not necessarily relate to a participants' ethnic background – and the challenge is to know when ethnicity makes a difference and when it does not. This reminds us, once again, how our approach to analysis is intrinsically linked to other decisions and concepts informing the rest of the research process.

Dissemination: using research to inform policy and practice

Dissemination of research findings represents the final stage of the research process and is especially important when working within a multiethnic society. As we have noted, offering an analysis of the problems facing ethnic minority populations is one thing; doing something about it is another. Often there is a gap between our understanding of the issues and our willingness to act on their implications to improve service delivery. A commitment to change, informed by critical insight is, therefore, essential in ensuring research informs policy and practice.

Practitioners, for example, often feel overwhelmed about providing care for people from diverse cultural and linguistic backgrounds (Qureshi *et al.* 2000). They are increasingly burdened by the volume of evidence reminding them of their failure to provide accessible and appropriate care. They are often presented with advice, emphasizing the importance of responding to cultural diversity and tackling discrimination, while providing no tangible framework with which to improve care (Atkin 2004).

A good dissemination strategy is not, therefore, simply about presenting research evidence, but also engaging with professional practice and the organizational context in which it occurs. Practitioners need to be empowered to respond to complex and diverse situations, without relying on programmatic responses laid out in fact files enabling them to make judgments about the most appropriate intervention for a person from a particular ethnic background. To support practitioners and produce helpful policy and practice guidance we, as researchers, need to provide an initial evidence base and critical insight into how the people from ethnic minority communities, themselves, experience health and social care on one hand; and how current discursive practices engage with their experience on the other. More generally, such a process also renders the basis and consequences of current discriminatory practices transparent, thereby providing opportunities to challenge these. This, in turn, requires a cultural shift in how practitioners and public agencies engage with ethnic minority populations – questioning the way they define problems and impose solutions.

While alternative (and sometimes radical) frameworks informing practice are possible (cf. Rojeck *et al.* 1988), we need to reiterate that social practices cannot simply be imposed, and reflective practice is only one of the mediating links for the required cultural shift under discussion. Professionals need to listen carefully and ask sensible questions in order to provide appropriate support. This requires health and social care professionals to constantly evaluate and reflect on their practice and focus on the *context of need*. In doing so, practitioners also need to question their own professional culture and the fundamental assumptions informing health and social care for ethnic minority populations.

Ethnic minority populations, for their part, are becoming increasingly disillusioned about contributing to research without seeing any tangible improvements in service delivery (Butt and O'Neil 2004). Research, itself, must be seen as part of a broader political process and can also be used as means of empowering ethnic minority populations to realize their citizenship rights. Ensuring the accountability and reflexivity within the research process, particularly given the emerging lack of trust between researchers and ethnic minority populations, is especially important. Dissemination activity, of course, needs to be culturally and linguistically sensitive in a way similar to the research design to ensure engagement and long term partnerships. This engagement, however, is helpful throughout the entire research process and genuine partnership between researchers and the people they do research with, especially when such populations are disadvantaged and subject to discrimination, is an important step forwards (see further discussions of this in Chapter 4).

Ethics

Research ethics are, of course, central to the research process, although a detailed discussion is outside the scope of this chapter. Many excellent guidelines exist (see Social Research Association and British Sociological Association). Nonetheless, it is perhaps worth making some general points. As we have mentioned, reflexivity is a key aspect of any research design. Obtaining informed consent, maintaining privacy, avoiding exploitation, and awareness of the potential harm to participants are key issues to consider when designing a research protocol. Consent may be more difficult to obtain for people who speak languages other than English (although this is not a reason for excluding such people from a study). In a study involving multi-stakeholders, such as service users, carers and practitioners, care needs to be exercised to ensure confidentiality is maintained between participants. This is sometimes far from straightforward. Reflexivity, however, is not simply about individual reflection on ethical practice, but an engagement with how institutional and discursive practices frame research in a particular way (see Alvesson 2002). The frequency of essentialized accounts, which pathologise and misrepresent the experience of minority ethnic populations, remind us of the political nature of the research process. Key questions, therefore, emerge (also see above). Is the research necessary? What assumptions does it make about ethnic differences? How will its findings be interpreted and acted up on? Is there a clear link between the research and improved outcomes?

Conclusion

This chapter, by exploring the process of doing qualitative research in a multi-cultural society, presents a reflexive account that emphasizes the importance of context, transparency, accountability and power relationships that come to define the area we work in. In doing so, our intention is to challenge simplistic approaches to qualitative research, by reflecting on the need for a method that is both rigorous and systematic and is able to explore the experience of ethnic minority populations without recourse to essentialized accounts of cultural practices based on assumptions about the "other." At the very outset, this involves a judicious understanding of the purpose of research and a critical appraisal of how the notion of ethnicity will be used; a strategy for engaging with ethnic minority populations; and a commitment to using research to inform policy and practice.

Following from above, practical issues related to the research process must be reconciled within an explicit theoretical framework. This is fundamental, since qualitative research is, otherwise, in danger of being reduced to presenting little more than descriptive accounts or comparisons, which are poorly contextualized and not informed by any theoretical understanding of broader issues, and fail to add to our understanding of the field of health and social care within a multiethnic society.

In this chapter, we have tried to provide a framework for qualitative research that introduces accountability in all aspects of the research design. We deliberately avoided presenting a "cook book" or "fact file" approach, which offers simplistic solutions. Rather, our concern is to raise issues that require reflection among those thinking of doing research with minority ethnic populations. In particular, we discussed some of the challenges of doing qualitative research that is theoretically informed, methodologically coherent and also committed to addressing disadvantage and inequity within a multiethnic society. We suggested that an ongoing process of reiterative questioning, involving both methodological and ideological reflexivity, is fundamental to a framework for presenting the experiences of ethnic minority populations as part of the larger society rather than as marginal to the whole.

Notes

1   We acknowledge the vast amount of research in ethnicity, which has been incredibly helpful in developing an "evidence" base. The existence of front-line academic journals, devoted to ethnicity, further demonstrate the interest and activity in the area. Our point about marginalization, however, is much broader than this and reflects the difficulty of ensuring debates about ethnicity and diversity influence the mainstream, everyday concerns of disciplines such as Social Policy, Sociology and Health Service Research. There is a danger that the ever-increasing sophistication of debates on ethnic differences takes place in isolation, with little impact on mainstream concerns. With one or two exceptions, a scan of the respective journals of these disciplines illustrates this potential marginalization.
2   This philosophical prologue is grounded in the Western intellectual tradition that does not engage with other older hermeneutic ideas popular in Chinese and Indian philosophical traditions. The dominance of Western philosophy in the development of qualitative methodologies, however, raises another important issue (see Marcus and Fisher 1986). To what extent do these philosophical influences embody Eurocentric thinking, framing the social world in a way that does not necessarily reflect alternative accounts of social reality? This is a question beyond the scope of this chapter and one that is extremely difficult to answer.
3   Interestingly, the origins of hermeneutics in the West lie in theology, in particular biblical studies, and a concern for looking into meaning beyond the text and interpret what was being said, as a means of understanding God's purpose. Such approaches proved influential in the more secular works of twentieth-century writers such as Edmund Husserl (1859–1938), Martin Heidegger (1889–1976) and Hans Georg Gadamar (1900–2002).
4   See, for example, John Gabbay and Andrée le May's article, "Evidence based guidelines or collectively constructed 'mindlines?' Ethnographic study of knowledge management in primary care" (the *British Medical Journal*, 7473, October 2004). They were helped by a third, part-time interviewer who carried out the "formal" interviews.

References

Ahmad, W.I.U. (1996) 'Family obligations and social change among Asian communities', in W.I.U. Ahmad and K. Atkin (eds) *Race and Community Care*, Buckingham: Open University Press.

Ahmad, W.I.U. (2000) 'Introduction', in W.I.U. Ahmad (ed.) *Ethnicity, Disability and Chronic Illness*, Buckingham: Open University Press.

Ahmad, W.I.U., Atkin, K. and Chamba, R. (2000) 'Causing havoc among their children: parental and professional perspectives on consanguinity and childhood disability', in W.I.U. Ahmad (ed.) *Ethnicity, Disability and Chronic Illness*, Buckingham: Open University Press.

Ahmad, W.I.U., Atkin, K. and Jones, L. (2002) 'Young Asian deaf people and their families: negotiating relationships and identities', *Social Science and Medicine*, 55: 1757–1769.

Alvesson, M. (2002) *Postmodernism and Social Research*, Buckingham: Open University Press.

Alvesson, M. and Sköldberg, K. (2000) *Reflexive Methodology: new vistas for qualitative research*, London: Sage.

Anionwu, E. and Atkin, K. (2001) *The Politics of Sickle Cell and Thalassaemia*, Buckingham: Open University Press.

Anthias, F. (1992) *Ethnicity, Class, Gender and Migration: Greek Cypriots in Britain*, Aldershot: Avebury.

Arber, S. (1994) 'Gender, health and ageing', *Medical Sociology News*, 20: 14–22.

Arber, S. and Ginn, J. (1991) *Gender and Later Life: a sociological analysis of resources and constraints*, London: Sage.

Atkin, K. (2004) 'Primary health care and South Asian populations: institutional racism, policy and practice', in S. Ali and K. Atkin (eds) *South Asian Populations and Primary Health Care: meeting the challenges*, Oxford: Radcliffe.

Atkin, K. and Rollings, J. (1996) 'Looking after their own? Family care giving in Asian and Afro-Caribbean communities', in W.I.U. Ahmad and K. Atkin (eds) *Race and Community Care*, Buckingham: Open University Press.

Atkin, K., Ahmad, W.I.U. and Anionwu, E. (1998) 'Screening and counselling for sickle cell disorders and thalassaemia: the experience of parents and health professionals', *Social Science and Medicine*, 47: 1639–1651.

Ballard, R. (1989) 'Social work and Black people: what's the difference?', in C. Rojeck, G. Peacock and S. Collins (eds) *The Haunt of Misery: critical essays in social work and helping*, London: Routledge.

Bauman, Z. (1992) *Intimations of Post Modernity*, London: Routledge.

Bhakta, P., Katbamna, S. and Parker, G. (2000) 'South Asian carers' experiences of primary health care teams', in W.I.U. Ahmad (ed.) *Ethnicity, Disability and Chronic Illness*, Buckingham: Open University Press.

Bhopal, R. (1997) 'Is research into ethnicity and health racist, unsound, or important science?', *British Medical Journal*, 314: 1751–1756.

Bhopal, R. (2001) 'Racism in medicine', *British Medical Journal*, 322: 1503–1504.

Bourdieu, P. (1977) *Outline of a Theory of Practice*, Cambridge: Cambridge University Press.

Bourdieu, P. (1990) *The Logic of Practice*, Cambridge: Polity Press.

Bowler, I. (1993) '"They are not the same as us: Midwives": stereotypes of South Asian maternity patients', *Sociology of Health and Illness*, 15: 157–178.

Bradby, H. (2003) 'Describing ethnicity in health research', *Ethnicity and Health*, 8: 5–14.

Bryman, A. and Burgess, R. (1994) *Analyzing Qualitative Data*, London: Routledge.

Burgess, R. (1984) *In the Field: an introduction to fieldwork*, London: George Allen & Unwin.

Bury, M. (1997) *Health and Illness in a Changing Society*, London: Routledge.

Butt, J. and O'Neil, A. (2004) *Let's Move On: Black and ethnic minority older people's views on research findings*, York: Joseph Rowntree Foundation.

Chamba, R., Hirst, M., Lawton, D. *et al.* (1999) *On the Edge: a national survey of ethnic minority parents caring for a severely disabled child*, Bristol: Policy Press.

Chamberlayne, P. and King, A. (2000) *Cultures of Care: biographies of carers in Britain and the two Germanies*, Bristol: Policy Press.

Chattoo, S. and Ahmad, W.I.U. (2003) 'The meaning of cancer: illness, biography and social identity', in D. Kelleher and G. Cahill (eds) *Identity and Health*, London: Routledge.

Clifford, J. (1988) *The Predicament of Culture: twentieth century ethnography, literature and art*, Cambridge, MA: Harvard University Press.

Clifford, J. and Marcus, G.E. (eds) (1986) *Writing Culture: the poetics and politics of ethnography*, Berkeley, CA: University of California Press.

Creswell, J.W. (1994) *Research Design: qualitative and quantitative approaches*, London: Sage.

Critical Appraisal Skills Programme (2002) *Ten Questions to Help you Make Sense of Qualitative Research*, Milton Keynes: Milton Keynes Primary Care Trust.

Darr, A. (1997) 'Consanguineous marriage and genetics: a model for genetic health service delivery', in A. Clarke and E. Parsons (eds) *Culture, Kinship and Genes*, London: Macmillan Press.

Denzin, N.K. and Lincoln, Y.S. (1998) *The Landscape of Qualitative Research*, London: Sage.

Geertz, C. (1973) *The Interpretation of Cultures: selected essays*, New York: Basic.

Gerhardt, U. (1989) *Ideas about Illness: an intellectual and political history of medical sociology*, London: Macmillan.

Giddens, A. (1991) *Modernity and Self Identity: self and society in late modern age*, Cambridge: Polity Press.

Gilman, S. (1985) *Difference and Pathology: stereotypes of sexuality race and madness*, Ithaca, NY: Cornell University Press.

Glaser, B.G. and Strauss, A.L. (1967) *The Discovery of Grounded Theory: strategies for qualitative research*, Chicago, IL: Aldine Press.

Green, J. and Murton, F.E. (1996) 'Diagnosis of Duchenne Muscular Dystrophy: parents' experiences and satisfaction', *Child Care, Health and Development*, 22: 113–128.

Gunaratnam, Y. (1997) 'Culture is not enough: a critique of multiculturalism in palliative care', in D. Field, J. Hockey and N. Small (eds) *Death, Gender and Ethnicity*, London: Routledge.

Gunaratnam, Y. (2001) 'We mustn't judge people . . . but: staff dilemmas in dealing with racial harassment amongst hospice service users', *Sociology of Health and Illness*, 23: 65–83.

Habermas, J. (1986) *Knowledge and Human Interests*, Cambridge: Polity Press.

Hammersley, M. (1996) 'The relationship between qualitative and quantitative research: paradigm loyalty versus methodological eclecticism', in T.E. Richardson (ed.) *Handbook of Qualitative Research Methods*, Leicester: British Psychological Society.

Hammersley, M. (2002) 'Ethnography and Realism', in A.M. Huberman and M.B. Miles (eds) *The Qualitative Researcher's Companion*, London: Sage.

Hammersley, M. and Atkinson, P. (1995) *Ethnography Principles in Practice*, London: Routledge.

Harrison, S. (2004) 'Equity, clinical governance and primary care', in S. Ali and K. Atkin (eds) *South Asian Populations and Primary Health Care: meeting the challenges*, Oxford: Radcliffe.

Hunter, J.D. and Killoran, A. (2004) *Turning Health Inequalities: turning policy into practice?* London: Health Development Agency.

Husband, C. (1996) 'Defining and containing diversity: community, ethnicity and citizenship', in W.I.U. Ahmad and K. Atkin (eds) *Race and Community Care*, Buckingham: Open University Press.

Hussain-Gambles, M. 2003 'Ethnic minority under-representation in clinical trials: whose responsibility is it anyway?', *Journal of Health Organisation and Management*, 17: 138–145.

Karlsen, S. and Nazroo, J.Y. (2002) 'Agency and structure: the impact of ethnic identity and racism in the health of ethnic minority people', *Sociology of Health and Illness*, 24: 1–20.

Kincheloe, J.L. and McLaren, P.L. (1998) 'Rethinking critical theory and qualitative research', in N.K. Denzin and Y.S. Lincoln (eds) *The Landscape of Qualitative Research*, London: Sage.

Lipsky, M. (1980) *Street Level Bureaucracy: dilemmas of the individual in public services*, New York: Russell Sage Foundation.

Mclean, C.A. and Campbell, C.M. (2003) 'Locating research informants in a multi-ethnic community: ethnic identities, social networks and recruitment methods', *Ethnicity and Health*, 8: 41–62.

Malterud, K. (2001) 'Qualitative research: standards, challenges, and guidelines', *The Lancet*, 358: 483–488.

Marcus, G.E. (1998) 'What Comes Just After "Post"? The Case of Ethnography', in N.K. Denzin and Y.S. Lincoln (eds) *The Landscape of Qualitative Research*, London: Sage.

Marcus, G. and Fischer, M. (1986) *Anthropology as Cultural Critique: an experimental moment in the human Sciences*, Chicago, IL: University of Chicago Press.

Marshall, S.L. (1994) 'Interviewing respondents who have English as a second language: challenges encountered and suggestions for other researchers', *Journal of Advanced Nursing*, 19: 566–571.

Mason, D. (2000) *Race and Ethnicity in Modern Britain*, Oxford: Oxford University Press.

Mason, J. (1996) *Qualitative Researching*, London: Sage.

Mays, N. and Pope, C. (2000) 'Qualitative research in health care, assessing quality in qualitative research', *British Medical Journal*, 320: 50–52.

Mir, G. and Tovey, P. (2003) 'Asian carers' experience of medical and social care: the case of cerebral palsy', *British Journal of Social Work*, 33: 465–479.

Modell, B. and Darr, A. (2002) 'Genetic counselling and customary consanguineous marriage', *Nature Reviews Genetics*, 3: 225–229.

Modood, T., Berthoud, R., Lakey, J. *et al.* (1997) *Ethnic Minorities in Britain: diversity and disadvantage*, PSI Report 843, London: Policy Studies Institute.

Nazroo, J. (1997) *The Health of Britain's Ethnic Minorities*, London: Policy Studies Institute.

Oakley, A. (1980) *Women Confined: towards a sociology of childbirth*, Oxford: Martin Robertson.

Oakley, A., Wiggins, M., Turner, H. *et al.* (2003) 'Including culturally diverse samples in health research: a case study of an urban trial of social support', *Ethnicity and Health*, 8: 29–40.

Oliver, M. (1990) *The Politics of Disablement*, London: Macmillan Education.

Outhwaite, W. (1986) *Understanding Social Life: the method called verstehen*, East Sussex: Jean Stroud.

Parekh, B. (2000) *Rethinking Multi-culturalism: cultural diversity and political theory*, Basingstoke: Palgrave.

Popay, J., Jadad, A., Nichol, G. *et al.* (1998) 'Rationale and standards for systematic review of qualitative literature in health services', *Qualitative Health Research*, 8: 341–351.

Pope, C. and Mays, N. (1995) 'Reaching the parts other methods cannot reach: an introduction to qualitative methods in health and health service research', *British Medical Journal*, 311: 42–45.

Qureshi, T., Berridge, D. and Wenman, H. (2000) *Where to Turn? Family support for South Asian communities: a case study*, London: Joseph Rowntree Foundation.

Richards, L. and Richards, T. (1991) 'The transformation of qualitative method: computational paradigms and research process', in N.G. Fielding and R.M. Lee (eds) *Using Computers in Qualitative Research*, London: Sage.

Rojeck, J., Peacock, G. and Collins, S. (1988) *Social Work and Received Ideas*, London: Routledge.

Rorty, R. (1988) *Contingency, Irony and Solidarity*, Cambridge: Cambridge University Press.

Ryan, M., Scott, D.A., Reeves, C. *et al.* (2001) *Eliciting Public Preferences for Healthcare: a systematic review of techniques*, London: Health Technology Assessment, 5(5).

Silverman, D. (2000) *Doing Qualitative Research – a practical handbook*, London: Sage.

Smaje, C. (1995) *Health, 'Race' and Ethnicity: making sense of the evidence*, London: King's Fund Institute.

Stacey, M. (1988) *The Sociology of Health and Healing*, London: Unwin Hyman.

Stanfield, J.H. (1998) 'Ethnic modeling in qualitative research', in N.K. Denzin and Y.S. Lincoln (eds) *The Landscape of Qualitative Research*, London: Sage.

Taussig, M.T. (1980) 'Reification and the consciousness of the patient', *Social Science and Medicine*, 14: 3–13.

Taylor, C. (2004) *Modern Social Imaginaries*, Durham, NC and London: Duke University Press.

Waterman, H., Tillen, D., Dickson, R. and de Koning, K. (2001) *Action Research: a systematic review and guidance for assessment*, London: Health Technology Assessment, 5(23).

Wengraf, T. (2001) *Qualitative Research Interviewing*, London: Sage.

Williams, G. (1993) 'Chronic illness and the pursuit of virtue in everyday life', in A. Radley (ed.) *Worlds of Illness: biographical and cultural perspectives on health and disease*, London: Routledge.

Willis, P. (2000) *The Ethnographic Imagination*, Cambridge: Polity Press.

Zola, I. (1972) 'Medicine as an institution of social control', *Sociological Review*, 20: 487–504.

Chapter 8

Conducting surveys among ethnic minority groups in Britain

Sally McManus, Bob Erens and Madhavi Bajekal

Introduction

This chapter discusses issues to do with carrying out a quantitative survey with a representative sample of ethnic minority groups in Britain. This may be a targeted survey among specific minority groups, or a boost sample to increase the number of ethnic minority respondents for a survey among the general population. The issues examined are those of particular concern to designing a survey of ethnic minority groups, so general survey design issues are not covered (for a more general discussion of survey methodology see Groves *et al.* 2004, Fowler 2001, Moser and Kalton 1985, Hoinville *et al.* 1978). While the discussion centres around surveys at a national level, the issues and principles are similar for locally based surveys.

The main topics covered include categorising and sampling ethnic minority groups, translating questionnaires, fieldwork issues (e.g. training interviewers, ethnic matching), and analysis and weighting. For a number of reasons, carrying out a survey among ethnic minority groups is more expensive (in unit cost terms) than a similar survey would be among the general population. While in all surveys there is a tension between costs and quality, this is particularly the case for surveys of special populations such as ethnic minority groups. This chapter aims to provide some useful tips for cost savings, while maintaining the representativeness and quality of the results.

Classifying the population of interest

Quantitative surveys require distinct categories for the purposes of sampling and analysis. However, as described in Chapter 2, creating an ethnic minority group classification that is universally accepted has proved elusive. This is not surprising given the multidimensional nature of defining 'ethnic groups'. Over time, 'ethnicity' has been defined using one or more of a combination of different characteristics, including country of birth (own or parents'), nationality, language, religion, skin colour, cultural traditions and ancestral origins. Moreover, definitions of particular 'ethnic' groups are fluid: they will vary from country to country and, within a single location, may also change over time in accordance with socio-political developments.

Agreeing an ethnic classification is just the beginning, not the end, of the problem. Methods need to be devised to assign individuals to the appropriate categories. This will vary according to the classification used. Some characteristics are easier to measure than others, such as country of birth (although even this can be problematic if borders change over time). Other characteristics, however, are much more subjective, whether self-defined or ascribed by a third party. In some cases, the questions may be difficult to phrase, such as questions to do with religious identity or practices, or with cultural traditions. In others, even if a question can be asked in a relatively straightforward way, responses may not be stable, i.e. they may vary over time or according to the context in which the question is asked. For these reasons, it has been suggested that ethnic 'origin' (that is family origins) is likely to lead to more stable responses than ethnic 'identity' (Aspinall 2001: 833).

Thus, no 'ethnic' classification system is perfect, and none is universally accepted, in Britain or elsewhere. This may not be a problem if, as some have argued, the definition of ethnic groups should, at any rate, reflect the purpose of the study and the hypothesis under investigation (e.g. McKenzie and Crowcroft 1996, BMJ 1996, Smaje 1995). While this approach may seem axiomatic, taken to an extreme it can lead to a different set of problems since, if every study were to employ its own unique classification suited only for its own needs, it would become difficult to make comparisons or explore links between studies. This is a fair summary of the current situation for making international comparisons, and it also applies to a large extent to studies within Britain (Bhopal 2004, Aspinall 2002).

In an attempt to introduce some conformity for studies within the UK, the Office of National Statistics (ONS) designed an ethnic classification system for the 1991 census of population. This classification was subsequently revised for the 2001 census, and a guide for collecting and classifying ethnicity data was issued towards the end of 2003 (ONS 2003). ONS has opted for self-defined ethnicity, arguing that since

> membership of an ethnic group is something that is subjectively meaningful to the person concerned ... we are unable to base ethnic identification upon objective, quantifiable information as we would, say, for age or gender. And this means that we should rather ask people which group they see themselves as belonging to.
>
> (ONS 2003: 9)

The guide provides 'harmonised' questions that are now widely used on national government-funded surveys in the UK, and ONS urges 'everyone who needs to collect data on ethnicity and national identity to adopt the principles and procedures set out in the guidance' (ONS 2003: 4).

The question used in the 2001 census is as follows:

What is your ethnic group? Choose ONE section from A to E, then tick the appropriate box to indicate your ethnic group.

A   White
British
Irish
Any other White background, please write in _____

B   Mixed
White and Black Caribbean
White and Black African
White and Asian
Any other Mixed background, please write in _____

C   Asian or Asian British
Indian
Pakistani
Bangladeshi
Any other Asian background, please write in _____

D   Black or Black British
Caribbean
African
Any other Black background, please write in _____

E   Chinese or other ethnic group
Chinese
Any other, please write in _____

This is the question that ONS recommends for collecting ethnic group data. The question would be asked in this way in a self-completion format. For a face-to-face interview, these categories would be included on a single show card. For a telephone interview, two questions need to be asked: the first to select the main category (White, Mixed, Asian or Asian British, Black or Black British, Chinese or other ethnic group), and the second to establish the detailed group (e.g. if the respondent says Black to the first question, the follow-up question would ask the person to choose between Caribbean, African or another Black background).

Thus, the ONS solution to categorising ethnicity is to combine a number of aspects of ethnicity (nationality, country of birth, geographical origin, skin colour) to form a single classification, and to limit individuals to selecting only one category from the alternatives provided.

In their guidance, ONS provide a more detailed list of how the 'write in' categories are allocated to the main census ethnic groups. Thus, if a person were to write in 'Nigerian' or 'Somali', they would be counted in the census as Black African. However, some write-in answers are not easily categorised, such as 'Arab', 'Jewish' or 'Sikh'. If a person had written 'Sikh' in the White main heading, they would be counted as 'Other White background'; but if the answer was recorded under the Asian or Asian British heading, they would be recorded as 'Other Asian background'.

Using the ONS classification in UK studies offers a number of benefits, most notably standardisation across surveys, or other data sources, which can then be compared with each other as well as with the results from the 2001 census. Another significant advantage is that census data are most likely to be used to design a cost effective sample for a survey of ethnic minority groups, and this would require the use of a classification system which reflects that used on the census. These arguments apply, of course, to the use of standardised census measures in other national contexts.

This classification, however, is also open to a number of criticisms. One of the more obvious problems is that, while it distinguishes three separate South Asian categories (Indian, Pakistani, Bangladeshi), all individuals from sub-Saharan Africa are covered by a single category, despite the fact that 'Black Africans' in Britain are a very heterogeneous group (Elam and Chinouya 2000). The rationale for not distinguishing between different African countries is explained by the relatively small number of residents of each country in Britain. While this is justifiable at a national level, specific locations may have a relatively high proportion of residents from a particular ethnic minority group which is not separately identified in the census categories (e.g. Somalis living in east London); in these circumstances, the census question alone is unlikely to be sufficient.

Despite the problems with the ONS harmonised ethnicity question, the advantage of being able to make comparisons with other surveys and with census results – particularly in terms of judging the representativeness of the achieved sample – is generally a sufficient reason for including this question on surveys interested in ethnic minority groups in Britain. In many surveys, however, it will also be necessary to include additional questions in order to collect more detailed data that would enable alternative classifications to be derived. Although the extra variables required will depend on the purpose of the survey, they could include questions on religion, country of birth, migration history and language spoken. Since the 2001 census also included questions on religion and country of birth, a survey that included the census questions will also have a good basis for making comparisons with population data on these two variables.

Which ethnic minority groups to include in a survey

Many studies will wish to focus on a health or social issue to do with specific ethnic minority groups. Other studies will be locally based and will wish to ensure that all of the ethnic minority groups within their area are sufficiently represented. However, there will be some surveys, especially those for which nationally representative results are required – perhaps to compare with data from the general population – where decisions about which ethnic minority groups should be included cannot be made a priori. Even where it is considered desirable to include all, or a wide range of, ethnic minority groups, the extent to which this will be possible is normally constrained by sample size requirements and the level of funding for the survey. Then, practical considerations to do with obtaining a probability sample of sufficient size and within the funds available will be a key factor. Over the past decade, when such considerations have been applied to a number of large national surveys of ethnic minority groups in Britain, the result has been to focus the surveys on the most populous ethnic minority groups in the country. For example, the Fourth National Survey of Ethnic Minorities in Britain, carried out in 1993–1994, limited its scope to six groups (Caribbean, Indian, African Asian, Pakistani, Bangladeshi, Chinese) (Smith and Prior 1996). The first ethnic minority boost sample included in the 1999 Health Survey for England was similarly limited to including six groups (Black Caribbean, Indian,

Pakistani, Bangladeshi, Chinese and Irish) (Erens *et al.* 2001a); the second time ethnic minority groups were boosted on the Health Survey for England, Black Africans were also included.

The reasons for limiting national surveys to covering only the most populous ethnic minority groups becomes apparent when one looks at the distribution of ethnic groups within the population (see Table 1.1 on p. 2 which shows the distribution of people from different ethnic minority groups in the UK from the 2001 population census).

It is clear from the census data that, by following usual sampling practice, even in a large national survey (in England and Wales) of, say, 10,000 adults, there would only be about 400 Asian respondents, of whom 200 would be Indian, 100 Pakistani and 40 Bangladeshi. The numbers for Black, Mixed and Chinese would be even lower. By contrast, there would be 9,250 White respondents. Except for the majority White group, these numbers are clearly insufficient for separate analysis by ethnic group, especially when most analysis will wish to look at results separately by gender, age and other analysis variables. (If the survey also includes Scotland, the proportion of White respondents would be slightly higher, since ethnic minority groups make up only two per cent of the Scottish population.)

Thus, a means must be found to 'boost' the number of people from ethnic minority groups in the achieved sample. Furthermore, the challenge is to do this in a way that ensures the sample is not biased and is fully representative of the ethnic minority groups included in the study. Various means of boosting samples of ethnic minority groups have been devised, and are described in the following section. When reaching a decision about which ethnic minority groups can be included in a national survey, it generally comes down to a combination of numbers (i.e. of particular ethnic minority groups) and whether they can be sampled in a cost-effective way. While it is possible to include some of the smaller ethnic minority groups in a national survey, it is generally expensive to do so, and for most of the smaller groups prohibitively so. This partly depends on their pattern of residence, since if they are highly clustered within particular locations, the costs of sampling will be lower.

The same principles apply to a survey carried out in a specific geographical area. The researcher will need to examine the proportion of ethnic minority groups within the survey area in order to determine which groups would be represented sufficiently by taking a probability sample in the usual way, and which groups can be boosted in a cost-effective way. For example, a survey carried out in Tower Hamlets in London would be able to easily boost Bangladeshis, since this group makes up 33 per cent of the population in that area (even though they are only 0.6 per cent of the population nationally); and, since the majority of the Bangladeshis are further clustered within parts of Tower Hamlets, the sample design would focus on the relevant wards or postcode sectors (whichever is the primary sampling unit).

Boosting ethnic minority groups

It is clear from the proportion of people describing themselves as members of ethnic minority groups at the 2001 census that a straightforward probability sample of the population will result in too few respondents from ethnic minority groups to enable separate analysis within particular groups. Therefore, the sample needs to be designed in such a way that it will increase the number of respondents from ethnic minority groups, and this needs to be done within budget while at the same time maintaining sample representativeness for each group. As Kalton and Anderson note: 'The design of an efficient sample for surveying a rare population is one of the most challenging tasks confronting the sampling statistician' (1986: 65).

The ideal solution would be to have a sample frame that listed every person in the country along with their ethnic group category. Obviously, no such list exists, nor would such a list be desirable in a democratic country. However, there are comprehensive lists that are publicly available for sampling purposes, some of which pertain to individuals and others to addresses.

Until about 10–15 years ago, the Electoral Register (ER) was the list most often used for sampling purposes in Britain. While it includes the names and addresses of the vast majority of the adult (i.e. aged 18 and over) population in Britain, even during the period when it was widely used it was estimated that the level of under-representation of eligible voters was about 16 per cent by the end of the year for which the ER was in force (Lynn and Lievesley 1991). Since October 2002, electors have been given the opportunity to opt-out of having their names included on the register that is made publicly available or passed to a third party. It was estimated that the publicly available ER in 2003 included only about 73 per cent of registered electors, so the ER is now no longer viable as a comprehensive national sampling frame. Even without the recently provided right to opt-out of having one's name included on the publicly available ER, the utility of the ER was always much reduced for sampling ethnic minority groups, both because non-registration of eligible electors was two to four times higher for Asian and Black groups than for Whites, but also because a proportion of Asian and Black residents are not British nationals and thus ineligible to register.

As well as incomplete coverage of ethnic minority residents, another problem with using the ER for sampling ethnic minority groups is that the sample can only be selected using name analysis to identify potential sample members via their surnames. This difficulty applies to using any other lists of individuals which may appear to be comprehensive in terms of coverage but which do not include reliable (or any) ethnic classificatory data (e.g. telephone directories, GP or patient lists). This method has been used in many studies in Britain and elsewhere. One such software package is Nam Pehchan, which was originally developed by Bradford City Council in the 1980s, and which has gone through several rounds of development. This package includes a database of several thousand known South Asian names, and is estimated to have a sensitivity and specificity score of more than 90 per cent (sensitivity = percentage of Asians with a surname on the list; specificity = percentage of non-Asians not on the list) and a positive predictive value (PPV) of around 60–70 per cent (PPV = percentage of people with Asian surnames who are actually Asian), depending on the geographic database of the reference dataset. The problem with name analysis is that it is more viable for some groups than others: for example, while Hindu and Sikh names are easily identifiable, as are some Chinese names (Aspinall 2001: 841), Muslim names, on the other hand, tend not to be country specific so are not useful for assigning individuals to their country of origin. Even when such an approach is adopted out of necessity, such as was the case when sampling Chinese residents on the Health Survey for England, it is recognised that this approach has been taken on grounds of cost effectiveness even though a significant proportion of Chinese residents have no chance of selection.

There are other obvious disadvantages of using a name matching approach including:

*   Women who have married men from a different background and changed their surname have no chance of selection. This approach, therefore, potentially biases the sample against women (and their children) living in mixed marriages, a situation that is not uncommon: an analysis of 1991 census data showed that 28 per cent of Chinese women were married or cohabiting with a White partner (Aspinall 2001: 841).
*   For other ethnic minority groups, such as Black Caribbean, a name matching approach will not work at all, since they have surnames that are common in the general population.
*   An electronic version of the ER or other list needs to be available for automated searching, and purchasing the lists and paying for the searches could be time-consuming and costly.

In general, therefore, lists that identify individuals, such as the ER, tend to be rejected as a sampling frame for national surveys of ethnic minority groups. They may, however, still have a useful role either for sampling particular ethnic minority groups (such as the Chinese, as described later in this chapter) or for locally based surveys with limited budgets which cannot afford screening.

An alternative list for sampling purposes is the Postcode Address File (PAF), which is now the most commonly used sampling frame for large general population surveys in Britain. Compared with the ER, it offers more complete coverage of households, it is regularly updated, and so enables flexible and efficient organisation of fieldwork. However, the PAF is an address-based list and contains no information about occupants at an address. For a survey of the general population without inclusion/exclusion criteria, this presents no problems; however, for a survey of ethnic minority groups, it means that some form of 'screening' is required to identify eligible individuals.

Screening is commonly used within general population surveys to identify a number of sub-groups within the population, either because they are the main focus of the study or in order to over-sample people from these groups; examples include selecting individuals in a particular age range or households with a particular composition (e.g. those with children). The principle of screening for individuals from specific ethnic minority groups is the same as in these other cases. The difficulty of screening for ethnic minority groups, however, is apparent from the population data shown in Chapter 1: that is, since they comprise less than 10 per cent of the population (and only 12 per cent of households include a person from a non-White ethnic minority group), screening involves considerable extra fieldwork simply to identify the potential sample, and this can have significant implications for survey costs. For national surveys, however, it is usually possible to improve the cost effectiveness of a screening exercise, first, by careful sample design and, second, by using a special screening technique referred to as 'focused enumeration'. The extent to which either of these approaches will be effective in identifying the sample and reducing costs depends on how rare the sub-group is in the population, how clustered it is, and whether focused enumeration is a possibility. The fact that many studies have now successfully used these approaches is a demonstration of their suitability for national surveys of the main ethnic minority groups, and there is no reason why these methods would not be suitable at more local levels. Both approaches are described in more detail below.

Designing a sample for boosting ethnic minority groups

In designing a sample of ethnic minority groups, whether it is to be the main sample or a boost to a general population sample, it is essential to make use of the fact that the population of most ethnic minority groups is concentrated within particular areas of the country. For example, an analysis of 2001 census data shows that it would be possible to identify a subset of just 23 per cent of all wards in England and Wales that between them would cover (at least) 91 per cent of the Black Caribbean, Black African, Indian, Pakistani and Bangladeshi population. Omitting a small percentage of the ethnic minority population from a survey may not lead to serious biases, in which case the sampling frame for the groups to be included can be restricted to the subset of wards that covers the vast majority of these groups. In other cases, it may be important to include those who live in less concentrated areas.

Nevertheless, by restricting the sampling frame in this way, it should be possible to generate a larger sample of members of ethnic minority groups than would be the case if the sampling frame covered the entire country. By taking this approach a step further and over-sampling within those areas where the density of ethnic minority groups is particularly high, the cost effectiveness of the design can be improved even further. This will lead to a higher 'strike rate' – i.e. the likelihood of finding a member of one of the target groups – than taking an equal probability sample of wards.

Thus, the first stage for a sample design that involves screening for individuals from ethnic minority groups is generally to divide the sampling frame containing the primary sampling units (PSUs) into strata based on the density of their ethnic minority population (preferably just of the groups of interest to the study), using, for example, data from the census. PSUs (such as wards or postcode sectors) are then sampled independently from each stratum, usually with variable sampling fractions (i.e. by taking a much higher proportion of PSUs from the high-density, compared with the lower-density, strata). Table 8.1 shows the distribution of the six largest non-White ethnic minority groups across five strata defined according to the proportion of residents (adults and children) of these six ethnic minority groups. So, in 2001, there were about 3.3 million individuals in England and Wales from these six ethnic minority groups, of whom 58 per cent were in stratum A (wards where ethnic minority groups comprised over 20 per cent of residents). As is apparent from Table 8.1, different groups have different distributions so that 68 per cent of Bangladeshis are in stratum A compared with only 23 per cent of Chinese.

Table 8.1 is shown for illustrative purposes only. The detailed strata definitions will vary according to the aims and coverage of each specific survey – for example, a survey that was sampling only South Asians would define its strata based on the proportion of the population in wards (or postcode sectors) that was South Asian (ignoring the other ethnic minority groups for this purpose). Moreover, the number of strata defined is not fixed at five, but will vary from survey to survey, as will their definitions. Factors influencing strata number and definitions include the geographical

Table 8.1 Percentage of six largest ethnic minority groups in England and Wales living within five strata (A–E) defined by proportion of residents in ward from these six ethnic minority groups* (%)

Ethnic minority group	Strata (figures in percentage of ward residents from these six ethnic minority groups)				
	A More than 20%	**B** 10–20%	**C** 5–10%	**D** 2.5–5%	**E** Less than 2.5%
Black Caribbean	60	19	9	6	7
Black African	63	19	8	4	6
Indian	55	18	11	7	9
Pakistani	64	18	8	5	5
Bangladeshi	68	12	8	4	7
Chinese	23	17	16	13	30
Total all six ethnic minority groups	58	18	8	6	9

* The table is based on data from the 2001 population census for England and Wales.

distribution of the ethnic minority groups being sampled as well as the variation in the density of the groups (e.g. some areas have a high density of Bangladeshis, other areas have a high density of Black Caribbeans, etc.).

Once the strata are defined, it is generally cost effective to over-sample PSUs from the areas with a higher density of ethnic minority populations (strata A–D); however, this over-sampling must be done carefully so as not to reduce sample efficiency (see later section on weighting the data). Generally, the stratum with the lowest ethnic minority population density is excluded from the survey. This inevitably reduces sample coverage and introduces potential bias since ethnic minority individuals living in those parts of the country that are nearly all White will be excluded. While their exclusion will carry implications that need to be considered in the context of study aims and questions, it is normally justified because of the very high cost of screening in such low-density areas.

Decisions also need to be made about the number of addresses to select in each PSU, which, in turn, depends on the number of eligible individuals at each selected address. For most social or attitude surveys, it is common to randomly select only one adult at each address, and to apply corrective weighting to adjust for the fact that individuals in multi-adult households are under-represented. This is done in order to reduce the possibility of 'contamination' due to respondents becoming aware of the content of the survey before they take part, reduce response burden in a single household and to keep design effects due to clustering to a minimum. In health surveys, by contrast, it is not unusual to include in the survey all adults living at an address. While this theoretically increases design effects due to extra clustering, this tends to be less problematic for health surveys, which will usually carry out their analyses separately for men and women and for different age groups. It also benefits from not having to carry out a further stage of weighting to adjust for sub-selecting one adult from all those living in the household. However, it has the disadvantage of increasing the burden within any one household, which could result in lower response rates. On any survey, the statistical, theoretical and practical advantages and disadvantages of including all, or selecting only one/some, individuals at an address need to be carefully weighed.

This issue is even more important for surveys of ethnic minority groups, since the average number of adults per address is larger among some ethnic minority groups than it is among Whites. The number of adults per household who are eligible for the survey will clearly influence the number of addresses selected for issue to interviewers. For example, it has been estimated that if only one Bangladeshi adult is selected in a household, then the number of addresses that need to be screened is 2.8 times as high as a sample where all Bangladeshi adults at an address are selected (Korovessis 2001).

Focused enumeration

As is apparent from the above discussion, screening for ethnic minority groups in an interview survey necessarily involves a door-to-door fieldwork operation. Focused enumeration (FE) was developed as a cost-effective means of screening in areas where the estimated 'strike rate' for finding eligible ethnic minority respondents is very low. FE was developed by the National Centre for Social Research and the Policy Studies Institute for the Third National Survey of Ethnic Minorities, carried out in 1982 (Brown and Ritchie 1981). It has since been used to boost numbers of ethnic minority groups on a large number of surveys, including the Fourth National Survey of Ethnic Minorities (Smith and Prior 1996), British Crime Survey (Hales *et al.* 2000), Health Survey for England (in 1999 and 2004) (Erens *et al.* 2001a), second National Survey of Sexual Attitudes and Lifestyles (Erens *et al.* 2001b), Crime and Justice Survey (Hamlyn *et al.* 2003), and others. A similar approach was developed in the US for sampling Black Americans in areas where they represented only a very small proportion of residents; this approach was termed by its developers as WASP, for 'Wide Area Sampling Procedure' (Hess 1985, Jackson 1991).

FE makes use of local knowledge by asking neighbours to identify members of ethnic minority groups living at adjacent addresses to their left and right. Hence, not only is the sampled address screened but also an additional fixed number of addresses. To improve accuracy, field experience has shown that the recognition distance should be no further than four doors away to the left or right of the sampled address, and it is quite common to restrict FE to two addresses on either side. In order not to bias the probabilities of inclusion, standard rules need to be set out to help screeners consistently identify the neighbouring addresses for diverse dwelling layout – e.g. blocks of flats, street corners, mixed commercial and residential areas, etc.

Where potentially positive identifications are made for adjoining addresses, interviewers visit each identified address in person in order to complete the screening process. False positives are eliminated when interviewers visit the address and find that it does not contain a member of one of the target ethnic minority groups. If the respondent at the sampled address says that none of the adjacent addresses include members of the target groups, the addresses are considered to be ineligible and are screened out. In instances where the respondent at the sampled address is unsure, refused information or could not be contacted in person, the interviewer obtains information from either house immediately adjacent to the sampled address in the first instance, followed by the next closest pair and so on, until a definite outcome is obtained for all addresses included in the defined block of FE addresses.

Evidence from the field suggests that FE works best in areas with a modest density of ethnic minority groups (Smith 1996). The precise cut-off for switching from screening all addresses to the use of FE will vary from survey to survey, and the decision will largely be dependent on cost considerations. For example, in the 2004 Health Survey for England, FE was used in postcode sectors with ethnic minority populations over two per cent but less than ten per cent of the target groups, while in the second National Survey of Sexual Attitudes and Lifestyles, FE was used for sectors where ethnic minority residents were between six and 12 per cent of the population.

There are several limitations of the FE method. One is that it includes the possibility of error in terms of false negatives. It was estimated on the Health Survey for England that the level of identification missed around one-third when two addresses either side were screened (varying somewhat by ethnic minority group and, of course, a much smaller proportion of the total eligible sample when higher-density areas, where FE is not used, are also considered). Thus, when deciding on an issued sample size, the number of addresses to be issued using FE should be about 50 per cent (1/0.66) higher than would be required with full screening. There is some evidence that the failure to identify all households with ethnic minority groups does not introduce any major biases into the sample: the Health Survey for England found no significant differences between the ethnic minority respondents sampled at selected addresses and those sampled at adjacent addresses, the two sources giving very similar distributions in terms of age, sex, economic status and a range of health indicators. A second limitation is that FE is more likely to work when screening for people of Black and Asian origin, and thus cannot be used to screen for all ethnic minority groups. Another is that it is only designed for surveys involving face-to-face interviewing, so is not suitable for telephone or postal surveys.

Obtaining an ethnic minority boost using other sampling methods

Even when using the approaches described above – i.e. a stratified sample design and FE screening methods – it can still be difficult to obtain a sufficient boost in numbers for some ethnic minority groups for analysis purposes. Therefore, it may be necessary to resort to other methods. We recommend that, if another method for sampling ethnic minority groups is used, probability sampling techniques should still be employed, even if it means there are some compromises on coverage or resorting to a different classification for some groups. Two examples that maintain known selection probabilities are described below.

The first example has to do with the difficulties of sampling members of the Chinese community in Britain. These difficulties arise for two reasons: first, compared with the other Black and South Asian ethnic minority groups, the Chinese community is relatively small (at around 220,000 adults, it is the smallest of the 'main' ethnic minority groups in Britain); second, unlike the other ethnic minority groups, the Chinese population is not clustered. Because of the small numbers and low density, a very large number of addresses would have to be screened to identify a reasonably sized sample, and such an approach would not be cost effective. Therefore, the approach that has been adopted in some other surveys of the Chinese, including a study of the health of the Chinese population in England (Sproston *et al.* 1999) and the Health Survey for England in 1999 (Erens *et al.* 2001a) and 2004, is to use the surname matching approach described earlier. For example, the sample design for the 2004 Health Survey for England stratified postcode sectors according to density of the Chinese population and sampled sectors where at least 0.1 per cent of the resident population was Chinese. For each selected sector, the ER was searched to identify addresses with at least one Chinese sounding surname, and a proportion (which varied according to the strata) of these addresses were selected for the sample. (The list of surnames used includes about 1,300 of the most common Chinese surnames, and was designed by ONS.) Each selected address was then screened using an interviewer, and all Chinese residents at the address were eligible for the survey. Although this approach has some inherent biases (i.e. excluding Chinese people with a non-Chinese surname unless they happen to live in a household with another person who has such a surname), it is the most cost-effective approach to achieve a reasonably representative sample of the Chinese in England, and it remains a probability sample since the chances of selection are known for all sample members.

The second example involves boosting the number of Irish residents in a sample. Although the second most populous ethnic minority group after Indian (third most populous after Indian and Pakistani if children are included), like the Chinese they are also not clustered geographically, nor is FE a suitable approach for boosting their numbers. The 1991 census did not include Irish as a separate category in the ethnic classification, so before the 2001 census there were no national data available estimating the number of residents who classified themselves as Irish. (The 1991 census collected country of birth, but this is clearly a much smaller group than those who classify themselves as having Irish ethnic identity.) Thus, the 1999 Health Survey for England adopted a different approach for screening for Irish residents than for the other ethnic minority groups. People were classified as Irish if they or one of their parents were born in the Republic of Ireland. So, instead of using self-identity for classifying Irish residents in England, country of 'origin' was used instead, which, however, allows the inclusion within the Irish category of some who do not self-identify as Irish.

Other methods have been discussed in the literature as a means of boosting extremely rare sub-groups, such as quota sampling or 'snowball' sampling. These could apply to a particularly small ethnic minority community in Britain, or to a sub-category of one of the larger communities. For example, while there has been a wealth of research into gay men and their sexual health needs, these studies have tended to under-represent gay men from ethnic minority groups (Fenton *et al.* 2000). Even the major national study of sexual behaviour in Britain, which boosted ethnic minority respondents, found only a small number of Black and Asian men reporting same-sex behaviour (McManus *et al.* 2002). In situations such as these, researchers may resort to snowball sampling. This technique requires the researcher to locate a few members of the group of interest, and to ask each of them to identify other members of the group; these new members are then contacted by the researchers, who in turn are asked to identify more members of the group. This continues until sufficient people are deemed to have been interviewed. This technique is often used for qualitative research, but is also often used for quantitative studies where there may be limited time and/or budgets to carry out a probability sample. For example, this was one of several sampling methods used in a health study of ethnic minority groups in the Bristol area, mainly to find Black respondents (Hughes *et al.* 1995).

The difficulty with snowball sampling is summarised by Kalton and Anderson:

> With this approach, those with many contacts with other members of the rare population are more likely to be included in the survey than those with few contacts . . . However, since the sample is not a probability sample, objective weighting adjustments cannot be employed in the analysis to compensate for this factor. Steps may be taken to make the sample conform to known or hypothesised distributions for certain background variables, as in quota sampling, but this cannot ensure that the sample produces unbiased estimates for other variables. Moreover, distributions of important background variables are seldom known for a rare population; the use of hypothesised distributions in place of known distributions introduces its own potential biases. Given the likelihood of substantial bias with this use of snowball sampling, the results from a snowball sample need to be assessed with considerable caution.
>
> (1986: 78)

Kalton and Anderson conclude that snowball sampling is 'more suited for exploratory and qualitative investigations . . . than for statistical surveys' (1986: 78). Despite the limitations of name matching for surveys, it appears a better option than snowball sampling in circumstances where it can be employed (e.g. for Chinese and some South Asian ethnic minority groups). For boosting ethnic minority groups in Scotland, the Scottish Executive recommends name matching from the ER in areas where the population of ethnic minority groups is under 1 per cent (which would be combined with full address screening in high-density areas and focused enumeration in medium-density areas) (System Three 2001). Given that only 2 per cent of Scotland's population is non-White, this seems a sensible solution to obtaining a sample using probability sampling methods.

Response rates among ethnic minority groups

When determining issued sample sizes for an ethnic minority boost sample, an estimate of the relative response rates of the different groups will also need to be incorporated into the calculation. A number of surveys have shown fairly consistent patterns in response, namely: Black Caribbean and Black African groups tend to have the lowest response rates, and are also generally lower than those that would be obtained for a general population sample; South Asians tend to have the highest response rates, with Bangladeshis usually considerably higher than response for Indians and Pakistanis (which are usually quite similar); response rates for Bangladeshis are usually higher than those for the general population, while Indian and Pakistani rates have been less consistent, sometimes being higher and sometimes lower than the general population; Chinese response rates tend to be similar to, or slightly lower, than response rates for Indians and Pakistanis. The difference between the lowest response rate for Black Caribbeans and the highest rate for Bangladeshis is usually at least 10 per cent, and has been more than 20 per cent in at least one survey (i.e. Health Education Authority 1994).

An example sample design to boost ethnic minority groups

As will be apparent from the preceding discussion, designing samples to boost ethnic minority groups is far from straightforward, and benefits from skilled input from sampling specialists, especially if they have designed boost samples in the past. Below we describe, by way of example, a sample design that was used to boost the numbers of four ethnic minority groups for the second National Survey of Sexual Attitudes and Lifestyles (NATSAL) (Erens *et al.* 2001b, Fenton *et al.* 2005). The aim was to achieve about 735 interviews with members of four ethnic minority groups within the age range of 16–44 years.

The main sample was a typical stratified multi-stage PAF sample, with 466 postcode sectors selected throughout Britain. The sample was designed to over-represent London, so that 64 sectors were selected in inner London, 50 in outer London and 352 in the rest of Britain (with the results being weighted to reflect the correct regional population distribution). In the London postcode sectors 90 addresses were selected per sector, and in the rest of Britain 84 addresses were selected in each sector. All addresses were screened for residents aged 16–44, and at screened-in addresses one person within this age range was randomly selected for the survey.

For boosting ethnic minority groups, 150 additional postcode sectors were selected as primary sampling units (PSUs). Before selection, all postcode sectors in Britain were assigned to one of three strata (A to C) based on the proportion of residents (using 1991 census data) who were Black African, Black Caribbean, Indian or Pakistani (the four groups being boosted). The strata were defined as follows:

A postcode sectors where more than 12 per cent of the resident population were from one of these four groups;
B not in stratum A, but where at least 6 per cent of the resident population were from one of these four groups;
C all other sectors.

Within each of the three strata, the sectors were sorted into region and population density bands, before 150 sectors were selected systematically with a probability in proportion to the number of addresses in the sector. In all, 72 sectors were selected in stratum A, and 78 sectors were selected from stratum B (with stratum C not being sampled). The final sample was weighted to take account of the different selection probabilities by stratum. (Ethnic minority groups living in stratum C were eligible for inclusion in the main general population sample, so the combined sample of the main plus the boost represented the four groups throughout the entire country. However, for stratum C to be represented in its correct proportion, ethnic minority respondents from this stratum would need to be given very large weights. This is not done because of the effect such weighting would have on standard errors; instead, the weights are trimmed to truncate large values and a certain degree of bias is accepted.)

In stratum A, 100 addresses were selected, and a full door-to-door screen was carried out by interviewers. In stratum B, focused enumeration was used. Interviewers were given 20 selected addresses to call at, and they screened the selected address plus two on either side. In total, the sample design for boosting the four ethnic minority groups involved screening 15,000 addresses.

The additional complication when designing a boost sample such as this is that the higher prevalence groups, in this case Indians and Black Caribbeans, will come up much more often in a screening exercise than the lower prevalence groups. It may not be necessary to achieve such a large boost with these two groups, so it is typical to divide the sectors into different 'sample types' and to screen for different groups in each sample type. NATSAL was aiming to achieve about equal numbers of each ethnic minority group, so Indians and Black Caribbeans were not screened for in all sectors. There were three samples types in NATSAL:

1   full screen for Black African, Black Caribbean, Indian and Pakistani (18 sectors in stratum A);
2   full screen for Black African and Pakistani only (54 sectors in stratum A);
3   screen for all four groups at sampled addresses, and at two addresses on either side using focused enumeration (all 78 sectors in stratum B).

At any screened-in addresses, the procedure was exactly the same as for the main general population sample, i.e. one adult member aged 16–44 of any of the relevant groups was randomly selected for inclusion in the survey.

By the end of fieldwork, interviews were achieved with 949 people in the boost sample. The reason for exceeding the target number of interviews (735) by more than 25 per cent highlights one of the difficulties of designing boost samples of this sort, i.e. the reliance on census data to stratify the sample and to estimate the strike rates in the PSUs. Since the census is carried out every ten years, the data on the distribution of ethnic minority groups – both at the national level and local levels – becomes more and more out of date during the course of the decade. Since the NATSAL sample was designed in 2000, and fieldwork was carried out in 2001, the census data from 1991 was ten years out of date by that time; hence, the estimates proved overly pessimistic, and the screening identified far more members of the four groups than anticipated. (Fuller details of this sample design may be found in Erens *et al.* 2001b.)

The NATSAL boost was a relatively straightforward sample design, because all four of the groups being boosted are relatively populous ones and are also quite clustered geographically. This design clearly demonstrates the scale of the task involved when using probability sampling methods for boosting ethnic minority groups: i.e. 15,000 addresses had to be screened in order to achieve fewer than 1,000 interviews. Depending on the survey, it is possible to increase the 'strike rate' of interviews in a number of ways: e.g. by interviewing more than one person in an eligible household or by reducing the coverage of the groups in the population by only sampling areas with a higher density of the groups of interest. On other surveys, however, the design may become more complex, combining several types of screening: e.g. by country of birth along with name matching (for the Chinese). The 1999 and 2004 Health Survey for England included these elements within its sample design (for details see Erens *et al.* 2001a).

Data collection issues

Questionnaire content

Chapter 5 dealt with the complex problems associated with asking standardised questions across a range of cultures and in different languages, issues to do with conceptual equivalence, semantic equivalence, measurement equivalence, etc. (Meadows and Wisher 2000, Pasick *et al.* 2001, Sproston and Nazroo 2002, Hunt and Bhopal 2004). In this section, we are mainly concerned to draw attention to additional questionnaire content that should be considered when surveying members of ethnic minority groups.

As mentioned in the section on ethnic classification and in Chapter 2, it is now widely recognised that asking self-identified ethnicity, while important, is not usually sufficient for analysis purposes and that additional variables allowing for alternative classifications are also likely to be required. For example, Modood noted that not asking parents' country of birth was a failing of the Fourth National Survey of Ethnic Minorities (Modood *et al.* 1997). As well as country of birth (for the respondent, parents and possibly grandparents), other domains that may be asked about include: languages spoken and read, main language spoken in the home, and respondents' self-perceived main language; religious identification and participation; year first moved to Britain and number of years living in Britain; ethnicity of other household members; age completed full-time education and educational qualifications obtained abroad; the extent of wearing traditional clothes; and questions on experience of discrimination in Britain.

As in any survey, it is, of course, essential that other socio-demographic variables that might confound associations also be collected, such as age, marital status, household size and composition, area of residence, economic activity, current or last occupation, education, details of accommodation, benefit receipt and household income. Using the 'harmonised' questions developed by ONS for many of these variables (which are available on its website: www.statistics.gov.uk/about/data/harmonisation/primary_standards.asp) would provide consistency across surveys (as well as allowing the verification of sample representativeness against census data).

There are also instances when culturally specific information may need to be collected as well as, or instead of, the usual survey information. An obvious example concerns questions on diet and eating habits, and the need to include relevant food types for ethnic minority groups. An instance of one of the questions in a food frequency questionnaire being modified in this way relates to fried food, which, in the general population questionnaire, includes as its example fried fish or chicken, chips or cooked breakfast; in the ethnic minority version, the examples were expanded to include West Indian soup or stew, fritters, fried potatoes, fried rice puris, bhajis and samosas. Another example concerns tobacco consumption: whereas a general population questionnaire would normally only include questions on cigarette and cigar consumption, the questions asked of South Asians should also refer to paan and other chewing tobacco and the use of a hookah.

Other issues have to do with the cultural acceptability of some topics or questions asked of ethnic minority groups. For example, a survey on the health and lifestyles of ethnic minority groups in England included questions on sexual health; however, after piloting, it was decided not to ask these questions of South Asian respondents

(Health Education Authority 1994). Other instances of 'sensitive' questions include tobacco or alcohol use, which are prohibited in some religions (e.g. drinking among Muslims, smoking among Sikhs) and may thus be underreported by particular ethnic groups. This is not to suggest that such questions cannot be asked of these groups, only that the questions need to be well designed and appropriately administered.

There have recently been suggestions that the use of anchoring vignettes may help to make comparisons between ethnic minority groups who may be interpreting identical questions in different ways (King *et al.* 2004). This involves describing hypothetical scenarios to respondents in order to tap into different dimensions of the concept under investigation. Vignette questions have been applied successfully in recent work on international comparisons of health and political efficacy (King *et al.* 2004, Saloman *et al.* 2004). The original King *et al.* (2004) model shows how vignettes can help to identify systematic differences in response scales between groups (or countries), making it possible to decompose observed differences in, for example, self-reported health into differences due to variation in the performance of the response scale (sometimes called Differential Item Functioning (DIF)) and genuine differences in health. King *et al.* (2004) show the potential of the vignettes to correct for DIF. For example, in a comparative study of political efficacy of Chinese and Mexican citizens, they found that without correction the Chinese seem to have more political influence than Mexicans, but that this conclusion is reversed once the correction is applied.

Interviews with non-English speakers

Issues to do with the extent to which translated questionnaires are culturally appropriate and how this affects their equivalence to the original English version were covered in Chapter 5, and have been the subject of much recent discussion in the literature (Hunt and Bhopal 2004, Bhopal *et al.* 2004, Pasick *et al.* 2001, Meadows and Wisher 2000).This section deals with more practical issues to do with translating the English questionnaire into other languages.

A proportion of people from some ethnic minority groups either do not speak, or are not fluent in, English. Fluency in English varies markedly by ethnicity, gender and age, with female and older immigrants being the least able to speak English. Therefore, it is important to have available both a (standardised) translated questionnaire and interviewer/translators who can speak and read the relevant languages, in order to maximise the quality of the information obtained and ensure that particular sub-groups of respondents (often the most marginalised) are not excluded altogether. Data quality would not be enhanced, rather the opposite, if bilingual interviewers were allowed to translate the questionnaire themselves while carrying out an interview with a non-English speaking respondent, since there would be no way of maintaining consistency across interviewers, or even across interviews carried out by the same interviewer. Whatever the temptation, and whatever an individual may think about the translated version of the questionnaire, it must be made very clear during training that interviewers are never permitted to improvise their own translation during the interview. Similar concerns apply to using other members within the respondent's household to improvise their own translation. However, in large national surveys, it is often not possible, including for funding reasons, to cover more than a few of the many languages spoken by the ethnic minority groups in Britain.

Whether or not translations are required, and the languages that will be needed, depends of course on the ethnic minority groups being included in the study. Although it may be obvious that a decision needs to be taken about which languages are appropriate for translation, the grounds for making such a decision are not always readily apparent and will depend on a number of factors including:

- which ethnic minority groups are included in the survey;
- the proportion of each group likely to be interviewed in a language other than English, and this could vary if the survey is concerned only with particular subgroups of the ethnic minority group (e.g. if only young people are sampled, the need for translations could be marginal, while if older people are the focus, the importance of having a non-English questionnaire will increase);
- the actual number of interviews likely to be carried out in each language;
- the research and 'political' implications of excluding non-English speakers;
- the practicalities of translating the questionnaire into certain languages (e.g. those that have no written form such as Sylheti);
- the practicalities of recruiting and training interviewers/translators who speak and read the language; and
- the cost of preparing and testing the translation in each language.

While translation costs are clearly dependent on the length of the questionnaire and the number of documents that need to be translated, these can be quite considerable for a typical survey, often running to £5,000 or more per language (for the translation agency) with additional costs for independent checking and piloting.

In national surveys in Britain, translations have generally focused on Asian languages. The main languages often used for translations are Hindi, Gujarati, Punjabi (Gurmukhi script), Urdu, Bengali, Mandarin and Cantonese. (A large group of Bangladeshis in Britain give Sylheti as their main language, but this cannot be easily translated for an interview since it is a dialect with no standard spoken form and has no written form, so Bengali script is used instead.) Translations tend not to be used for Black ethnic minority groups because nearly all of them speak English. Further, in the case of Black Africans, while there are many 'community' languages, few Black African people are literate in them. Also, English is considered a 'neutral' language that does not reflect tribal affiliations (as languages such as Yoruba, for Nigerian people, might) or particular institutions (such as the association between Swahili and the military for Ugandans) (Elam and Chinouya 2000). In local surveys, questionnaires may be translated into other languages to accommodate a particular ethnic minority group which is an important part of the local community (e.g. Somali in East London) (Erens 1993).

To help inform a decision, it is useful to have an idea of the proportion of interviews likely to be carried out in each language, as this varies considerably by ethnic group. Data on English (spoken) fluency from the Fourth National Survey of Ethnic Minorities in Britain showed that: Asian men are more likely to be fluent than Asian women; Indian respondents were the most fluent, closely followed by Chinese and Pakistani respondents, with Bangladeshi respondents the least fluent of these groups;

nearly all individuals aged under 25 from all groups were fluent in English, except for Pakistani and Bangladeshi women; and recent migrants were the least likely to be fluent (Modood *et al.* 1997). These findings are consistent with those from the 1999 Health Survey for England, which found that, of people classified as Indian 55 per cent identified English as their main spoken language, compared with 45 per cent of Pakistanis, 41 per cent of Chinese and 20 per cent of Bangladeshis. The proportion of adults in each group which carried out the Health Survey interview wholly in English was 85 per cent for Indians, 70 per cent for Pakistanis, 69 per cent for Chinese and 34 per cent for Bangladeshis (Erens *et al.* 2001a). The main (non-English) languages were Bengali/Sylheti, Urdu, Punjabi and Cantonese, with smaller numbers being carried out in Gujarati or Hindi. When interviewing a younger cohort, however, the need for translations is likely to be less; for example, the second National Survey of Sexual Attitudes and Lifestyles included individuals aged 16–44, and 99 per cent of Indian and 89 per cent of Pakistani respondents in the ethnic minority boost sample were interviewed wholly in English (Erens *et al.* 2001b).

The number of interviews carried out in any particular language will depend on the groups being sampled and the relative size of each group. For example, in a survey of 10,000 interviews with the general population, there are likely to be 40 Bangladeshis selected, of whom about 25 would be interviewed in Bengali/Sylheti; and, while the majority of the 190 sampled Indians would be interviewed in English, about 30 would require an interview in Gujarati or Punjabi. The merits of translating the interview into these languages would need to be weighed against the costs of doing so. If the Bangladeshi group was to be boosted in the survey, then the balance of factors may be tilted in favour of translating the questionnaire into Bengali/Sylheti. The merits of translating the interview into Hindi also need to be considered, given that so few Indians in Britain mention Hindi as their main language (Erens *et al.* 2001a); having a Hindi translation may be justified more for reasons to do with equity in the way South Asian groups are treated than with necessity for the survey.

The process of translating and then checking the translated questionnaire is a long and complex one. Bhopal *et al.* (2004) have argued that the ideal format for adapting a questionnaire into another language is to:

1   have a panel of bilingual people individually translate the questionnaire and then discuss the various translations to negotiate a 'best fit';
2   discuss the translation with people who are monolingual in the translated language to assess the meaning and acceptability of the translation (and to make any changes required);
3   field test the questionnaire;
4   if a questionnaire has been translated into more than one language, each language version should be compared with every other (as well as with the English version, perhaps through back-translation);
5   finally, carry out tests of validity, reliability and responsiveness in each language.

The authors acknowledge that, of the 15 studies they examined, most met only one or two of these guidelines, and usually only partially. This is unsurprising given not only the cost implications of this process, but also the practical difficulties (e.g. of finding a person who can speak both Cantonese and Sylheti to compare these two versions) and the usual need of surveys to work to an agreed, and often tight, timetable. With respect to timing, it is not unusual for a survey questionnaire to be finalised shortly before piloting, so the scope for carrying out lengthy discussions between a panel of bilingual people followed by further discussion with monolingual people before a field test, with the need to get the translated questionnaire into a format that can be issued to interviewers, may be limited.

The best that (some, but not all) well-funded national surveys usually manage is to use a specialist agency to translate the questionnaire into one or more South Asian languages (a process that is likely to require 2–4 weeks, depending on interview length). The agency should have had the translation checked by another individual independent of the person first doing the translation. The 'final' agency translation should then be checked against the questionnaire by the survey organisation using an independent translator. Ideally, this person should be a researcher or interviewer who is familiar with the English questionnaire and aware of the meaning of the questions, and who is able to judge if the agency translators have interpreted the question appropriately and whether the language used is relatively colloquial and acceptable to respondents (since a common complaint of translated questionnaires is that the language used is 'too formal'). Any queries this process throws up should be agreed in discussion between the agency and the independent translators (which is likely to add another week or more to the process). The questionnaire is then tested in the field in the different languages, which provides feedback from a larger pool of bilingual interviewers. This procedure has been found to be cost effective and to work better than using a second specialist agency to carry out a back-translation or a second independent translation, since it can be difficult to get (rival) agencies to negotiate and agree a 'best fit' translation. This process partly meets steps (a) to (c) (see p. 134) even if the 'panel' of bilingual people at the first step consists of only two bilinguals from the agency and one from the survey organisation, and the discussion with monolinguals only happens during the field test. It is very rare indeed for steps (d) and (e) to be carried out on a typical survey, and doing so would require significantly more resources and time than is normally available. Steps (d) and (e) seem appropriate for validating standardised survey instruments that are intended to be used in many surveys over time; but work validating such an instrument should be a project in its own right, as it will often be too much to expect a researcher working on an ad hoc survey to a tight timescale and budget (which has other competing priorities such as maximising sample size) to undertake this work.

Most large surveys in Britain are now carried out using Computer Assisted Personal Interviewing (CAPI), where the interviewer enters responses directly on a laptop computer. If the CAPI software package is able to handle the different character sets for the appropriate languages, it should also be possible for the translated questionnaires to be done in CAPI. However, this is often not possible (since many CAPI packages will only display Roman characters), and to date it has been much more common to have translated questionnaires in a paper format, even if the English questionnaires are done using CAPI. Even with a paper translated questionnaire, however, the interviewer can still key in the answers in the (English) CAPI questionnaire on the laptop. This, of course, requires considerable care in cross-referencing the CAPI questions with the paper documents. To minimise the scope for error, it is recommended that the paper translation mirror the CAPI screen exactly, using the same screen 'page numbers' and same 'question names' as the CAPI variables. Preparing this translated document is very time-consuming, potentially taking up to a week for each language. The effort is, however, essential in order to minimise errors during fieldwork. (This approach is also appropriate for telephone interviews, whether on paper or computer assisted.)

On self-completion questionnaires, or if the English questionnaire is also on paper, it is more usual to have the translation just below (or next to) the English question and the response categories, as was the case for the Fourth National Survey of Ethnic Minorities (Modood *et al.* 1997).

Self-completion questionnaires

The use of self-completion questionnaires and show cards during face-to-face interviews, has some additional problems for non-English respondents due to, first, the fact that some languages do not have a written version (e.g. Sylheti) and, second, there is limited literacy among some ethnic minority groups, especially among women. A survey carried out in the early 1990s found illiteracy rates of 5 per cent for Indian respondents (aged 16–74, which was the age range for the survey), 11 per cent for Bangladeshis and 17 per cent for Pakistanis (Health Education Authority 1994). Women aged 50–74 had the highest rates of illiteracy (25 per cent Indian, 52 per cent Bangladeshi, 68 per cent Pakistani women). This survey measured self-reported illiteracy, so that the proportion who are unable to read sufficiently well to complete a questionnaire is likely to be even higher. Even if a face-to-face interview survey does not involve a self-completion questionnaire, there are often show cards that need to be read by respondents. On the second National Survey of Sexual Attitudes and Lifestyles, the proportion of respondents (who were aged 16–44) who needed the show cards read out to them by the interviewer was 3 per cent for Whites, 7 per cent for Black Caribbeans, 13 per cent for Black Africans, 12 per cent for Indians and 19 per cent for Pakistanis (although show cards may be read out because of problems other than reading difficulties, such as poor eyesight) (Erens 2001b).

Surveys which involve both a face-to-face interview and a self-completion questionnaire provide an opportunity to look at literacy among different groups. For example, on the 1999 Health Survey for England, despite the self-completion questionnaires being translated into Punjabi, Urdu and Bengali, Pakistani and Bangladeshi respondents were the least likely to have completed them: 83 per cent and 81 per cent (respectively) of those interviewed, compared with 96 per cent of the general population who usually do so.

The use of audio-CASI, in which the questions are read out to respondents who listen through headphones and key their answers directly into the laptop, is an exciting development which is increasingly being used on large-scale surveys, and offers a potential solution to problems of illiteracy among both the general population and ethnic minority groups, since the questions can be read out in any number of languages. In fact, longer term, the use of audio-CASI may be used instead of bilingual interviewers in some circumstances – e.g. in areas where there is going to be little demand for a particular language, it would potentially be more cost effective to allow that respondent to do the interview using audio-CASI than paying for an interviewer from another location to visit that respondent.

Using bilingual interviewers and translators in the field

Carrying out non-English interviews can be done in a number of ways. In a general population survey, where there are likely to be only a handful of non-English interviews, the research team may decide that having translations done would not be cost effective and it would be acceptable to allow another person in the respondent's household to translate the questions and answers. (This scenario might also apply to a survey of ethnic minority groups where the questionnaire was translated into some languages, but not all.) This situation was more often encountered a decade ago than it is today; and, when it was allowed, it was generally for surveys collecting factual and non-sensitive data. Currently, however, few survey organisations, if any, would allow another person in the household to improvise their own translation, because of concerns about ethics and about data quality. (As mentioned already, concerns about consistency and data quality would mean that even fully trained bilingual interviewers would also not be permitted to improvise their own translation during an interview.)

In cases where a translation of the questionnaire is available, there are two strategies currently available for carrying out non-English interviews. The most common, and preferred, option is to recruit and train bilingual interviewers who can speak and read both English and one of the translated languages. These interviewers would undergo the survey organisation's full training and briefing procedures (and would therefore be available to work on projects that did not involve ethnic minority boosts). While working as any other interviewer, for logistic reasons during a survey which is boosting ethnic minority groups, the pool of bilingual interviewers may be held back from interviewing English-speaking respondents so their interviewing capacity could be concentrated on non-English speakers.

The second option is to have a bilingual translator accompany the survey organisation's English-speaking interviewer and to read out the translated questions to the respondent, and interpret the answers for the interviewer. The translator would not be a trained interviewer, although it is recommended that s/he is given some brief training in interview techniques and a broad description of the aims of the survey and the questionnaire. Using translators instead of bilingual interviewers may be necessary if recruiting bilingual interviewers proves difficult, or when it is not cost effective to do so (e.g. in areas where interviews in a language are likely to be few in number).

Ethnic matching and cultural issues in the field

While language matching of interviewers with non-English speaking respondents is necessary to include them in the survey, the argument for ethnic matching interviewers and respondents when carrying out surveys in English is less clear-cut (see the discussion in Chapter 5). One potential benefit of using interviewers from the same ethnic minority groups as respondents is an increase in the perceived legitimacy of the survey, which may lead to a higher response rate. The evidence also shows that ethnic matching may be beneficial for certain topics, such as when racial discrimination is being examined, however it also shows that there are few or no interviewer effects in other circumstances (Aspinall 2001, Rhodes 1994, Weeks and Moore 1981).

In fact, matching interviewer and respondents according to national, religious or cultural criteria may create problems since both individuals may feel bound by the same social norms and values. For example, it could be difficult for a young Muslim interviewer to ask an elder Muslim respondent about their smoking or drinking behaviour, and it may be more difficult for a Muslim respondent to confess to having an alcoholic drink to a Muslim than to a non-Muslim interviewer. For some groups, gender matching may be more important than ethnic matching, and this could vary according to the topic of the survey. In some households among some ethnic groups, the husband is perceived to be the head of the household, and it can be difficult to convince the household head that he was not selected for the survey and that it is his wife's or daughter's views that are being sought. In such circumstances when a female member of the household has been randomly selected, it may be necessary to match the interviewer along gender lines (although the authors are familiar with a recent case in which a male interviewer was permitted to carry out an interview with a female respondent by having the two of them sit in separate rooms and speak to each other through a closed door).

There are also practical difficulties when matching the ethnicity of interviewers and respondents. It is costly to recruit, train and maintain a team of bilingual interviewers throughout the country. Ethnic matching also complicates fieldwork and is likely to significantly increase the length of the fieldwork period.

Since ethnic matching creates practical difficulties in the field, and in general is not likely to affect the results, it is not often carried out. What is important, then, is ensuring that interviewers are sufficiently briefed on potential sensitivities in the questionnaire for particular ethnic groups (e.g. on religious taboos to do with drinking, smoking and diet) as well as on general cultural issues (e.g. conventions regarding first names and surnames, dates of important festivals, forms of greeting, acceptable dress and behaviour in people's homes, appropriateness of eye contact). There are additional problems for health surveys that involve taking physical measurements and blood or urine samples. Issues relating to culturally competent research are discussed further in Chapter 6 of this volume.

Finally, some ethnic minority groups tend to have larger households, on average, than the majority White population and/or to live in over-crowded conditions. This can make it difficult to carry out an interview without distraction or, for a survey on sensitive topics, in private.

Data analysis

Weighting the data from a boost sample of ethnic minority groups

As is apparent from the earlier discussion, sample designs for boosting ethnic minority groups tend to be quite complex, and simple random sampling (SRS) is rarely, if ever, used in Britain, at least for surveys involving face-to-face interviews. (SRS may be used for postal surveys, but this would require a sampling frame that would allow selection on the basis of ethnicity, and this is only likely to be achieved if comprehensive administrative records are available for the survey.) Some of the complexities of a typical sample design using the PAF will involve over-sampling geographical areas with high proportions of ethnic minority groups, selecting a different number of addresses in postcodes from different strata, combining boost samples with ethnic minority respondents interviewed as part of a general population core sample, and sub-selecting individuals within households. For all of these reasons, selection probabilities will not be equal for sample members, and this has a number of implications including the need for weighting to adjust for the different probabilities of selection, as well as an increase in variance which reduces the precision of the results.

Before the data can be used as a representative sample of the ethnic minority groups included in the boost sample, the imbalances created by the use of different probabilities of selection must be removed. Often the weighting scheme will have a similar complexity to the sample design, with several sets of weights, for example, to correct for the unequal probabilities of selection of the PSUs (usually postcode sectors), the unequal probabilities of selection for addresses within the PSUs, and the varying probabilities of selection of adults within households. The corrections at each of these levels are made by applying weights that are inversely proportional to the selection probabilities for the relevant postcode sectors, addresses and number of adults. (If some respondents have extremely high weights relative to the average for a particular ethnic group, it is common practice to 'trim' the weights.) Weights calculated in this way would give gross estimates of the actual population members within each ethnic minority group. The weights would usually be scaled by a constant factor so that the weighted sample size across the ethnic minority groups would be the same as the unweighted sample size. One of the effects of using a complex sample design is that standard errors are generally higher than the standard errors that would be derived from a simple random sample of the same size. The calculation of the standard errors also requires the use of specialist software packages that can handle such complex sample designs (such as STATA).

Age standardisation

Ethnic minority groups in Britain tend to have very different age distributions from each other and from the general population, with Asian and Black groups tending to have a younger age profile than White British residents (see Chapter 1).

The different age profile of the different ethnic groups may partly explain differences in their social behaviours/lifestyles, health status, and attitudes/experiences. One way of removing the age element of the difference when comparing ethnic groups is to use age standardisation. There are various ways to do this, all of which increase the standard errors of the estimates. Rather than standardising to a real age distribution (e.g. of the general population), some studies have standardised to an artificial age distribution in order to minimise the increase in standard errors that the standardised weighting introduces (e.g. Erens *et al.* 2001a).

Concluding remarks

Obtaining high quality representative data from ethnic minority groups is one of the most challenging tasks facing researchers and survey organisations. This chapter aimed to cover the key issues encountered by researchers when trying to operationalise a survey of ethnic minority groups in Britain. In the event, the resulting survey will inevitably be a compromise between what the researcher ideally would wish to achieve and what is practical and achievable within funding restraints. Using examples from some recent surveys focusing on ethnic minorities, we have sought to describe how operational, quality and cost considerations impact on the decisions made at the various stages of the research process: from the classification, inclusion and sampling of ethnic minority groups, through topics to do with questionnaire content, translations and data collection, to data analysis issues of weighting and standardisation. By addressing topics such as the uneven population distribution of ethnic minority groups, the impact of culture on participation rates, and variations in language and literacy, researchers need to consider what is achievable within a realistic budget, without compromising the representativeness and validity of the results.

References

Aspinall, P.J. (2001) 'Operationalising the collection of ethnicity data in studies of the sociology of health and illness', *Sociology of Health and Illness*, 23: 829–862.

Aspinall, P.J. (2002) 'Collective terminology to describe the minority ethnic population: the persistence of confusion and ambiguity in usage', *Sociology*, 36: 803–816.

Bhopal, R. (2004) 'Glossary of terms relating to ethnicity and race: for reflection and debate', *Journal of Epidemiology and Community Health*, 58: 441–445.

Bhopal, R., Vettini, A., Hunt, S. *et al.* (2004) 'Review of prevalence data in, and evaluation of methods for cross cultural adaptation of, UK surveys on tobacco and alcohol in ethnic minority groups', *British Medical Journal*, 328: 76–80.

BMJ editorial (1996) 'Style matters: ethnicity, race, and culture: guidelines for research audit, and publication', *British Medical Journal*, 312: 1094.

Brown, C. and Ritchie, J. (1981) *Focussed Enumeration: the development of a method for sampling ethnic minority groups*, London: Policy Studies Institute and Social and Community Planning Research.

Elam, G., Chinouya, M. and the Joint Health Surveys Unit (2000) *Feasibility Study for Health Surveys Among Black African Populations Living in the UK: Stage 2 – Diversity among Black African communities*, London: Department of Health.

Elam, G., McMunn, A., Nazroo, J. *et al.* (2001) *Feasibility Study for Health Surveys Among Black African People Living in England: Final Report – Implications for the Health Survey for England 2003*, London: Department of Health.

Erens, B. (1993) *The Residents of Bethnal Green*. London: National Centre for Social Research.

Erens, B., Primatesta, P. and Prior, G. (eds) (2001a) *Health Survey for England: the health of minority ethnic groups 1999, (Volume 1: Findings, Volume 2: Methodology and Documentation)*, London: The Stationery Office for the Department of Health.

Erens, B., McManus, S., Field, J. *et al.* (2001b) *National Survey of Sexual Attitudes and Lifestyles II: technical report*, London: National Centre for Social Research.

Erens, B., McManus, S., Prescott, A. *et al.* (2003) *National Survey of Sexual Attitudes and Lifestyles II: Reference tables and summary report*, London: National Centre for Social Research.

Fenton, K., White, B. and Weatherburn, P. (2000) *What Are You Like? Assessing the sexual health needs of Black gay and bisexual men*, London: Big Up.

Fenton, K., Mercer, C.H., McManus, S. *et al.* (2005) 'Ethnic variations in sexual behaviour in Great Britain and risk of sexually transmitted infections: a probability survey', *The Lancet*, 365: 1246–1255.

Fowler, F. (2001) *Survey Research Methods*, Newbury Park: Sage Publications.

Groves, R.M., Fowler, F.J., Couper, M.P. *et al.* (2004) *Survey Methodology*, Hoboken: John Wiley & Sons.

Hales, J., Henderson, L., Collins, D. and Becher, H. (2000) *2000 British Crime Survey (England and Wales) Technical Report*, London: National Centre for Social Research.

Hamlyn, B., Maxwell, C., Hales, J. *et al.* (2003) *2003 Crime and Justice Survey (England and Wales) Technical Report*, London: National Centre for Social Research and BMRB Social Research.

Health Education Authority (1994) *Health and Lifestyles: black and minority ethnic groups in England*, London: HEA.

Hess, I. (1985) *Sampling for Social Research Surveys 1947–1980*, Ann Arbor, MI: University of Michigan.

Hoinville, G., Jowell, R. and Associates (1978) *Survey Research Practice*, London: Heinemann.

Hughes, A.O., Fenton, S. and Hine, C.E. (1995) 'Strategies for sampling black and ethnic minority populations', *Journal of Public Health Medicine*, 17: 187–192.

Hunt, S.M. and Bhopal, R. (2004) 'Self report in clinical and epidemiological studies with non-English speakers: the challenge of language and culture', *Journal of Epidemiology and Community Health*, 58: 618–622.

Jackson, J.S. (ed.) (1991) *Life in Black America*, Newbury Park: Sage Publications.

Kalton, G. and Anderson, D.W. (1986) 'Sampling rare populations', *Journal of the Royal Statistical Society A* 149, Part 1: 65–82.

King, G., Murray, C.J.L., Salomon, J.A. *et al.* (2004) 'Enhancing the validity and cross-cultural comparability of measurement in survey research', *American Political Science Review*, 98: 567–583.

Korovessis, C. (2001) 'Sampling minority ethnic populations in the UK general population', *Survey Methods Newsletter*, 21: 12–19.

Lynn, P. and Lievesley, D. (1991) *Drawing General Population Samples in Great Britain*, London: SCPR.

McKenzie, K. and Crowcroft, N. (1996) 'Describing race, ethnicity, and culture in medical research', *British Medical Research*, 312: 1054.

McManus, S., Field, J., Prescott, A. and Erens, B. (2002) *National Survey of Sexual Attitudes and Lifestyles II: topic report one: sexual behavior*, London: National Centre for Social Research.

Meadows, K. and Wisher, S. (2000) 'Establishing cross-cultural validity in health surveys', *Survey Methods Centre Newsletter*, London: National Centre for Social Research.

Modood, T., Berthoud, R., Lakey, J. *et al.* (1997) *Ethnic Minorities in Britain: diversity and disadvantage*, PSI Report 843, London: Policy Studies Institute.

Moser, C.A. and Kalton, G. (1985) *Survey Methods in Social Investigation*, London: Heinemann.

Office of National Statistics (2003) *Ethnic Group Statistics: a guide for the collection and classification of ethnicity data*, London: HMSO.

Pasick, R.J., Steward, S.L., Bird, J.A. *et al.* (2001) 'Quality of data in multiethnic health surveys', *Public Health Reports 2001, Supplement 1*, 116: 223–243.

Rhodes, P.J. (1994) 'Race-of-interviewer effects: a brief comment', *Sociology*, 28: 547–558.

Saloman, J.A., Tandon, A. and Murray, C. (2004) 'Comparability of self-rated health: cross-sectional multi-country survey using anchoring vignettes', *British Medical Journal*, 328(7434): 258–260.

Smaje, C. (1995) *Health, 'Race' and Ethnicity: making sense of the evidence*, London: King's Fund Institute.

Smith, P. (1996) 'Methodological aspects of research amongst ethnic minorities', *Survey Methods Centre Newsletter*, 16: 20–24.

Smith, P. and Prior, G. (1996) *The Fourth National Survey of Ethnic Minorities: technical report*, Social and Community Planning Research.

Sproston, K. and Nazroo, J. (eds) (2002) *Ethnic Minority Psychiatric Illness Rates in the Community*, London: The Stationery Office.

Sproston, K., Pitson, L., Whitfield, G. and Walker, E. (1999) *Health and Lifestyles of the Chinese Population in England*, London: Health Education Authority.

System Three (2001) *Scoping Study for a National Survey of Scotland's Minority Ethnic Population*, Edinburgh: Scottish Executive Central Research Unit.

Weeks, M.F. and Moore, R.P. (1981) 'Ethnicity-of-interviewer effects on ethnic respondents', *Public Opinion Quarterly*, 45: 245–249.

Chapter 9

Ethnicity and research evaluating health interventions

Issues of science and ethics

Ann Oakley

The scientific purpose of ethnicity and health research, as noted by Bhopal and Donaldson (1998: 1304) is 'elucidating the causes of diseases and the interplay between cultural factors and health'. Its practical purpose is 'ensuring that services and policies are appropriate'. The element missing from this definition is the requirement that research also identifies those interventions that promote health most effectively. This is the focus of the present chapter.

Health services and health promotion research include a wide range of research questions and study designs, as does social care research and social research more generally. A key component of research concerns the effectiveness of interventions aimed at promoting health and wellbeing. While most such interventions are undeniably well-intentioned, the real possibility of harm or ineffectiveness can only be ruled out by well-conducted evaluations. With the growth of evidence-based medicine in the UK and elsewhere, the findings from these evaluations are increasingly seen as pivotal in guiding health professionals' best practice and establishing 'state-of-the-art' understandings of the treatment and prevention of disease. This approach also applies to other areas of intervention research, including social care, education, criminal justice, transport and the environment, and public policy generally (Davies *et al.* 2000, Macdonald 1997, Thomas and Pring 2004). The importance of rigorous intervention evaluation research means that there are critical issues, not only about the extent to which such evaluations have been carried out, but about who takes part in evaluation research: how 'representative' are the samples included in such studies, and why does representativeness matter?

This chapter examines some of the key issues in the relationship between ethnicity as a socio-cultural variable and the conduct of evaluation research. It focuses on evaluation research which is designed to measure the impact of interventions implemented by health care or health promotion practitioners, or others, and aimed at improving the health and wellbeing of individuals and communities.

Other chapters in this volume provide full discussions of theories, concepts and definitions of race and ethnicity, so these are not repeated here. The perspective taken in the chapter is to view the treatment of ethnic minority people in health intervention evaluation research as part of a general phenomenon of social exclusion. This is a societal phenomenon that is reflected in the practices of evaluation researchers. Studies of the social production of scientific knowledge show how the dominant beliefs and values of a society shape the training, funding and practices of researchers, including the questions asked and the methods used to answer these (Krieger 1992).

As Dieppe and colleagues (2004) have noted, there is a complex overlap between different factors associated with social exclusion generally, including socio-economic disadvantage, age, and ethnic minority and gender status, and the social characteristics of those who take part in intervention evaluation research. Ethnic minority groups are more likely to be living in poverty, to live in overcrowded households and to have high rates of unemployment (Modood *et al.* 1997).

Evaluation research: some general design issues

The key questions about interventions aimed at improving health are whether or not the intervention achieves its aims, and whether there are anticipated and/or undesirable effects. Questions about the *outcomes* assessed in the evaluation of interventions need to be supplemented by others relating to the *processes* involved in the design, implementation and evaluation of health-related interventions (Oakley *et al.* 2004, Wight and Obasi 2002). Process data can help to explain outcome effects (or the lack of these), and also provide valuable information about intervention implementation, delivery and social context.

Ideally, all health interventions should be evaluated before being introduced into practice. However, the world is far from ideal, although the advent of the Cochrane Collaboration (www.cochrane.org) has done much to promote the message that synthesised evidence from well-conducted experimental studies is the best way of reaching the most reliable answers about intervention effects. 'Well-conducted' experiments are those that measure intervention effects against the standard of what happens to one or more 'no-intervention' control groups, using a prospective design with assignment of research participants to intervention and control groups on a random basis (randomised controlled trials (RCTs)). Randomisation is the preferred method for assigning people to experimental and comparison groups in evaluation research simply because it is the most efficient way of ensuring socially equivalent groups (Kunz *et al.* 2003). This minimises the risk of confusing intervention effects with the consequences of differences between intervention recipients and those in the comparison group. For this reason, prospective controlled studies using random allocation are preferable to attempts to 'match' on potentially confounding factors, an exercise that requires accurate knowledge (rarely attainable) of what all these factors are.

Put the other way round, the best way of practising on the basis of biased evidence is *not* to subject interventions to evaluation at all, and the next best way is to use evaluation designs that inefficiently control for bias. The most popular of these designs are 'observational' or 'qualitative' studies which collect selective experiential data about an intervention's effectiveness (for example, by asking samples of people providing or receiving an intervention what they think about it); experimental studies in which the outcome of interest is measured before and after intervention (pre- and post-test studies) but without any comparison group; and controlled trials, where assignment of research participants to intervention and comparison groups is on a non-random basis. In all these cases, it may be impossible to attribute reliably any apparent difference in health outcomes observed to the effects of the intervention itself, because we have no way of knowing about the effects of time or of assessing the impact of the particular characteristics of the research participants who provided data. The fact that most interventions, whether clinical or social, have very modest effects (Berge and Sandercock 2002), and the social systems into which interventions are introduced are by their nature complex, underscores the importance of rigorous design in all evaluation research.

The hallmarks of a 'good' RCT have been described as: trialling a high quality intervention; answering important and relevant questions; incorporating an ethical control group; measuring outcomes with proven high validity; having adequate sample size and statistical power; including adequate evaluation of the intervention and its delivery; documenting external factors that could influence trial outcomes; and using culturally sensitive intervention and evaluation designs (Ross and Wight 2002: 45–47).

The importance of sound evaluation design raises two immediate questions: how common this is, and whether ethnic minority people are included in such studies as often as majority populations, compared with less reliable ones. Both questions are difficult to answer in the present state of knowledge.

Probably the bulk of health care interventions in common use today have not been properly evaluated. In health promotion research, sound evaluation design is not the norm. For example, a review in 1990 of health education interventions in developing countries showed that only 11 per cent of 500 studies included any kind of evaluation and only four were RCTs (Loevinsohn 1990). In 1996 Peersman reviewed research related to health promotion for young people in the areas of mental health, nutrition, physical activity, sexual health and substance abuse and found that many interventions were not evaluated and most that were did not use RCTs. In five recent systematic reviews of health promotion research in the areas of children's and young people's healthy eating and physical activity and young people's mental health, most studies that evaluated the outcome of one or more health promotion interventions did not use an RCT design, and one in four used a design with no control group (Brunton *et al.* 2003, Harden *et al.* 2001, Rees *et al.* 2001, Shepherd *et al.* 2001, Thomas *et al.* 2003, 2004).

The second question, whether ethnic minority people are more likely to be included in methodologically flawed intervention evaluation research, is almost impossible to answer because there is simply very little information available. There are certainly some well-known examples of ethnic minorities having been included in trials without having been asked for informed consent (see e.g. Coney 1988, Jones 1993). Table 9.1 shows the reporting of ethnicity in a sample of health promotion trials divided into those that were assessed as methodologically 'sound' and 'flawed'. Data on sex and social class are also shown. There is a tendency for those studies in which ethnicity, sex and social class are not reported to be less methodologically robust than the others.

Inclusivity: why it matters

Inclusivity matters on grounds of both science and ethics.

From a scientific point of view, the most fundamental point is that non-inclusivity interferes with generalisability, by limiting the external validity of a study (Anderson 1983, Hall 1999). Internal validity may be high, because the groups exposed and not exposed to the intervention may be very similar, and steps may have been taken to ensure high study retention and response rates, but this is not enough to warrant generalising the research findings to the general population. For example, in a drug

Table 9.1 Reporting of ethnicity, sex and social class in methodologically 'sound'* and 'flawed' health promotion trials (N = 215 studies)

	Sound (%)	(N)	Flawed (%)	(N)	Total (%)	(N)
Ethnicity						
Mainly 'other'	28	(8)	72	(21)	100	(29)
Mainly 'White'	32	(13)	68	(28)	100	(41)
Mixed	21	(5)	79	(19)	100	(24)
Not reported	23	(28)	77	(93)	100	(121)
Sex						
Females	5	(1)	95	(19)	100	(20)
Males	22	(5)	78	(17)	100	(23)
Mixed	28	(43)	72	(109)	100	(152)
Not reported	24	(5)	76	(16)	100	(21)
Social class						
Mainly 'working class'	17	(5)	83	(24)	100	(29)
Mainly 'middle class'	22	(4)	78	(14)	100	(18)
Mixed	33	(22)	67	(41)	100	(61)
Not reported	23	(25)	77	(85)	100	(110)

* Defined as reporting on all the study aims, giving baseline and outcome data for all participants, and demonstrating the use of socially comparable intervention and control groups.

Source: Oakley *et al.* 1998; Health promotion databases of the Evidence for Policy and Practice Information and Co-ordinating Centre 2004.

trial where participants are restricted to White men aged 20–45, it would be unwise and possibly dangerous to argue that the observed effectiveness of the drug in this group meant that it was equally effective in women, older people, or those from ethnic minorities.

Exclusion of minorities from research may mean that we simply have no information about such differential patterns. A strong argument for inclusivity in trials of interventions is thus that heterogeneous research samples enable us to answer questions about the possibly differential impact on different population subgroups of the intervention being evaluated. But this only applies if there is a 'reasonable' hypothesis that there will be differential impact. Reasons for differential impact may be biological (Krecic-Shepard *et al.* 2000), but even where some biological basis for differential risk exists, there may be other, equally important, social factors. For example, the ADH2*2 gene is believed to protect against alcoholism. It is relatively common among Maori people in New Zealand but is not found in New Zealand Europeans. However, alcohol-related health problems are more common among Maori people, suggesting that the hypothesised protective effect of genetic factors is being outweighed by the impact of cultural factors (Pearce *et al.* 2004). Another example is anaemia. Haemoglobin levels differ between South Asian and Chinese ethnic groups and between men and women in these groups. Genetic explanations in terms of sickling or thalassaemia genes are unlikely to explain most of the anaemia observed, but diet is likely to be relevant, as anaemia is more common among vegetarians and most British Indians (who make up a large part of the British South Asian group) do not eat meat (Fischbacher *et al.* 2001a).

So far as trials of interventions are concerned, some have argued that disease/condition-specific prevalence is more appropriate as an eligibility criterion than representativeness in the population. Thus, differences by ethnic group in the prevalence of diseases such as insulin-dependent and non-insulin-dependent diabetes, coronary heart disease, stroke and cancer may be relevant in some trials of health care or health promotion interventions (Smaje 1995). Researchers planning a trial of a health promotion intervention to prevent accidental injury might want to take into account the fact that mortality ratios for accidents in people under the age of 15 and over the age of 65 are greater in migrants from Ireland and the Indian subcontinent than those born in England and Wales (Balarajan 1995). In a trial of an intervention to decrease alcohol use, investigators would need to consider the generally lower levels of alcohol use among all ethnic minorities in the UK, and might want to exclude the Pakistani and Bangladeshi communities, since total abstinence is common among Muslims (Nazroo 1997). The situation in trial design and reporting is currently highly confused on these issues. In a review of the reporting of race/ethnicity in clinical trials in areas of health disparities, Corbie-Smith and colleagues (2003) found that many trials of interventions for diseases with known ethnic disparities did not report the ethnicity of trial participants, and almost none analysed outcome data by ethnicity. Trials of HIV/AIDS interventions were most likely, and those in the area of cancer were least likely, to report ethnicity.

Hypotheses relating to differential findings for ethnic minorities in trials, or to the need for purposive sampling by ethnicity, must be carefully documented, supported by good evidence, and specified in advance of the trial being conducted. As an example of good practice, an RCT of a specialist nurse intervention to reduce unscheduled asthma care which was carried out in a deprived multiethnic area, hypothesised a differential effect by ethnicity: hospital admission rates and morbidity from asthma are considerably higher among ethnic minority groups and improving asthma outcomes among such groups is a 'global challenge'. When analysed, the results of the RCT were, indeed, consistent with greater benefit for White than South Asian and other ethnic minority patients (Griffiths *et al.* 2004). Without such careful specification of hypotheses relating to ethnic differences, research may suggest a racist view of ethnicity as a biological construct (Rathore and Krumholz 2003), and may fuel the search for biological explanations while ignoring strong social evidence (Anand 1999).

One dimension of trial design that has received little attention from this point of view is the calculation of sample size. This is commonly made on the basis of the numbers needed to show an effect of the intervention under test. For example, the sample size for an RCT of postnatal social support was partly calculated using a figure for the prevalence of maternal depression derived from an earlier study of social support. This showed a prevalence of 40 per cent, but the study included English-speaking women only (Oakley *et al.* 1990). Baseline prevalence in a second trial, which had a more culturally diverse population, was significantly lower (Wiggins *et al.* 2004). This may have reflected a pattern of lower levels of depression among some ethnic minority mothers (Lloyd 1998). Alternatively, it could have been due to the use of standardised instruments for measuring depression that have not been validated for most ethnic minority groups. Where power calculations are derived from samples that differ significantly from those actually used, a trial may be significantly under-powered and thus unlikely to yield useful information.

The second argument for inclusivity is on grounds of ethics. People have an equal right to take part in research designed to inform public policy, including the provision of health and social care. If such research is not democratic in its methods, it cannot be democratic in its conclusions. Non-inclusive research practices in this area, as in others, are a form of 'institutional racism' (Hussain-Gambles 2004). A further twist to this argument is provided by the evidence that people who take part in trials generally have better health outcomes than those who do not, regardless of which group they are in (Edwards *et al.* 1998). If this is a causal, rather than selection, effect, excluding ethnic, or other, minorities, from participation in trials denies them this benefit. Equally important is the argument that excluding minorities means that the state-of-the-art evidence contributed by such trials may not be relevant to them, and this limitation may mean that they lack access to effective and appropriate treatment and care.

What is the state of the evidence about the inclusion of ethnic minority people in evaluation research?

Many clinical trials are restricted to middle-class, married White males (Swanson and Ward 1995); the 'default' practice of using the most homogeneous populations possible has effectively filled medical libraries with data on middle-aged white men (Cotton 1990). Analysis of the national research register held by the English Department of Health in 2003 found over 1,000 RCTs, of which only nine referred to ethnic minority or non-English speaking groups (Johnson and Szczepura 2003). The extent to which ethnic minorities are included in intervention evaluation studies more generally is difficult to gauge, since the major problem is missing information (Bartlett *et al.* 2003, Dieppe *et al.* 2004, Grady *et al.* 2003). There are two linked issues here: reporting of inclusion/exclusion criteria and reporting of sample characteristics.

The evidence relating to reporting of inclusion/exclusion criteria in RCTs was summarised by Prescott and colleagues (1999). They concluded that restrictive trial entry leading to poor generalisability is a major problem in the design and conduct of many RCTs. Reviewing trials of adjuvant therapy for breast cancer in the US, Begg and Engstrom (1987) showed a median of 23 exclusion categories, the rationale for which was often unclear. This is a common pattern (Britton *et al.* 1999, Hunninghake *et al.* 1997, Wiederman *et al.* 1996). Many of the arguments about inclusivity in relation to ethnicity in intervention evaluation research parallel those relating to sex and age. For example, Bayer and Tadd (2000) examined the exclusion of older people from studies submitted to research ethics committees. Out of 155 studies that were of relevance to older people, over half had an upper age limit that was unjustified. Interestingly the ethics committees had not requested a justification.

'Unspecified cultural differences' are sometimes offered as a reason for exclusion (Geiger 1996). Commonly, the exclusion is implicit rather than explicit; a recent review by Mason and colleagues (2003) of six clinical trials conducted by a centre in northern England found that none of the trials specified exclusion criteria relating to ethnicity, but all had patient information sheets and consent forms in the English language only. Frayne and colleagues (1996) reviewed the exclusion of non-English-speaking people in medical research and found that the most common reason was that investigators had simply 'never thought about the issue': this applied to 51 per cent of the 40 per cent of investigators who had excluded non-English speakers. Interestingly, the evidence is that increased sensitivity to 'race' or ethnicity as a variable in health research does not necessarily lead to fewer unjustified exclusions. In an analysis of papers published in the *American Journal of Epidemiology* between 1921 and 1990 Jones and colleagues (1991) showed that the proportion of papers containing a reference to 'race' rose steadily from 1975, but those reporting inclusion of 'non-White' subjects did not increase over this period.

Table 9.1, which gives reporting data in 215 health promotion studies, shows that the ethnicity of research participations was not reported in the majority (56 per cent – 121/215 studies). Non-reporting of the social characteristics of trial participants, including ethnicity, is the major issue here. This unsatisfactory practice is supported by the current version of the CONSORT guidelines for reporting trials, which specifies only that 'baseline demographic and clinical characteristics' of each group in a trial should be reported; no further guidelines are given about how this is to be handled (Moher *et al.* 2001). Sometimes reports of research give almost no information about the source of the sample; Silagy and Jewell (1994) found no mention of how the study population had been obtained in 22 per cent of 90 RCTs published in a general practice journal. Other studies give figures for the reporting of ethnicity as a social characteristic of trial participants that vary from 17 per cent to 27 per cent (Bartlett *et al.* 2003, Clay *et al.* 2002, Sheikh *et al.* 2004). In a review of 65 studies conducted in the US and published in 1993–1995 that gave information on participation recruitment, Ness and colleagues (1997) found that only one study reported the ethnicity of potential study participants, and only one gave information about the ethnicity of those who refused. The ethnicity of successfully recruited participants was less likely to be reported than either age or gender (59 per cent versus 91 per cent and 80 per cent, respectively). These findings accord with the pattern shown in Table 9.1. The omission of information about cultural diversity, including ethnicity, is particularly striking in areas such as research on communication skills (Fellowes *et al.* 2004) or dietary interventions (Ammerman *et al.* 2001), where cultural factors are likely to have a high impact.

Information about the extent to which the profiles of populations included in trials reflect those of wider populations can sometimes require extensive detective work, as in the study by Mason and colleagues (2003) where ethnic origin could only be established for participants in some trials through detailed analysis of names. This exercise showed that the participation of South Asian people in the trials underrepresented by 50 per cent (1.7 per cent versus 3.4 per cent) their prevalence in the population. In Waldenström and Turnbull's (1998) review of 12 RCTs of continuity of midwifery care, none of the trials described the population from which the trial sample was drawn (and five did not do so for the trial population either). In an analysis of 25 trials of non-steroidal anti-inflammatory drugs in osteoarthritis, Dieppe and colleagues (2004) found that the profile of trial participants particularly underrepresented people at risk of adverse effects, minority groups and older people (those over 75 were excluded from most trials).

Lack of information about how research samples are made up, including the representation of ethnic minorities, has the further important limitation of restricting the information about effective and appropriate care that is available as a result of systematic reviews of primary studies – the main methodological tool of evidence-based medicine. Thus, a systematic review of four key topics related to coronary heart disease in women stratified by ethnicity had to omit many eligible studies because these lacked information about gender or ethnicity or both; only one of the four review questions could be addressed in relation to ethnicity (Grady *et al.* 2003). Most commonly, however, systematic reviews of primary studies either give no information about the ethnicity of participants or note that 'narrow ranges' have been included (Parker *et al.* 2002). An analysis by Tsikata and colleagues (2003) of the extent to which Cochrane systematic reviews contain useful information about health equity reviewed a random 10 per cent sample of the Cochrane Library from 2000 to 2003 to examine the reporting of socio-economic gradients. Using PROGRESS, an acronym for Place of residence, Race/ethnicity/culture, Occupation, Gender, Religion, Education, Social capital and Socio-economic status, they found that only 22 per cent of 95 review groups considered these aspects of participants' circumstances. Out of a 10 per cent sample of 120 primary trials only 29 per cent provided relevant information.

Ethnicity, recruitment and consent to take part in intervention evaluation research

Barriers to equitable representation of ethnic minorities in intervention evaluation research can operate at many different levels. These include: study design; researcher or practitioner bias; concern on the part of ethnic minority people about taking part in trials; inadequate consent procedures; problems in developing and implementing effective and appropriate recruitment strategies; and costs.

There is an important distinction to be made between bias in eligibility criteria, on the one hand, and selective agreement to participate in research, on the part of those asked, on the other. A US study of a multicentre maintenance trial in schizophrenia found that women, Black people and older people were more likely to be defined as not meeting eligibility criteria, and women and older people were more likely, and Black people less likely, to refuse study participation (Robinson *et al.* 1996). Ashcroft and colleagues' (1997) review of the implications of socio-cultural contexts for the ethics of trials importantly uncovered no evidence that any cultural groups have specific objections to the approach of evaluating interventions using RCTs. A limitation here is that general research on attitudes to trial recruitment tends to be insensitive to ethnic and other cultural diversity (Featherstone and Donovan 1998). A significant example is the piloting of a standardised instrument – the Attitudes to Randomised Trials Questionnaire (ARTQ) – in samples for which no information is given about ethnicity; consequently, the validity of the instrument in ethnically diverse populations is unknown (Fallowfield *et al.* 1998, Jenkins and Fallowfield 2000). A recent qualitative study by Hussain-Gambles reports the first UK-based research exploring the attitudes of South Asian patients to taking part in trials. She found that negative factors cited by patients included: the practical burden of trial participation; language and discriminatory practices of the NHS; mistrust of health professionals; and a preference on the part of some women for female trial staff. However, the similarities with the attitudes of White patients were more pronounced than the differences (Hussain-Gambles 2004).

Deficient information about the opportunities for entering patients into trials and lack of minority investigators were given as reasons for low minority recruitment rates in another US study of cancer trials (McCaskill-Stevens *et al.* 1999). The perceptions of health care providers that ethnic differences in attitudes to trials exist can be very influential (Stone *et al.* 1998), and can significantly misread some of the factors that may operate as barriers to full participation. For example, in an Australian midwifery trial reported by Homer (2000), questionnaire response rates were lower among Arabic-speaking than English- or Chinese-speaking women; process data suggested that one reason for this was that the former group was more likely to see childbirth as a normal life event and thus an inappropriate topic for formal evaluation. Careful documentation of research processes may be required to reveal some critical sources of bias. In a pilot study evaluating the use of 'informed choice' leaflets for women using the maternity services, midwives in antenatal clinics were asked to identify the main language spoken and the literacy level of all eligible women. Some midwives just transferred this (often inaccurate) information directly from the hospital notes, without asking women themselves. Some did not understand that 'literacy' meant literacy not just in English, but in the main language spoken. Others were reluctant to hand out the leaflets to women whom they considered would not benefit from them, and such women were therefore excluded from taking part in the study (Oliver *et al.* 1995).

There has been little formal evaluation of strategies for recruiting minority populations to trials (Prescott *et al.* 1999, Swanson and Ward 1995). A number of observational studies suggest that developing 'culturally appropriate' strategies can raise minority recruitment figures (Lewis *et al.* 1998, Preloran *et al.* 2001), although the evidence is mixed (Thompson *et al.* 1996).

Examples of trials that have set out to be inclusive in their recruitment strategies include several in the area of maternal and child health. In an RCT of a community-based model of midwifery, Homer (2000) reported the use of health-care interpreters, translation of trial materials into common community languages and engaging the local community in promoting the relevance of the trial. Wiggins and colleagues (2004) evaluated two different strategies for providing postnatal support to mothers in a disadvantaged urban area with an ethnic minority population of 22 per cent (compared to around 9 per cent nationally). The Social Support and Family Health (SSFH) Study aimed to be inclusive in its recruitment procedures, and to this end employed a team of 11 researchers, materials translated into six languages, and interpreters speaking 25 different languages. As a result, 42 per cent of the women recruited self-identified as 'non-White' and 39 per cent did not have English as their first language. Table 9.2 shows some of the differences between the groups of women recruited with and without interpreters. More of those recruited using interpreters were socially disadvantaged. The only exception is shown in the last line of Table 9.2; fewer non-English-speaking women were smokers, reflecting differences by ethnicity and gender in smoking behaviour.

A conclusion with important implications for evaluation research practice was that the inclusive practices used in the SSFH Study raised the costs of conducting the research; for example, the cost per women recruited for those who needed interpreters was £135 compared with £80 for those who did not (Oakley *et al.* 2003). Other evidence supports the increased costs of trials using inclusive recruitment strategies.

Table 9.2 Characteristics of English-speaking and non-English-speaking participants in the Social Support and Family Health Study (N = 731)

	% English speakers	% non-English speakers
Ethnicity 'not White'	35	86
Partner had paid work in the last month	77	47
Weekly income <£200	49	94
Rented accommodation	66	92
Left full–time education <16	6	30
Smoker	29	10

Source: Oakley *et al.* 2003: 35.

Cost calculations for two well-known American studies, the Physicians' Health Study and the Multiple Risk Factor Intervention Trial (MRFIT), show that including women and minorities would have almost doubled the costs of both studies (Meinert 1999). Not surprisingly, the costs of being inclusive are sometimes cited by investigators as reasons for excluding non-English-speaking people from research (Frayne *et al.* 1996). An environment in which inclusivity is not the norm, and the implications of restricted samples for the generalisability of research evidence are not widely discussed, is one in which research funders are not likely to criticise the excuse of higher cost as a reason for non-inclusive recruitment practices.

The extent to which participants in experimental studies of health interventions are asked for informed consent is another area where issues of science and ethics collide. The tension is between the scientific desirability of recruiting as many people as possible to trials, and the ethical requirement of providing for fully informed consent. The infamous Tuskegee study in Alabama, in which African American men with syphilis were given no treatment, remains an influential part of the background to current discussions of the ethics of experimental health research involving ethnic minority groups (Jones 1993).

A report commissioned by the Health Technology Assessment programme of *Ethical Issues in the Design and Conduct of Randomised Controlled Trials* comprehensively reviews the literature in the area of consent (Edwards *et al.* 1998). It identifies many problems with current trial consent practices, though there is little explicit discussion in the report of ethnic inclusivity as a design or conduct issue. Like the ethnicity of research participants, whether or not informed consent was obtained is an under-reported aspect of evaluation research. In an analysis of RCTs published in the *Archives of Diseases in Childhood* from 1982 to 1996, 45 per cent (112) of 249 trial reports said nothing about informed consent. Of the remainder, 81 per cent (111/137) worryingly quoted consent rates of 100 per cent (Campbell *et al.* 1997). Out of 182 evaluations of health promotion interventions held in the database of the Evidence for Policy and Practice Information and Coordinating (EPPI) Centre, 58 per cent did not report or give clear information about whether consent was sought; among the subset of 70 RCTs, this figure was 50 per cent. Interestingly, the figures for the non-reporting of consent in the domain of educational research studies included in the EPPI-Centre database were higher: 81 per cent of 203 evaluations, and 85 per cent of 54 RCTs. This suggests that practice in the health care and health promotion fields may be ahead of that in the evaluation of other social interventions.

Consent to participate in trials is increasingly formal, with research ethics committees playing a key role as guardians of proper consent procedures. In order to provide valid consent, people must be given information about the trial that they can understand in their own language. In the UK, some Multi-centre Research Ethics Committees acknowledge the 'problem' of non-English speakers, and advise that 'special arrangements' should be made to seek consent in these situations, without any guidelines as to the nature of these arrangements. The background here is the vast increase in the bureaucracy of research ethics committees in recent years, and the diminishing relevance of many of the questions asked by these committees to important ethical issues such as who is regarded as eligible to take part in research, and what kinds of information and consent procedures should be used (Wald 2004).

Direct translation (either verbal or written) of informed consent materials does not address the issue of cultural diversity in the meanings attached to those concepts that are key to current dominant understandings of informed consent. These include the idea of individual autonomy, which is intrinsic to the liberal-individualistic Western rights-based approach of the ethical framework underlying RCTs (Ashcroft *et al.* 1997). Cultural values and practices relating to autonomy differ, and for some people the normal consent-forming process includes the family and community (Berg 1999, Cullinan 1997, Wiggins *et al.* 2004). The notion of informed consent depends on principles of human rights, which some minority people may not assume, especially when they are refugees from oppressive political regimes (Yu 1994).

Ethnicity and trial retention/response rates

The problem of differential drop-out in trials and follow-ups to trials and other longitudinal studies is well known. Generally, drop-out and non-response rates are highest in the most socially disadvantaged groups, which includes many people from ethnic minorities. The reasons why people decline to be recruited to trials or drop out of these are many and varied, including problems with additional medical appointments and painful medical procedures, lack of time, travel costs, anxiety and excessive study demands. However, few studies of these barriers to participation in trials have considered ethnicity or other social characteristics. Where they have, the evidence is equivocal: some studies suggest higher 'compliance' rates among the socially advantaged, while others report the reverse pattern (Prescott *et al.* 1999). Michie and Marteau (1999) explored this issue in an RCT of screening in antenatal care. They concluded that the sampling strategy (only including literate English-speaking women), long questionnaires and the use of White researchers all helped to explain the ethnic bias in the women recruited to and retained in the study.

Cultural appropriateness of interventions

A major issue in the design of evaluation research relates to the choice of the intervention to be tested: what is the scientific basis for selecting one type of intervention rather than another, and does this include consideration of the intervention's appropriateness in a culturally diverse population? 'Type' of intervention here includes not only its content (drug, counselling, education, etc.), but the materials that are used and how the intervention is implemented and by whom. For example, in the SSFH trial referred to earlier, there was a lower uptake of both interventions evaluated (support from home-visiting health visitors and from community groups) among women whose first language was not English. Process data collected during the study suggested that in the health visitor intervention group the model of one-to-one support provided in repeated home contacts may have been less appropriate for some ethnic minority mothers than for others. These mothers had stronger family and community ties (not all of which were experienced as supportive), were less comfortable with the one-to-one model of the support provided by the health visitors, and had greater basic health and social care needs. An RCT in Nepal of postnatal health education which used a similar intervention had no significant impact on maternal or infant health outcomes. In commenting on this finding, the investigators suggested that a more appropriate focus would be interactions within the family, peer groups or communities (Bolam *et al.* 1998). Among women in the SSFH Study allocated to be offered support by local community groups, there were problems not only with language but with cultural inappropriateness – for instance, in relation to women visiting groups outside their homes and mixing with strangers (Wiggins *et al.* 2004).

The importance of culturally tailored interventions has been identified in other areas, for example diabetes and exercise awareness programmes (Simmons *et al.* 1996), though including different interventions within the same trial clearly poses problems for evaluation design, and the approach of emphasising cultural differences may be to the detriment of the health and social care needs shared by minority and majority populations (Qureshi *et al.* 2004). Evaluations of health promotion interventions in populations that include ethnic minority groups rarely describe the use of culturally sensitive approaches (Rees *et al.* 2001). This reflects the fact that many are not designed with ethnic minorities in mind. For example, only 17 of 345 studies in the area of mental health promotion for young people identified ethnic minorities as relevant target groups (Harden *et al.* 2001). In a cluster RCT of free smoke alarms to reduce fire-related injuries in a deprived (18 per cent ethnic minority) urban population, DiGiuseppi and colleagues (2002, Rowland *et al.* 2002) identified some cultural factors that may help to explain the apparent failure of the intervention to reduce fires or injuries. While the researchers used 'foreign' language brochures and local ethnic minority recruiters to explain the trial, most of the 20,050 smoke alarms distributed had not been installed or maintained properly: investigators noted a common lack of tools to install these; worries about landlords objecting to installation; the small physical size of households producing 'false' alarms; and possible difficulties in comprehending the intervention among those to whom the alarms were distributed. However, and despite a *British Medical Journal* Editorial describing the report of the trial as 'flawless' (Pless 2003: 979) no data about ethnicity in relation to the outcome or processes of the trial were given, making it impossible to judge how much of a difference these factors made to the apparent failure of the intervention, and how it might have been adapted to increase its usefulness to ethnic minority groups.

Translation and cultural (non-)equivalence

Non-proficiency in oral or written English overlaps, but is not synonymous with, ethnic minority group status. For example, around 23 per cent of immigrants to Britain born in China, Bangladesh, India and Pakistan have no functional skill in English, and 70 per cent are unable to function fully in an English-speaking environment; but this means that most do have some functional English-speaking skill and a third are fully functional in English (Free and McKee 1998).

As discussed elsewhere in this volume, the translation of information or intervention materials and of questionnaires or interview questions to collect baseline, process or outcome data in trials raises critical issues about linguistic equivalence and the impact of translation on research findings. This is another area in which relatively little research has been done. Translations can fail to achieve equivalence in terms of appropriateness and meaning of questions originally framed in English (Stewart and Napoles-Springer 2000). Examples include the term 'feeling blue' used in the American version of the short form health questionnaire 36 (SF-36) and other instruments measuring mental health: this term has different connotations in different languages (Bullinger *et al.* 1998); 'check up' and 'Pap smear' have no conceptual equivalent in any Chinese language (Pasick *et al.* 2001). The midwifery trial reported by Homer (2000) identified an unanticipated difficulty in using questionnaires translated into Arabic: the nuances of spoken Arabic meant that the gender and region of origin of the reader altered the interpretation of the text in the questionnaires so that it was offensive to some women, but not to others. Such difficulties are compounded where the written and spoken languages are not the same (for example Arabic and Cantonese) and where data are collected from non-English speaking trial participants by translating questionnaires in face-to-face interviews. In a small study exploring the translation of interview material into Chinese, Twinn (1997) reported differences in findings according to whether Chinese or English transcriptions of the interviews were used. Bilingual interviews take more time; questions asked via a third party require translation time, but also the time taken by the task of ensuring that questioner and questioned understand one another and agree on the meaning of terms and expressions (Turner 1996). These issues of translation and cultural equivalence may be critical when communication is central to the definition of the intervention, as, for instance in counselling, information- or skills-giving interventions, or in the case of the social support interventions discussed above.

Most research to date has focused on the translation of standardised instruments, not on issues of psychometric equivalence (Anderson *et al.* 1985). Most standardised instruments are developed using English-speaking White populations. They may thus have lesser validity for some ethnic groups, and this can bias evaluation findings (Fischbacher *et al.* 2001b). For example, instruments such as the Edinburgh Postnatal Depression Scale (Cox *et al.* 1987) and the General Health Questionnaire (Goldberg and Williams 1988) are problematic for populations, such as Asian and African Caribbean women, for whom the 'meanings' and prevalence of outcomes such as depression and health service use are different from those in the groups for which these instruments were originally developed. The types of life events included in the commonly used Holmes and Rahe life-event scale may inadequately reflect those that are important to different ethnic groups (Chalmers 1981). The sensitivity of such instruments may vary across populations, and different cut off points may be needed (Bradley *et al.* 1998).

These are issues that require careful research, especially since the lack of valid and reliable cross-cultural measurements may be given as a reason for not including minority groups in clinical trials and epidemiological studies (Bartlett *et al.* 2003).

Standardised guidelines for the cross-cultural adaptation of health-related quality of life measures have been produced which include many useful suggestions (Guillemin *et al.* 1993). An interesting development that attempts to overcome the cultural specificity of questionnaires is the 100-item World Health Organization Quality of Life Assessment (WHOQOL). Rather than developing the questionnaire in one culture, and then translating it to others, concepts and questions were developed in 15 countries and then synthesised (WHOQOL Group 1993).

The broader context of health need

Evaluation research in health and social care takes place in a context in which people from ethnic minorities are not treated equally. Patterns of health service use show problems of access to primary care and a lower incidence of referrals to secondary and tertiary care (Nazroo 1997, Rudat 1994, Smaje and LeGrand 1997). Such differences in health care utilisation could partly explain lower rates of ethnic minority access to trials, since the centres used by trial investigators may themselves under-represent ethnic minorities. There may also be very different levels of information about treatments and services among different ethnic groups, and these can affect both recruitment to research and research findings. For example, in a pilot study evaluating the use of 'informed choice' leaflets in maternity care, the main issue that arose in relation to the ethnic minority women who took part in the research was the enormous unmet need for basic information about pregnancy, childbirth and maternity care; this swamped the detailed questions that were the focus of the study, about the acceptability of information relating to the evidence-base for routine ultrasound screening and the best positions to use during labour (Turner 1996).

Challenges to ethnic inclusiveness: towards a more inclusive future

Current and past practices in evaluation research are clearly deficient in many different ways in relation to the goal of including ethnic minorities. Similar issues exist in relation to including the 'minorities' of women and older people. An ethnically inclusive approach to health and social care intervention evaluation research means confronting a number of challenges. The presumption that trials need only be conducted and reported in the English language, and that systematic reviews of the evidence need only survey the literature in English (Moher *et al.* 2003), are both implicitly forms of racism. Less often mentioned, and sometimes confused with linguistic diversity, is the broader issue of differences in cultural values and belief systems relating to health and health care. Conceptions of the body and of the meanings of health and illness are culturally patterned; the assumed conceptual universality underlying standardised health measures and many structured questions can be false and thus socially exclusive (Staniszewska *et al.* 1999). 'Culture', here, includes religion, language, kinship, diet, clothing, health beliefs, and birth and burial practices, all of which may be relevant to intervention evaluation research – and to health research more generally (Helman 1985, McPherson *et al.* 2003, Rack 1991).

In the US, inclusion of minorities in RCTs in proportion to their representation in the population was mandated by the 1993 National Institutes of Health Revitalization

Act. The same legislation required the inclusion of women in health research in sufficient numbers to allow for analyses of any differential effects of drug treatments and
other interventions. In neither case is the cost of being inclusive considered a permis-
sible reason for being exclusive. Proposals for increasing the sensitivity of health
intervention evaluation research to ethnic and other cultural diversity in the UK include
following the US example and mandating such diversity as a condition for commissioning research (Mason *et al.* 2003). The unequal treatment that occurs as a result
of policies being based on research evidence from which ethnic minority people are
unjustifiably excluded can already be construed as unlawful under the 1976 UK Race
Relations Act. The Race Relations (Amendment) Act of 2000 placed a new duty on
public authorities to take the initiative in working towards the elimination of unlawful
discrimination and promoting equality of opportunity. This could be interpreted as
placing a new obligation on public bodies that fund research to ensure ethnically
inclusive practice. However, this interpretation does not yet appear to have been taken
up by research commissioners and funders. Judging from the US example, legislation on its own is unlikely to achieve equity (Ramasubbu *et al.* 2001); although
American RCTs are five times more likely than European RCTs to report ethnicity,
three-fifths still do not do so (Sheikh *et al.* 2004).

Other strategies for promoting inclusivity include developing educational programmes for trial investigators and funding bodies to increase their awareness of the
under-representation of ethnic minority people in trials, and ensuring that ethics
committees take a more systematic and rigorous approach to issues of inclusivity in
research (Hussain-Gambles 2003). Modification of the CONSORT guidelines for
reporting trials to specify more detailed socio-demographic descriptions of samples
at baseline would also be an important step forward. Similar sets of guidelines need
to be established for social intervention trials, including those in social care and
education.

Trial researchers should collect and report information on their recruitment processes (Prescott *et al.* 1999, Robinson *et al.* 1996). There needs to be more research
on recruitment strategies. The potential for increasing recruitment by embedding trials
in qualitative research as described by Donovan and colleagues (2002) for men eligible
for prostate cancer trials may be considerable. In this study, in-depth pre-recruitment
interviews with potential participants ironed out many obstacles to researchers' understanding of participants' perspectives and participants' understanding of trial design
and rationale. However, the value of this strategy to the recruitment of ethnic minority
people to trials is as yet untested.

Issues of language and cultural meaning need to be addressed by a participatory
approach, whereby representatives from the groups to be included in the research
work with the investigators to develop appropriate questions and measures; language
differences should be seen as challenges and not as obstacles (Hunt and Bhopal 2003).
As discussed in Chapter 4, more effort needs to be made to include different ethnic
groups in the whole process of designing evaluation research, including the questions to be studied, and the measures and research procedures to be used. Sometimes
the policy, academic and research communities which commission, design and carry
out research invoke practices of tokenism whereby junior ethnic minority researchers
are included in some studies to make these look more representative; this is not necessarily a useful advance (Sehmi 2003). While there has been a sustained move towards

more user or 'consumer' involvement in the design and analysis of intervention evaluation research, there is little discussion in this literature of the importance of ethnic
and cultural diversity (see e.g. Goodare and Lockwood 1999, Sakala *et al.* 2001).

There has been surprisingly little attention paid in the methodological literature to
the fundamental question raised at the beginning of this chapter: the extent to which
inclusive or exclusive practices in relation to evaluation research may be biasing the
evidence drawn from such research about effective approaches to promoting health
and wellbeing. Differences in the findings of different studies may be explained by
the different samples included. For example, the findings from the SSFH trial, which
was inclusive in its approach, were broadly that there was little basis on which to
recommend routine use of either of the support interventions tested. This contrasts
with the conclusions of a trial of supportive midwifery-led postnatal care conducted
around the same time, which excluded non-English-speaking women, and which
concluded that the intervention had positive effects and should be put into routine
practice (MacArthur *et al.* 2003). It is possible that some such interventions work
better for some populations than for others.

Conclusion

This chapter has reviewed some of the key issues relating to the inclusion of ethnic
minorities in evaluation research in order to identify some significant research gaps
and practical strategies to further the goal of inclusiveness. The norm of middle-class
male, English-speaking whiteness has dominated the field of research evaluating interventions to promote health and wellbeing, just as it has characterised other forms of
domination (Cotton 1990, Mastroianni *et al.* 1994). Health researchers cannot ignore
the political dimensions of their work (Smaje 1995). This includes the obligation to
consider how conventional practices for evaluating health and social care interventions may systematically ignore the experiences of ethnic minority people. Many
research practices in this area demonstrate the kinds of confusion about what ethnicity
'is' and how it is relevant to health issues that are common in other areas of health
research (Comstock *et al.* 2004). While unwarranted exclusion of ethnic minority
people from health intervention evaluation research constitutes a form of 'institutional
racism', it is also important to 'look beyond ethnicity' at the ways in which different
social and economic factors are associated with socially exclusive practices applied
to minorities, including their treatment in health intervention research. Ethnicity should
be studied simultaneously with socio-economic status and class (Senior and Bhopal
1994). In particular, a too-narrow focus on ethnicity is likely to downplay the important relations between ethnicity, gender and social inequality which are relevant to the
development and evaluation of many health interventions (Lloyd 1998).

The issues about inclusivity and exclusivity in health intervention evaluation
research raised in this chapter extend to other policy domains and to a wide range
of social interventions. There are, for example, important questions to be asked about
the ways in which programmes aimed at improving the behaviour of children and
young people are evaluated, and these include questions about the social profiles of
those who have taken part in evaluation research (Roberts *et al.* 2004).

Inadequate evaluation is a general problem in much ethnicity and health intervention research. Interventions targeted at the general population may be more likely

to be evaluated than those targeted at ethnic minority groups. There is a specific need for more well-designed evaluations of interventions to improve health service access for ethnic minority groups (Atkinson *et al.* 2001). But many of the methodological issues identified in this chapter relate to the need to improve evaluation design more generally (Oakley 2005, Ross and Wight 2002).

Socially inclusive research is sounder science and better ethics, enabling the evidence that feeds into policy and practice to reflect the cultural diversity and complexity that characterise many societies today. To summarise the main pointers referred to in this chapter for improving practice relating to the inclusion of ethnic minorities in evaluation research:

* evaluations of health and social care interventions should be well designed to answer important questions of concern to minority as well as majority populations;
* inclusion/exclusion criteria should be clear and scientifically based; the 'default' assumption should be one of inclusivity, and the practice of excluding non-English speaking people on the conventional grounds of practical difficulty and cost should be abandoned;
* research funders should *require* inclusivity unless there are sound scientific reasons for an exclusive approach, and they should be prepared to find any additional costs;
* more attention should be given to developing and evaluating culturally appropriate interventions;
* where analyses of outcome data by ethnicity are carried out, these and their rationale should be pre-specified;
* published reports should contain information about the social characteristics of trial participants and of the population from which they were drawn to aid reliable conclusions about generalisability;
* more research should be undertaken of different approaches to recruitment; and
* the choice and measurement of outcomes in trials should be informed by more research on the perspectives of ethnic and other minority groups, including the development or adaptation of appropriate standardised instruments.

References

Ammerman, A., Lindquist, C., Hersey, J. *et al.* (2001) *The Efficacy of Interventions to Modify Dietary Behavior Related to Cancer Risk, Volume I Evidence report and appendices,* Rockville, MD: Agency of Healthcare Research and Quality.

Anand, S. (1999) 'Using ethnicity as a classification variable in health research: perpetuating the myth of biological determinism, serving socio-political agendas, or making valuable contributions to medical sciences?', *Ethnicity and Health*, 4: 241–244.

Anderson, J.M. (1985) 'Perspectives on the health of immigrant women: a feminist analysis', *Advances in Nursing Science*, October, 8: 61–76.

Anderson, R.T., Aaronson, N.K. and Wilkin, D. (1993) 'Critical review of the international assessments of health-related quality of life', *Quality of Life Research*, 2: 369–395.

Ashcroft, R.E., Chadwick, D.W., Clark, S.R.L. *et al.* (1997) 'Implications of socio-cultural contexts for the ethics of clinical trials', *Health Technology Assessment*, 1(9).

Atkinson, M., Clark, M., Clay, D. *et al.* (2001) *Systematic Review of Ethnicity and Health Service Access for London*, Warwick: Centre for Health Services Studies.

Balarajan, R. (1995) 'Ethnicity and variations in the nation's health', *Health Trends*, 27: 114–119.

Bartlett, C., Davey, P., Dieppe, P. *et al.* (2003) 'Women, older persons and ethnic minorities: factors associated with their inclusion in randomised trials of statins 1990 to 2001', *Heart*, 89: 327–328.

Bayer, A. and Tadd, W. (2000) 'Unjustified exclusion of elderly people from studies submitted to research ethics committee for approval: descriptive study', *British Medical Journal*, 321: 992–993.

Begg, C.B. and Engstrom, P.F. (1987) 'Eligibility and extrapolation in cancer clinical trials', *Journal of Clinical Epidemiology*, 5: 962–968.

Berg, J.A. (1999) 'Gaining access to under-researched populations in women's health research', *Health Care for Women International*, 20: 237–243.

Berge, E. and Sandercock, P. (2002) 'The nuts and bolts of doing a clinical trial', in L. Duley and B. Farrell (eds) *Clinical Trials*, London: BMJ Publishing.

Bhopal, R.S. and Donaldson, L.J. (1988) 'Health education for ethnic minorities: current provision and future directions', *Health Education Journal*, 47: 137–140.

Bhopal, R.S. and Donaldson, L.J. (1998) 'White, European, Western, Caucasian, or what? Inappropriate labelling in research on race, ethnicity and health', *American Journal of Public Health*, 88(9): 303–7.

Bolam, A., Manandar, D.S., Shrestham P. *et al.* (1998) 'The effects of postnatal health education for mothers on infant care and family planning practices in Nepal: a randomised controlled trial', *British Medical Journal*, 316: 805–811.

Bradley, K.A., Boyd-Wickizier, J., Powell, S.H. and Burman, M.L. (1998) 'Alcohol screening questionnaires in women: a critical review', *Journal of the American Medical Association*, 280: 166–171.

Britton, A., McKee, M., Black, N. *et al.* (1999) 'Threats to applicability of randomised trials: exclusion and selective participation', *Journal of Health Services Research and Policy*, 4: 112–121.

Brunton, G., Harden, A., Rees, R. *et al.* (2003) *Children and Physical Activity: a systematic review of barriers and facilitators*, London: EPPI-Centre, Social Science Research Unit, Institute of Education.

Bullinger, M., Alonso, J., Apolone, G. *et al.* (1998) 'Translating health status questionnaires and evaluating their quality', *Journal of Clinical Epidemiology*, 51: 913–923.

Campbell, H., Boyd, K.M. and Surry, S.A.M. (1997) 'Journals should require routine reporting of consent rates' (letter), *British Medical Journal*, 315: 247.

Chalmers, B. (1981) 'Development of a life event scale for pregnant, white South African women', *South African Journal of Psychology*, 11: 74–79.

Clay, D.L., Mordhorst, M.J. and Lehn, L. (2002) 'Empirically supported treatments in pediatric psychology: where is the diversity?', *Journal of Pediatric Psychology*, 27: 325–337.

Comstock, R.D., Castillo, E.M. and Lindsay, S.P. (2004) 'Four-year review of the use of race and ethnicity in epidemiologic and public health research', *American Journal of Epidemiology*, 159: 611–619.

Coney, S. (1988) *The Unfortunate Experiment*, Auckland: Penguin Books.

Corbie-Smith, G., St George, D.M.M., Moody-Ayers, S. and Ransohoff, D.F. (2003) 'Adequacy of reporting race/ethnicity in clinical trials in areas of health disparities', *Journal of Clinical Epidemiology*, 56: 416–420.

Cotton, P. (1990) 'Is there still too much extrapolation from data on middle-aged white men?', *Journal of the American Medical Association*, 263: 1049–1050.

Cox, J.L., Holden, J. and Sagovsky, R. (1987) 'Detection of postnatal depression: development of the 10-item Edinburgh Postnatal Depression Scale (EPDS)', *British Journal of Psychiatry*, 150: 782–786.

Cullinan, T. (1997) 'Other societies have different concepts of autonomy' (letter), *British Medical Journal*, 315: 248.

Davies, H.T.O., Nutley, S.M. and Smith, P.C. (eds) (2000) *What Works? Evidence-based policy and practice in public services*, Bristol: The Policy Press.

Dieppe, P., Bartlett, C., Davey, P. *et al.* (2004) 'Balancing benefits and harms: the example of non-steroidal anti-inflammatory drugs', *British Medical Journal*, 329: 31–34.

DiGiuseppi, C., Roberts, I., Wade, A. *et al.* (2002) 'Incidence of fires and related injuries after giving out free smoke alarms: cluster randomised controlled trial', *British Medical Journal*, 325: 995–997.

Donovan, J., Mills, N., Smith, M. *et al.* for the Protect Study Group (2002) 'Improving design and conduct of randomised trials by embedding them in qualitative research: ProtecT (prostate testing for cancer and treatment) study', *British Medical Journal*, 325: 766–770.

Edwards, S.J.L., Lilford, R.J., Braunholtz, D.A. *et al.* (1998) 'Ethical issues in the design and conduct of randomized controlled trials', *Health Technology Assessment*, 2.

Fallowfield, L.J., Jenkins, V., Brennan, C. *et al.* (1998) 'Attitudes of patients to randomised clinical trials of cancer therapy', *European Journal of Cancer*, 34: 1554–1559.

Featherstone, K. and Donovan, J.L. (1998) 'Random allocation or allocation at random? Patients' perspectives of participation in a randomised controlled trial', *British Medical Journal*, 317: 1177–1180.

Fellowes, D., Wilkinson, S. and Moore, P. (2004) 'Communication skills training for health care professionals working with cancer patients, their families and/or carers' (Cochrane Review), in *The Cochrane Library*, issue 2. Chichester: John Wiley & Sons.

Fischbacher, C.M., Bhopal, R., Patel, S. *et al.* (2001a) 'Anaemia in Chinese, South Asian, and European populations in Newcastle upon Tyne: cross sectional study', *British Medical Journal*, 322: 958–959.

Fischbacher, C.M., Bhopal, R., Unwin, N. *et al.* (2001b) 'The performance of the Rose angina questionnaire in South Asian and European origin populations: a comparative study in Newcastle', *International Journal of Epidemiology*, 54: 786.

Frayne, S.M., Burns, R.B., Hardt, E.J. *et al.* (1996) 'The exclusion of non-English-speaking persons from research', *Journal of General Internal Medicine*, 11: 39–43.

Free, C. and McKee, M. (1998) 'Meeting the needs of black and minority ethnic groups', *British Medical Journal*, 316: 380.

Geiger, H. (1996) 'Race and health care – an American dilemma?', *New England Journal of Medicine*, 335: 815–816.

Goldberg, D. and Williams, P. (1988) *A User's Guide to the General Health Questionnaire*, Windsor: NFER-Nelson.

Goodare, H. and Lockwood, S. (1999) 'Involving patients in clinical research', *British Medical Journal*, 319: 724–725.

Grady, D., Chaput, L. and Kristof, M. (2003) *Diagnosis and Treatment of Coronary Heart Disease in Women: a systematic review of evidence on selected topics*, Rockville, MD: Agency for Healthcare Research and Quality.

Griffiths, C., Foster, C., Barnes, N. *et al.* (2004) 'Specialist nurse intervention to reduce unscheduled asthma care in a deprived multiethnic area: the east London randomised controlled trial for high risk asthma (ELECTRA)', *British Medical Journal*, 328: 144–147.

Guillemin, F., Bombardier, C. and Beaton, D. (1993) 'Cross-cultural adaptation of health-related quality of life measures: literature review and proposed guidelines', *Journal of Clinical Epidemiology*, 46: 1417–1432.

Hall, W.D. (1999) 'Representation of blacks, women, and the very elderly (aged > or = 80) in 28 major randomized clinical trials', *Ethnicity and Disease*, 9: 333–340.

Harden, A., Rees, R. Shepherd, J. *et al.* (2001) *Young People and Mental Health: a systematic review of research on barriers and facilitators*, London: EPPI-Centre, Social Science Research Unit, Institute of Education.

Helman, C. (1985) *Culture, Health and Illness*, Bristol: John Wright & Sons.

Homer, C. (2000) 'Incorporating cultural diversity in randomised controlled trials in mid-wifery', *Midwifery*, 16: 252–259.

Hunninghake, D.B., Darby, C.A. and Probstfield, J.L. (1997) 'Recruitment experience in clinical trials: literature summary and annotated bibliography [review]', *Controlled Clinical Trials*, 8: 6–30.

Hunt, S. and Bhopal, R. (2003) 'Self reports in research with non-English speakers', *British Medical Journal*, 327: 352–353.

Hussain-Gambles, M. (2003) 'Ethnic minority under-representation in clinical trials: whose responsibility is it anyway?', *Journal of Health Organisation and Management*, 17: 138–143.

Hussain-Gambles, M. (2004) 'South Asian patients' views and experiences of clinical trial participants', *Family Practice*, 21(6): 636–642.

Hussain-Gambles, M., Atkin, K. and Leese, B. (2004) 'Why ethnic minority groups are under-represented in clinical trials: a review of the literature', *Health & Social Care in the Community*, 12(5): 382–388.

Jenkins, V. and Fallowfield, L. (2000) 'Reasons for accepting or declining to participate in randomized clinical trials for cancer therapy', *British Journal of Cancer*, 82: 1783–1788.

Johnson, M.R.D. and Szczepura, A. (2003) 'Population's ethnic profile should be recorded in all medical data' (letter), *British Medical Journal*, 327: 394.

Jones, C.P., LaVeist, T.A. and Lillie-Blanton, M. (1991) 'Race in the epidemiologic literature: an examination of the *American Journal of Epidemiology*, 1921–1990', *American Journal of Epidemiology*, 134: 1079–1083.

Jones, J.H. (1993) *Bad Blood: the Tuskegee syphilis experiment*, Glencoe, IL: Free Press.

Krecic-Shepard, M.E., Park, K., Barnas, C. *et al.* (2000) 'Race and sex influence clearance of nifedipine: results of a population study', *Clinical Pharmacology and Therapeutics*, 68: 130–142.

Krieger, N. (1992) 'The making of public health data: paradigms, politics and policy', *Journal of Public Health Policy*, Winter: 412–417.

Kunz, R., Vist, G. and Oxman, A.D. (2003) 'Randomisation to protect against selection bias in healthcare trials' (Cochrane Methodological Review), in *The Cochrane Library*, Issue 1, Oxford: Update Software.

Lewis, C.E., George, V., Foaud, M. *et al.* (1998) 'Recruitment strategies in the women's health trial: feasibility study in minority populations', *Controlled Clinical Trials*, 19: 461–476.

Lloyd, K. (1998) 'Ethnicity, social inequality and mental illness', *British Medical Journal*, 316: 1763–1770.

Loevinsohn, B.P. (1990) 'Health education interventions in developing countries: a methodological review of published articles', *International Journal of Epidemiology*, 19(4): 788–794.

MacArthur, C., Winter, H.R., Bick, D.E. *et al.* (2003) 'Redesigning postnatal care: a randomised controlled trial of protocol-based midwifery-led care focused on individual women's physical and psychological health needs', *Health Technology Assessment*, 7(37).

Macdonald, G. (1997) 'Social work: beyond control?', in A. Maynard and I. Chalmers (eds) *Non-random Reflections on Health Services Research*, London: BMJ Publishing Group: 122–146.

Mason, S., Hussain-Gambles, M., Leese, B. *et al.* (2003) 'Representation of South Asian people in randomised clinical trials: analysis of trials' data', *British Medical Journal*, 326: 1244–1245.

Mastroianni, A.C., Faden, R. and Federman, D. (eds) (1994) *Women and Health Research: ethical and legal issues of including women in clinical studies*, vol. 1, Washington, DC: National Academy Press.

McCaskill-Stevens, W., Pinto, H., Marcus, A.C. *et al.* (1999) 'Recruiting minority cancer patients into cancer clinical trials: a pilot project involving the Eastern Cooperative Oncology Group and the National Medical Association', *Journal of Clinical Oncology*, 17: 1029.

McPherson, K., Harwood, M. and McNaughton, H.K. (2003) 'Ethnicity, equity and quality: lessons from New Zealand', *British Medical Journal*, 327: 443–444.

Meinert, C.L. (1999) 'Redesign of trials under different enrolment mixes', *Statistics in Medicine*, 18: 241–251.

Michie, S. and Marteau, T. (1999) 'Non-response bias in prospective studies of patients and health care professionals', *International Journal of Social Research Methodology*, 2: 203–212.

Modood, T., Berthoud, R., Lakey, J. *et al.* (1997) *Ethnic Minorities in Britain: diversity and disadvantage*, PSI Report 843, London: Policy Studies Institute.

Moher, D., Schulz, K.F. and Altman, D.G. for the CONSORT Group (2001) 'The CONSORT statement: revised recommendations for improving the quality of reports of parallel-group randomised trials', *The Lancet*, 357: 1191–1194.

Moher, D., Pham, B., Lawson, M.L. and Klassen, T.P. (2003) 'The inclusion of reports of randomised trials published in languages other than English in systematic reviews', *Health Technology Assessment*, 7(41).

Nazroo, J. (1997) *The Health of Britain's Ethnic Minorities*, London: Policy Studies Institute.

Ness, R.B., Nelson, D.B., Kumanyika, S.K. and Grisso, J.A. (1997) 'Evaluating minority recruitment into clinical studies: how good are the data?', *Annals of Epidemiology*, 7: 471–478.

Oakley, A. (2005) 'Design and analysis of social intervention studies in health research', in A. Bowling and S. Ebrahim (eds) *Handbook of Health Research*, Maidenhead: Open University Press, 246–265.

Oakley, A., Peersman, G. and Oliver, S. (1998) 'Social characteristics of participants in health promotion effectiveness research: trial and error', *Education for Health*, 11: 305–317.

Oakley, A., Rajan, L. and Grant, A. (1990) 'Social support and pregnancy outcome: report of a randomised controlled trial', *British Journal of Obstetrics and Gynaecology*, 97: 155–162.

Oakley, A., Wiggins, M., Turner, H. *et al.* (2003) 'Including culturally diverse samples in health research: a case study of an urban trial of social support', *Ethnicity and Health*, 8: 29–39.

Oakley, A., Stephenson, J., Forrest, S. and Monteiro, H. (2004) 'Evaluating processes: a case study of a randomised controlled trial of sex education', *Evaluation*, 10: 440–462.

Oliver, S., Rajan, L., Turner, H. and Oakley, A. (1995) *A Pilot study of 'Informed Choice' Leaflets on Positions in Labour and Routine Ultrasound*, London: Social Science Research Unit, Institute of Education.

Parker, G., Bhakta, P., Lovett, C.A. *et al.* (2002) 'A systematic review of the costs and effectiveness of different models of paediatric home care', *Health Technology Assessment*, 6(35).

Pasick, R.J., Steward, S.L., Bird, J.A. and D'Onofrio, C.N. (2001) 'Quality of data in multi-ethnic health surveys', *Public Health Reports 2001, Supplement 1*, 116: 223–243.

Pearce, N.B., Foliaki, S., Sporle, A. and Cunningham, C. (2004) 'Genetics, race, ethnicity and health', *British Medical Journal*, 328: 1070–1072.

Peersman, G. (1996) *A Descriptive Mapping of Health Promotion Studies in Young People*, London: Social Science Research Unit, Institute of Education.

Pless, B. (2003) 'Smoke detectors and house fires' (editorial), *British Medical Journal*, 325: 979–980.

Preloran, H.M., Browner, C.H. and Lieber, E. (2001) 'Strategies for motivating Latino couples' participation in qualitative health research and their effects on sample construction', *American Journal of Public Health*, 91: 1832–1841.

Prescott, R.F., Counsell, C.E., Gillespie, W.J. *et al.* (1999) 'Factors that limit the quality, number and progress of randomised controlled trials', *Health Technology Assessment*, 3(20).

Qureshi, T., Berridge, D. and Wenman, H. (2004) *Where to Turn? Family support for South Asian communities*, London: National Children's Bureau.

Rack, P. (1991) *Race, Culture and Mental Disorder*, London: Tavistock/Routledge.

Ramasubbu, K., Gurm, H. and Litaker, D. (2001) 'Gender bias in clinical trials: do double standards still apply?', *Journal of Women's Health and Gender Based Medicine*, 10: 757–764.

Rathore, S.S. and Krumholz, H.M. (2003) 'Race, ethnic group, and clinical research', *British Medical Journal*, 327: 763–764.

Rees, R., Harden, A., Shepherd, J. *et al.* (2001) *Young People and Physical Activity: a systematic review of research on barriers and facilitators*, London: EPPI-Centre, Social Science Research Unit, Institute of Education.

Roberts, H., Liabo, K., Lucas, P. *et al.* (2004) 'Mentoring to reduce antisocial behaviour in childhood', *British Medical Journal*, 328: 512–514.

Robinson, D., Woerner, M.G., Pollack, S. and Lerner, G. (1996) 'Subject selection biases in clinical trials: data from a multicenter schizophrenia treatment study', *Journal of Clinical Psychopharmacology*, 16: 170–176.

Ross, D.A. and Wight, D. (2002) 'The role of randomized controlled trials in assessing sexual health interventions', in J. Stephenson, J. Imrie and C. Bonell (eds) *Effective Sexual Health Interventions: issues in experimental evaluation*, Oxford: Oxford University Press.

Rowland, D., DiGiuseppi, C., Roberts, I. *et al.* (2002) 'Prevalence of working smoke alarms in local authority inner city housing: randomised controlled trial', *British Medical Journal*, 325: 998–1001.

Rudat, K. (1994) *Black and Minority Ethnic Groups in England: Health and Lifestyles*, London: Health Education Authority.

Sakala, C., Gyte, G., Henderson, S. *et al.* (2001) 'Consumer-professional partnership to improve research: the experience of the Cochrane Collaboration's Pregnancy and Childbirth Group', *Birth*, 28: 133–137.

Sehmi, K.S. (2003) 'Lack of good data results in ineffective health policy for South Asians' (letter), *British Medical Journal*, 327: 394.

Senior, P. and Bhopal, R. (1994) 'Ethnicity as a variable in epidemiological research', *British Medical Journal*, 309: 327–330.

Sheikh, A., Netuveli, G., Kai, J. and Panesar, S.S. (2004) 'Comparison of reporting of ethnicity in US and European randomised controlled trials', *British Medical Journal*, 329: 87–88.

Shepherd, J., Harden, A., Rees, R. *et al.* (2001) *Young People and Healthy Eating: a systematic review of research on barriers and facilitators*, London: EPPI-Centre, Social Science Research Unit, Institute of Education.

Silagy, C.A. and Jewell, D. (1994) 'Review of 39 years of randomized controlled trials in the British Journal of General Practice', *British Journal of General Practice*, 44: 359–363.

Simmons, D., Fleming, C., Cameron, M. and Leakehe, L. (1996) 'A pilot diabetes awareness and exercise programme in a multiethnic workforce', *New Zealand Medical Journal*, 109: 373–376.

Singh, G. and Johnson, M.R.D. (1998) 'Research with ethnic minority groups in health and social welfare', in C. Williams, H. Soydan and M.R.D. Johnson (eds) *Social Work and Minorities: European perspectives*, London: Routledge.

Smaje, C. (1995) *Health, 'Race' and Ethnicity: making sense of the evidence*, London: King's Fund Institute.

Smaje, C. and LeGrand, J. (1995) 'Ethnicity, equity and the use of health services in the British National Health Service', *Social Science and Medicine*, 45: 485–496.

Staniszewska, S., Ahmed, L. and Jenkinson, C. (1999) 'The conceptual validity and appropriateness of using health-related quality of life measures with minority ethnic groups', *Ethnicity and Health*, 4: 51–63.

Stewart, A.L. and Napoles-Springer, A. (2000) 'Health-related quality of life assessments in diverse population groups in the United States', *Medical Care*, 38(9) (suppl): II102–124.

Stone, V.E., Mauch, M.Y. and Steger, K.A. (1998) 'Provider attitudes regarding participation of women and persons of color in AIDS clinical trials', *Journal of AIDS and Human Retrovirology*, 19: 245–253.

Swanson, G.M. and Ward, A.J. (1995) 'Recruiting minorities into clinical trials: towards a participant-friendly system', *Journal of the National Cancer Institute*, 87: 1747–1759.

Thomas, G. and Pring, R. (eds) (2004) *Evidence-based Practice in Education*, Maidenhead: Open University Press.

Thomas, J., Harden, A., Oakley, A. *et al.* (2004) 'Integrating qualitative research with trials in systematic reviews', *British Medical Journal*, 328: 1010–1012.

Thomas, J., Sutcliffe, K., Harden, A. *et al.* (2003) *Children and Healthy Eating: a systematic review of barriers and facilitators*, London: EPPI-Centre, Social Science Research Unit, Institute of Education.

Thompson, E.E., Neighbors, H.W., Munday, C. and Jackson, J.D. (1996) 'Recruitment and retention of African American patients for clinical research: an exploration of response rates in an urban psychiatric hospital', *Journal of Consulting and Clinical Psychology*, 64: 861–867.

Tsikata, S., Robinson, V., Petticrew, M. *et al.* (2003) 'Do Cochrane systematic reviews contain useful information about health equity?' [abstract], *XI Cochrane Colloquium: Evidence, Health Care and Culture*, 26–31 October, Barcelona, Spain: p. 77.

Turner, H. (1996) *Informed Choice in Pregnancy and Childbirth: what this means for black and ethnic minority women*, London: Social Science Research Unit, Institute of Education.

Twinn, S. (1997) 'An exploratory study examining the influence of translation on the validity and reliability of qualitative data in nursing research', *Journal of Advanced Nursing*, 26: 416–423.

Wald, D.S. (2004) 'Bureaucracy of ethics applications', *British Medical Journal*, 329: 282–284.

Waldenström, U. and Turnbull, D. (1998) 'A systematic review comparing continuity of midwifery care with standard maternity services', *British Journal of Obstetrics and Gynaecology*, 105: 1160–1170.

WHOQOL Group (1993) 'Study Protocol for the World Health Organisation project to develop a quality of life assessment instrument (WHOQOL)', *Quality of Life Research*, 2: 153–159.

Wiederman, M.W., Maynard, C. and Fretz, A. (1996) 'Ethnicity in 25 years of published sexuality research: 1971–1995', *The Journal of Sex Research*, 33: 339–342.

Wiggins, M., Oakley, A., Roberts, I. *et al.* (2004) 'The Social Support and Family Health Study: a randomised controlled trial and economic evaluation of two alternative forms of postnatal support for mothers living in disadvantaged inner city areas', *Health Technology Assessment*, 8(32).

Wight, D. and Obasi, A. (2002) 'Unpacking the "black box": the importance of process data to explain outcomes', in J. Stephenson, J. Imrie and C. Bonell (eds) *Effective Sexual Health Interventions: issues in experimental evaluation*, Oxford: Oxford University Press.

Yu, E.S.H. (1994) 'Legal and ethical issues relating to the inclusion of Asian/Pacific Islanders in clinical studies', in A. Mastroianni, R. Faden and D. Federman (eds) *Women and Health Research: ethical and legal issues of including women in clinical studies*, vol. 2, Washington, DC: National Academy Press.

Chapter 10

Secondary analysis of administrative, routine and research data sources

Lessons from the UK

Peter J. Aspinall

Introduction

The purpose of this chapter is to investigate the potential for secondary analysis of ethnically coded administrative, routine and research data sources in the UK context. Historically, official sources of such information have been few. However, the situation is now changing with the adoption by government of 'mainstreaming' as a fundamental principle of its race[1] and equal opportunities programmes (Alexander 1999). Such an agenda necessitates measures that are capable of uncovering disadvantage and racism where such processes may be insidious, hidden or identifiable only through analytic work. The implementation of race equality policies and assessment of their outcomes can only properly be undertaken if such policies are linked to appropriate ethnic data collection, making the mainstreaming of ethnic monitoring a logical extension of mainstreaming race equality. Recently, the Department of Health in England has made a commitment to the collection of ethnic origin information using the 2001 Census categories for all statistical datasets collected from the NHS (UK Parliament 2004). It states that this will be achieved by incorporating the collection of additional ethnic data items within existing collections.

The main stimulus to instituting and improving ethnic group data collection in the UK, the Race Relations (Amendment) Act 2000, gives public authorities a new statutory duty to promote race equality. This encompasses a general duty to make the promotion of racial equality central to their work, including the promotion of equality of opportunity and good race relations and the prevention of unlawful discrimination, and also places specific duties on many public (including health) authorities. These require them to assess whether their functions and policies are relevant to race equality, to monitor their policies to see how they affect race equality, assess and consult on new policies, publish the results of their consultations, monitoring and assessments, and to ensure that the public have access to the information and services they provide. Clearly, ethnic monitoring data will be required across all service delivery and other policy areas to demonstrate that the general duties to eliminate unlawful racial discrimination and the promotion of equality of opportunity and good race relations have been met.

In addition, other national legislation may determine what data are collected and how they are used. The confidentiality of data about living individuals ('personal data') is protected in law. The Data Protection Act 1998, the Human Rights Act

1998 and the Freedom of Information Act 2000 give rights to privacy and access to information held by public authorities. Strict conditions are specified for the collection, processing and use of sensitive personal data, even for research purposes. Further, the Department of Health's Caldicott guidelines (Department of Health 1997) require that the purposes for which patient information is used are 'robustly justified', patient-identifiable information in this context being defined to include 'ethnic group'. Despite these imperatives, the importance accorded to ethnicity data collection has so far been limited, uneven and disappointing. In most cases implementation is either in the planning stage or at the start of data collection, so it will be some time before quality data accrue.

Using administrative data sources

Ethnically coded administrative and routine data sources contain substantial potential for secondary analysis. However, there are drawbacks to their use, because such collections were designed to meet government information needs rather than those of the research community. This section will preview the range, quality and utility of the ethnicity data currently collected, highlighting problems related to usage and how they can be addressed.

Range of data sources

Patient contacts with particular services

The ethnicity data collected by the Department of Health and its organisations fall into a number of main categories (Table 10.1). The largest single generic category of data is that relating to patient contact with services. The most important of the administrative collections of such patient data in terms of the volume of records (over 13 million annually) is the Hospital Episode Statistics (HES), which is discussed further later. Information is collected and reported centrally on every patient who receives treatment in an NHS hospital as a day case or ordinary admission through completion of a contract minimum dataset on the patient's discharge. Ethnicity data has been a mandatory part of the collection since 1995.

The availability of ethnically coded data in primary care is much more limited. Unlike that for hospital in-patients, it is not mandatory to collect this data at patient registration and, until recently, coverage has been very patchy and largely confined to a small number of inner city practices. The potential of ethnically coded general practice data is substantial as such coding could be linked to computerised morbidity recording and prescribing data; in practice, however, few Primary Care Trusts are likely to be able to provide more than a profile of their registered patients.

Third, there is a range of sources that provide information on patient contacts for particular disease or condition-specific areas, such as drug services. According to the Department of Health (2003a) all submissions relating to patients and the services provided to patients or to NHS staff should include consideration of the case for collecting ethnic origin information as part of the data collection. However, an examination of these 'central returns' shows that ethnic data is missing from many.[2]

Table 10.1 The main ethnically coded administrative and routine data sources and their utility

Topic area/data source	Year started	Current status	Ethnic coding issues
Patient contact with services			
Hospital in-patient care: hospital episode statistics (HES)	1 April 1995 (collection mandatory)	Ongoing	64% records coded (2002–3), improving to 72% (2003–4)
Hospital out-patient attendances	Varies (collection optional)	Few hospital trusts collect ethnicity data	The few reports indicate very low levels of coding
Hospital A & E attendances	Varies (collection optional)	Few hospital trusts collect ethnicity data	The few reports indicate very low levels of coding
Primary Care Trusts' patient registration data for general practices	Varies (collection optional)	Increasing but currently geographically very patchy in coverage	No comprehensive information but completeness targets in London
Preventive health care	Varies (collection optional)	No comprehensive ethnic data on cervical and breast screening and vaccinations	Not reported
Drug misusers, users of AIDS/HIV services, children in need, etc.	Various	Ongoing	'Not known' coding variable: currently 16% (drug misusers), 3% (AIDS/HIV) and 8% (children in need)
Incidence and prevalence of particular conditions			
Disease registers (mainly primary care based)	Varies	Current developments do not address ethnicity	Most general practice-based registers lack ethnic coding
Cohort studies	Varies	Research-based rather than routine data source	Most European cohort studies in specific areas (e.g. cardiovascular disease) omit ethnicity
Mortality data			
Death registration data	(collection mandatory)	Only country of birth	Data quality high
ONS Longitudinal Study (LS)	(Cohort updated with decennial census and vital registration data)	2001 Census data added	Loss to follow-up at older ages up to 30% for some groups
Hospital case fatalities (part of HES dataset)	1 April 1995 (collection mandatory)	Ongoing	As for HES; hospital deaths not repre-sentative of all mortality

So, many different organisational areas, such as cancer registration, mental health and sexually transmitted infections have developed their own specific collections.

Incidence and prevalence of particular conditions

Studies of ethnicity and health require data that measure the frequency of diseases, that is, which ethnic groups get the disease and in what quantity, and also how these ethnic-specific frequencies compare with other populations. Disease registers and cross-sectional surveys can supply information on disease prevalence. However, the number of such ethnically coded accurate information sources is very limited (other than special collections).

Disease registers, usually computerised, are databases created to demonstrate quality of care in managing chronic diseases, such as asthma, diabetes, CHD and hypertension. They generally record diagnostic and health status information, family histories and, sometimes, other information such as hospital letters and medications. When combined with census denominator data, these registers can yield information on incidence and prevalence. However, they vary in the extent to which they can provide an accurate estimate of incidence or prevalence of the conditions they record, a consistent finding being that quality of recording varies between morbidities (better for diabetes than asthma, for example). A major drawback is that most of these registers lack ethnic coding.

Nevertheless, there are a number of major new developments in primary care trusts for collecting such disease data. A new non-financial database (Quality Prevalence and Indicator Database) has been extracted from the new payment system for GP practices for planning, public health and other purposes. Such data can give practice prevalence for a range of chronic diseases, intervention data and data on risk factors. However, the database currently lacks ethnic coding.

Mortality data

The lack of ethnic coding at death registration is a major drawback for the analysis of ethnic differentials in mortality. Mortality rates can only be compiled by country of birth, which is now a poor proxy for some ethnic groups. The 2001 Census showed that only about half of all persons in ethnic minority groups were migrants. The other drawbacks of stratifying deaths by country of birth have long been recognised. They include definitional problems (with respect to changing geographies historically, especially in the Indian subcontinent); the fact that some country of birth groups, such as Indian, East African, and others, may be ethnically heterogeneous and include members of the White group; and, as a proxy measure, country of birth groups substantially undercount the full size of the ethnic groups they represent and migrants within these groups may be very different from non-migrants, the consequent problems of small numbers resulting in the aggregation of groups and, therefore, concealment of heterogeneity. For example, the most recent analyses of mortality by country of birth aggregate the Indian, Pakistani and Bangladeshi groups into a pan-ethnic 'South Asian' group. However, ethnicity is needed in addition to country of birth, the latter enabling first-generation migrants and people born in the UK to be distinguished in the different ethnic communities.

Quality and completeness of ethnic coding and implications for analysis

One of the key factors affecting the use of administrative and routine data is their quality and completeness. In many parts of the UK ethnic minority groups comprise only a small percentage of the population and, given also the diversity of this population, any loss of numbers through lack of ethnic coding constitutes a serious drawback to use for research purposes. Until recently, the perception has been that the quality and completeness of most of this official data has been too poor to merit use for the intended purpose. This, of itself, has prevented any further improvement in quality, a process largely dependent upon and driven by use. It is only in the last few years that this situation has begun to change, largely in response to new legal requirements, but also because of new methods of analysis. As Table 10.1 shows, there are few datasets where completeness of ethnic coding exceeds 90 per cent. Clearly, the main drawback for analysis of incomplete data is the reduced utility of the data, including the possibility that the count for small groups will need to be suppressed.

Access to datasets

Another factor affecting the utility of administrative and routine data for secondary analysis is ease of access. This varies substantially with respect to the different datasets. As HES records relate to individual admitted patients and the associated consultant, the Department of Health does not allow open and direct access to them. Requests for ethnically coded admitted patient data are subject to confidentiality and other commissioning constraints. Primary care data other than in aggregate form are likely to be subject to similar conditions, and the lack of indexing in terms of key variables such as ethnic group is likely to present a major barrier to use. What the research community and practitioners in service settings are currently lacking is comprehensive documentation of the different sources, of the kind that has been provided for health and social surveys by the CASS Question Bank and the Economic and Social Data Service (ESDS).

The use of demographic data as denominators for administrative data

Epidemiology and health services research requires accurate information on the numbers of cases, people with the risk factors, or users of services – comprising the *numerator* – and the population from which they come – the *denominator* – to derive rates, ratios and proportions. The foregoing sections have addressed the accuracy of data collection in the numerator and the problems associated with achieving this in the various administrative collections. The need for quality and compatibility of data on the denominator, that is, those at risk, is equally essential. This population is often specifically captured in administrative systems. Where it is not, the denominator in investigations of social inequalities in health is most frequently derived from census data. Also GP practice populations and population estimates and projections developed by the Office for National Statistics (ONS) and other agencies have been used.

As discussed in Chapter 2 of this volume, defining and measuring an appropriate denominator is not always straightforward.

Indeed, with respect to ethnic/racial disparities in health, the availability of denominator data is limited. The 1991 Census was the first decennial census in Great Britain to include a question on ethnic group, although a number of Government social surveys had collected such data in the late 1970s and 1980s. In the 2001 Census Scotland used a somewhat different ethnic group question to that used in England and Wales and ethnic group was asked for the first time in Northern Ireland, using a question similar to that used in the 1991 Great Britain Census. A number of organisations have developed population projections by ethnic group, including the Greater London Assembly and some local authorities, and a feasibility study for deriving such projections nationally has been undertaken by the ONS (Haskey 2002). However, comprehensive data on the ethnicity of patients registered with GP practices is not available and the figures held centrally and accessed via computer links omit ethnic group.

There are a number of key issues to be addressed in using ethnicity data from the census as denominators for administrative data: compatibility with respect to the question asked and the defined categories; bridging between the 1991 and 2001 census where data series are required; consistency in method of assigning ethnic group; the number of separate fields used to collect information on ethnicity and other 'cultural factors' (notably, country of birth, language and religion), permitting such data to be cross-classified in both numerator and denominator and, thus, enriching the categorisation of ethnic/racial data; and generic concerns about completeness of the denominator. These are discussed next.

With respect to categorisation, there were a number of innovations in the 2001 Census classifications used, but also some continuing problems (Aspinall 2000c). It captured the rapidly growing 'Mixed' group, through free-text options in Scotland and Northern Ireland and a combination of free-text and predesignated categories in England and Wales. In the two Great Britain censuses the White group was broken down (unlike in the 1991 Census) to encompass, in England and Wales, 'British', 'Irish' and an open response 'Any other White background' and, in Scotland, 'Scottish', 'Other British', 'Irish' and 'Any other White background'. The failure to include 'Welsh' as a White 'cultural background' option in Wales resulted in much grassroots opposition, a subsequent enumeration in the Labour Force Survey, and the development by the ONS of a national identity classification for use with that on ethnic group (Office for National Statistics 2003). These two same censuses used the term 'Asian' for the first time on a census form – in England and Wales with respect to South Asian groups and in Scotland to refer to continental Asia (through including 'Chinese') – the interpretation of which is now feasible using the Samples of Anonymised Records. Finally, conceptualisations of increasingly popular bi-cultural identities were incorporated into the labels for the pan-ethnic groups, such as 'Black or Black British' in England and Wales, and 'Asian, Asian Scottish or Asian British' in Scotland.

The introduction of a question on religion for the first time in the England and Wales and Scotland Censuses – including options of 'Buddhist', 'Hindu', 'Jewish', 'Muslim' and 'Sikh' – has enabled the size of some of these larger religious communities, about which there had been much uncertainty concerning numbers, to be established (Aspinall 2000a). Also, the religion question findings should permit a much more sensitive breakdown of the South Asian groups for the purposes of exploring ethnic disparities in health and health care; the ONS 2001 Census standard tables include a breakdown of ethnic group by religion. Clearly, the utility of these more detailed denominator data is limited by the absence of such collection in numerators.

Of course, where administrative systems do collect information on these additional census variables, data can be cross-classified in ways that are compatible with census-derived counts, thus capturing the heterogeneity of the ethnic minority population. Some of these issues, including how groups should be combined when sample size requires some aggregation to conduct meaningful analyses, have been comprehensively addressed in recent guidance published by the ONS (2003).

This new set of classifications of ethnicity has brought both opportunities and problems for users, including the public health community. First, since the classifications for the 1991 and 2001 Censuses differ, there are likely to be data compatibility problems in using census denominator data for Department of Health collections for the year 2001–02. On 1 April 2001 all such collections changed to the 2001 Census classification, the Department recognising that for this and possibly subsequent data years both categorisations would be used. It is axiomatic that the same questions and categorisation must be used for numerators (cases) and denominators (population), unless an algorithm for conversion exists.

Given that the 2001 Census ethnicity classifications for Great Britain differ from those used in the 1991 Census, there is the problem of bridging between the two counts for the derivation of trends. Surprisingly little attention has been afforded this issue in Britain compared with the 'industry' that has grown around bridging and fractional assignment for the US 2000 Census. There is some evidence derived from the Quarterly Labour Force Survey (with follow-ups at quarterly intervals for a maximum of five quarters, thus bridging the two census classifications) that enables mapping between 1991 and 2001 ethnic categorisations. Further comprehensive evidence has recently become available through a mapping of responses to the 1991 and 2001 Census questions in the same individuals using the ONS Longitudinal Study dataset that should enable an algorithm to be developed to convert between the two (Simpson 2004). It is clear, however, that – with no simple read-across from one to the other, with the possible exception of the 'Indian', 'Pakistani', 'Bangladeshi' and 'Chinese' categories – the development of time series spanning the two censuses will be problematic.

In the 1991 and 2001 Censuses self-report was used to classify ethnic group data, although the extent to which the form-filler entered data on a proxy basis for other adult and child members of the household is unknown. It has been reported that around half of census questions are filled in by someone else (Cornish 1993) and that respondents 'mainly' choose to answer on behalf of other household members (Rainford 1997). In a majority of cases the head of household or first listed household member is likely to be the form-filler and the parent of the child(ren) in households with co-resident dependent children, as households containing relatives outside the nuclear family are very few, though more frequent in some ethnic groups.

However, it is known that in administrative collections a range of methods of assignment are used, including self-assignment, assignment by next of kin, observer-assignment by officials and data collectors, and the extraction of ethnic group from medical and personal records, or a mixture of several of these methods. In a survey of NHS trusts' implementation of the mandatory requirement to collect ethnic group data in the first reporting years, a quarter of trusts reported that staff matched the patient's response to categories, and in a further quarter that ethnic group was assigned by staff observation (in contradistinction to the recommended process of self-assignment) (Aspinall 2000b). Furthermore, assignment might be through the use of closed format questions (as in the standard for HES 'ethnos' data), census questions, or open response. Clearly, the different approaches to assigning ethnic group across different data collections will all affect compatibility with census denominator data.

Indeed, a major problem that occurred with respect to the use of the 1991 classification – and one that is likely to recur with that for 2001 – is that some collections excluded the write-in provision for the 'Black Other' and 'Any other ethnic group' options. In 1991 the OPCS used a complex algorithm to redistribute free-text responses to the predesignated categories on the census form and to create the new 'Other Asian' group (Aspinall 1995). Of the 0.75 million persons who used free-text options, 14.9 per cent were reassigned from the category they ticked to produce the output categories (even when 'Other Asian' and 'Other-other' were treated as one). Only four of the ten output categories (Indian, Pakistani, Bangladeshi and Chinese) contained counts consistent with those given by respondents in the census question. Given the increase in free-text responses in the 2001 Census (from two to five tick boxes) and the reassignment of responses judged incongruent by ONS, these difficulties are likely to surface in the use of the 2001 classification for denominator data. The scale of reassignment in the 1991 Census was such that it would have impacted on rates/ratios and, when not adjusted for, resulted in unexpectedly large counts for the 'Other' group.

The opportunities that ethnicity monitoring data hold and how they might be improved

There is clearly a substantial amount of ethnically coded data now being collected by government. As quality data accrue, the potential of some of these datasets to investigate ethnic disparities in health and health care is being realised and, once high levels of ethnic coding are achieved, this will be substantial. At present, however, much of this potential is not being realised. There are valid reasons in some cases for such underuse. Undoubtedly, the major current constraint is both the poor level of ethnic coding on many of the datasets and the widespread perception that the data are not of quality and, therefore, do not merit use.

Clearly, opportunities for the exploitation of administrative data might be improved by the dissemination of skills and experience in the analysis of such data and a Department of Health commissioned toolkit is now in development that should facilitate usage. There are two areas where such skills are needed: addressing problems of data quality and using the data to identify disparities and to assess equity of access to services. Both these areas require expertise that may not readily be available to the family of health care organisations. The solution lies in democratising access to such knowledge and tools rather than centralising analysis or contracting it out, as experience shows that where organisations remain close to and use the data its quality increases commensurately.

Once assessment of data coverage and quality has been undertaken, there may be other technical barriers, such as the complex technical process of identifying a hospital catchment population given substantial overlaps in some areas. Moreover, compatible denominator data may be unavailable, inaccurate or difficult to compile, especially downstream from the decennial census. Where this is the case, that is, when the only reliable data are on cases, proportional admissions (and mortality) ratios – which compare the number of admissions (or deaths) from individual causes as a proportion of all admissions (deaths) within a given group – can be used. This approach overcomes the problem of having to identify population denominators and has been used by the Health of Londoners Project (Bardsley *et al.* 2000) and London Health Observatory and, more recently, the Healthcare Commission, to examine ethnic differentials in hospital admissions and mortality. Bhopal (2004) has questioned the utility of this ratio for risk data presentation, other than as a preliminary or corroborative analysis tool, as its magnitude depends not only on the number of deaths from the cause under study but also the number of deaths from other causes. However, Aveyard (1998) suggests that the bias is small, amenable to reduction by several methods and of no practical importance. Indeed, recent analyses of ethnic differentials using proportional admission ratios and age standardised rates indicate that they yield stable measures of ethnic disparities.

A further drawback is the lack of other measures of cultural background and of socio-economic position on most administrative datasets, which may be a limiting factor to wider utilisation. Ethnic monitoring systems are set up for specific administrative purposes and often cannot answer the questions of interest to the wider research community about both ethnic disparities and the more complex issues of inequity. Given the focus on administrative use, for example, the precise conceptual base or set of associated variables used in the collection may not be the most appropriate to answer particular research questions (see Chapter 2 for further discussion of this). With respect to ethnicity, the salient concept is self-ascribed 'ethnic group' following practice in the 1991 and 2001 Censuses. Apart from the Princes Park Liverpool development site, little use has been made of other concepts such as that of 'family origins' used in the 1999 Health Survey for England (Erens *et al.* 2001) and the Policy Studies Institute (PSI)'s Fourth National Survey (Nazroo 1997), arguably somewhat more stable than ethnic group that is characterised by selective attribution. However, the Policy Studies Institute's mapping of responses to similar classification questions using concepts of 'family origins' and 'ethnic group' suggests that many survey respondents may be interpreting such questions as accessing the same semantic domain (Nazroo 1997) and there is, indeed, evidence of commonality of interpretation in other survey settings.

Among the set of variables collected in administrative systems, the lack of data on socio-economic group or position is one of the most important. There is a substantial evidence base that documents the relationship between socio-economic status or position and health. As this relationship also holds within particular ethnic groups, it is important to be able to assess the contribution to overall ethnic variations in health and access to health and social care made by socio-economic differences. In health and social surveys this relationship can be explored through the collection of specific data on socio-economic position, such as occupationally based social class/socio-economic group, housing tenure, educational attainment and standard of living. The PSI survey, for example, has been particularly innovative in this respect in exploring the utility of a range of indicators. This important relationship is especially difficult to assess using administrative data as much of this does not include indicators of socio-economic status. Given that some of these datasets are now yielding usable data to standard reporting categories, the lack of access to socio-economic measures to assess their contribution to ethnic disparities and socio-economic gradients in health is a severe limitation. Although recent government reports on race equality have urged the collection of individual socio-economic measures on major databases such as HES, the experience since the early 1990s of agreeing and implementing ethnic coding suggests that there are likely to be limits to adding other variables to public health surveillance datasets.

One solution (besides record linkage, which is technically demanding and often only feasible through probabilistic methods) that could be utilised for any administrative health and population data that is geo- or postcoded is the use of small-area census-derived socio-economic and deprivation measures. However, such measures provide only a partial picture and, while important in their own right, are different from individual level social class or socio-economic position. In Britain this area of research is poorly developed with respect to both the type of area-based socio-economic measures that might be most useful in specific contexts and to the appropriate levels of geography. A major US empirical study (Krieger 2002, Krieger *et al.* 2003) to examine these questions for the purposes of population-based health investigations found:

> absolutely no consensus on which area-based socioeconomic measures (ABSMs), at which level of geography should be used. The literature, instead, is incredibly eclectic, with myriad studies using different measures at different geographic levels, thereby precluding meaningful comparison across studies or over time.

To capture the diverse domains of economic position, the US study used a total of 11 single variable and eight composite measures pertaining to occupational class, income and income inequality, poverty, wealth, education and residential crowding, and combinations of these variables. One key finding is the robust impact of socio-economic position on health with respect to most of the ABSMs used, preliminary findings indicating that these results hold for different racial/ethnic and gender groups as well as the total population. As such US research cannot necessarily be extrapolated to Britain because of differences in patterns of residential segregation and other factors, similar empirical research should be a priority here to provide an evidence base regarding choice of area-based measures of socio-economic status and geographical levels.

In Britain, a range of area-based deprivation measures has been developed from census variables and other data. In recent years the 'Indices of Deprivation' (Office of Deputy Prime Minister 2004) have become salient. This is a composite measure comprising such components as employment and income and presented as scales covering different dimensions and in different statistical formats. However, the research has not been undertaken on the relative merits of the different approaches, including the use of composite methods. The time is now propitious to undertake such work as 2001 Census data has been released for new geographies (including the micro-spatial scale) and very high levels of completeness of postcode of residence – required for area-based linkage – on most datasets, including Hospital Episode Statistics, have been achieved. As ABSM data is census-based, it, too, is substantially complete. However, the simultaneity of measurement of the area-based measures and the health outcomes is important as policy needs to address where the main burdens of disease *are* located. Given the complexities of this kind of work, often requiring multi-level modelling and invoking problems such as spatial correlation, it is likely that collaborative development work between statutory health organisations and university-based researchers will be needed ahead of arguing for the addition of standard area-based socio-economic measures to public health datasets. This is likely to prove the most feasible method in the foreseeable future of *routinely* assessing the contribution of socio-economic and deprivation factors to ethnic disparities in health. However, the availability of standardised questions for the measurement of socio-economic status at the individual level which can be included in computer systems does offer scope to record this, too.

There will remain some specific dimensions of social life, notably, the impact of racism, that will not be satisfactorily reflected in these area-based measures. It is likely that the contribution of such factors to health disparities and some specific hypotheses will only effectively be measured through customised surveys where data collection is specifically designed to meet study needs. This area is currently underdeveloped. McKenzie (2003) has argued that in the UK, work on the effects of racism upon health is still in its infancy. Only a few studies have investigated this relationship. Using data from the fourth national survey (FNS), Karlsen and Nazroo (2002) have reported marked independent associations between the experience of racism and various mental and physical health indicators that were reasonably consistent across the different ethnic groups. They have also found that even the worry about racism was independently associated with poorer health experience among ethnic minority groups (Karlsen and Nazroo 2004).

Coverage of existing data sources: population and data categories

This section will primarily address the coverage of various datasets, of both population and data categories.

Primary care

Until recently, ethnic data collection in primary care has comprised ad hoc collections among practices located mainly in metropolitan areas and a number of ongoing pilot projects (Aspinall 1999, Aspinall and Anionwu 2002). One of the most notable national development sites for patient profiling is the Princes Park Health Centre, Liverpool, serving around 8,000 patients. A form was designed to collect information on self-ascribed ethnicity and patients' family origins and other supplementary information, such as access to a car and telephone, language spoken and written, requirements for interpreting, specific illnesses, and patient satisfaction. Differences in morbidity profiles and satisfaction for patient groups defined by ethnicity and socio-economic status have been reported, bringing about changes in service delivery. Patient profiling has now been extended to other local practices by Central Liverpool PCT, enabling around 25,000 patients to be profiled (Department of Health 2003b). However, in most practices that have introduced 'population profiling', the number of data items is likely to be far fewer: ethnic group only or, at most, the addition of preferred spoken/written language and religion. At a national level, comprehensive information on the range of data collected, its quality/completeness, and date of introduction is lacking. Recent reviews suggest that even London PCTs are facing considerable challenges in facilitating the collection of ethnicity data in primary care (Mitchell 2004).

While general practice data offers substantial potential as a source of population-based information on health care utilisation, morbidity, treatment and outcomes (because most contacts with the NHS take place in primary care), the frequent absence of ethnic coding from the data collected substantially reduces its utility. This absence is also reflected in the primary care databases, which derive their data from volunteer practices – such as QResearch, the General Practice Research Database and the IMS Mediplus system – and in sources such as PRIMIS and the Royal College of General Practitioners' Weekly Returns Service. One of the main UK sources of ethnic data remains the decennial surveys of morbidity statistics from general practice. Although now 15 years out of date (last undertaken in 1991–1992 (McCormick *et al.* 1995)) and with an under-representation of ethnic minority groups (reflecting the fact that few inner-city practices participated in the survey), but with good quality socio-demographic data, the dataset remains important and has recently been used by Gill *et al.* (2003) and Shah *et al.* (2001) for ethnicity analyses. In addition, some information is available on the patient experience from the first of the NHS Patient and User Experience Surveys which addressed general practice (Airey *et al.* 1998) and from the more recent surveys of PCTs undertaken by the Healthcare Commission.

Secondary care

The main source of ethnically coded data in secondary care – that for in-patients admitted to NHS hospitals – is the HES dataset. The mandatory collection of ethnic group data for NHS hospital in-patients is now in its tenth year of collection. The main advantage of this dataset is the comprehensiveness of the data items collected. It contains details of all patients admitted to NHS hospitals in England (there are similar independent organisations for Wales, Scotland and Northern Ireland) whatever the specialty of treatment, and includes private patients treated in NHS hospitals. Data items reported include diagnoses, operations, healthcare resource groups, NHS trusts, Health Authority areas, length of stay, waiting times, admission and discharge methods (the latter including hospital case fatalities), age and sex of patients, and detailed information on maternity and psychiatric care. However, it excludes information on drugs used in hospitals and information on out-patients, including those treated in A & E departments and then discharged immediately.

The main drawback of the dataset is incompleteness of ethnic coding, resulting in only limited use of HES data by both practitioners and the research community. Data for the HES year 2002–2003 shows that of the total of 12.15 million finished consultant episodes in England only 64.0 per cent had a valid ethnic code (Department of Health 2005). Of the total of 404 primary care and hospital trusts reporting these episodes, 42 (10.4 per cent) achieved 95+ per cent valid coding and a total of 79 trusts (19.6 per cent) achieved 90+ per cent valid coding. Two hundred and eighty-seven trusts (71 per cent) reported 50+ per cent valid coding, but 57 trusts (14.1 per cent) had less than 30 per cent valid coding. Incompleteness has been a persistent problem and improvements have been small with a marked improvement only in the most recent year (2003–2004).

The reasons for differing levels of valid coding across trusts are likely to be complex. An analysis by Fitzgerald (2004) on 2002–2003 data showed that children (0–14 year olds) have the poorest level of coding and the elderly (75–79 year olds) the best. Excluding hospital birth episodes, the different admission methods have similar percentages of missing ethnic codes. Day cases have a slightly higher percentage of Finished Consultant Episodes (FCE) with missing codes than ordinary admissions. The Main Specialty Groups of Nursing and Mental Health and Illness have the lowest proportion of FCEs with missing codes, and Dental Medicine, Histopathology, Dermatology, Mental Handicap, Medical Ophthalmology, Clinical Neurophysiology, and Oral Surgery the worst. Interestingly, when the 30 top and bottom trusts were compared in 2001–2002, difficulties in collecting the ethnic code for children were apparent in both, possibly because of uncertainties about who should assign ethnicity. Objection by hospital patients to collection does not appear to be a barrier, with refusals making up only 0.25 per cent of coded FCEs in a sample of Thames data (Aspinall 2000b). The ethnic composition of the NHS Trusts' catchments also did not appear to be a key determinant.

Moreover, a number of problems with data quality have been identified (Aspinall 2000b). These include the incorrect mapping by NHS trusts of local ethnic codes (an optional set of more detailed codes for local use) to the standard reporting categories and disproportionately large number of records coded to the residual 'Other ethnic group' compared with the 1991 Census data (Bardsley *et al.* 2000, Lowdell *et al.* 2000), although some of this excess may be explained by ONS's use of a complex algorithm to redistribute free text responses in 1991 Census data. Also, although the mandatory requirement specified that ethnic group must be obtained by asking the patient (except in a few specific circumstances), it is clear that in some trusts the assignment is made by staff (Aspinall 2000b).

These difficulties have had important repercussions upon the use of the data. With respect to NHS maternity services in England, for example, the most recently reported data (for 2001–2002) show that ethnic group was recorded in only about 62 per cent of delivery records (Department of Health 2003c). While estimates are published by broad ethnic group (Asian, Black, Chinese and other, and White) for methods of onset of labour and of delivery, and birthweight, the 'maternity tail' (a special extension of the HES record that provides additional information and covers home births and the private sector as well), covers only 70 per cent of NHS hospital deliveries and just 13 per cent of home deliveries, which sets limits to our ability to measure ethnic differences relating to the pregnancy and delivery. The non-reporting of ethnic coding for newborn babies (and the fact that this is not collected through the Birth Registration system) further limits our ability to investigate deliveries and outcomes.

Our ability to identify ethnic differences in access to, and use of, acute care services is similarly compromised by issues of incompleteness. For example, in reporting findings from the appropriateness of coronary revascularisation (ACRE) study undertaken in 1996–1997, Feder *et al.* (2002) pointed out the lack of a mechanism to monitor ethnic differences in invasive management of coronary disease in the NHS. More recently such audits have become possible; Abubakar and Kanka (2002) reported an audit of all patients admitted with unstable angina or acute myocardial infarction for 1999–2000 using data with ethnic coding 92.8 per cent complete. The ability of trusts to conduct such audits will increase as completeness improves and, in response to such shifts in data quality, substantial use has been made of HES data in the last year or so to present ethnic differentials by diagnosis and procedure usage. HES data have also been used to derive measures of the fertility of ethnic groups in London (Klodawski 2003).

These data quality issues aside, the HES dataset does have structural drawbacks for those who may wish to use the data for analytical or other research purposes. First, the information collected is for FCEs, defined as a period of patient care under one consultant in one health care provider. The figures do not represent the number of patients, as one person may have several episodes within the year, making it difficult to distinguish between first admissions and readmissions. Second, the dataset presents only one point in a frequently complex pathway of care; while there is information on referring GP, there is none on out-patients or patients treated in A & E departments and then discharged home immediately. Third, although the HES dataset is a rich source containing over 50 items of data for each record, it has no patient information on socio-economic position, although individual records can be linked to area-based measures of deprivation through the patient's postcode. Finally, it does not include data from private healthcare providers, which represents a varying proportion of activity regionally and by diagnosis or procedure.

Preventive services

Reporting of activity on breast and cervical screening programmes provides details of the women invited to attend, the coverage of the programmes by age group, and test results. Statistical bulletins are published annually summarising information from the computerised call and recall systems but these, and returns from pathology laboratories and from colposcopy clinics, omit consideration of ethnicity and there appear to be no plans to alter this in the near future. Although there are some ad hoc collections of ethnicity in Breast Screening Services, a lack of comprehensive ethnicity data is clearly a disadvantage in efforts to improve the coverage of these programmes for some ethnic minority groups (especially South Asian women) who underutilise them (Sutton *et al.* 2001).

Immunisation statistics obtained from COVER (Coverage of Vaccination Evaluated Rapidly), collected by the Communicable Disease Surveillance Centre of the Health Protection Agency, and from the Department of Health also do not include data on ethnic group. In the longer term, comprehensive ethnicity data collection by PCTs will remedy this situation but there is currently a dearth of information (nothing at all on flu vaccination, for example). Research studies have found immunisation rates among South Asian children to be the same as, or higher than, the White population, although some ethnic groups have been reported with significantly lower rates. A range of high and low rates has been reported for refugees and a recent Department of Health commissioned report on routine data and health impact assessment (Hansell and Aylin 2000) argued that it might be more useful if information on immunisations was available locally on hard to reach groups such as refugee populations. This is now being achieved by the introduction of a standardised health needs assessment form for all new refugees and asylum seekers.

Specific disease outcomes

Coronary heart disease

Information on coronary heart disease, the commonest cause of death in the UK, has recently been described as 'frequently patchy, obsolete, or simply not available' and for ethnic minorities 'particularly scarce, exacerbating inequalities' (Unal *et al.* 2003). Ethnically coded information on patient numbers undergoing coronary artery bypass graft (CABG) surgery and angioplasty is available from the HES dataset, but, as described above, it is of variable quality. Moreover, there are few data sources on cardiological treatments in primary care and what limited prescription and uptake data as are available from Prescription Analysis and Cost Tabulate (PACT) are not ethnically coded. However, the position is better with respect to cardiovascular risk factor data sources. Data on smoking, cholesterol levels, blood pressure, physical activity, obesity and diabetes were collected in the 1999 Health Survey for England, which focused on ethnic groups, and in several other national surveys.

The lack of any single comprehensive source of information to support CHD prevention and treatment strategies was addressed in the National Service Framework (NSF) (National Service Frameworks are long-term strategies for improving specific areas of care that set measurable goals within set time frames) for coronary heart disease. Ethnic coding is now available for two of the four priority datasets to support the NSF (Acute Myocardial Infarction, Paediatric Cardiac Care, Angioplasty, and Adult Cardiac Surgery); however, information is not yet available to explore the CHD patient journey, to define a core CHD dataset, and those needed to study heart failure and cardiac rehabilitation.

Cancer

ONS mortality data by country of birth and HES ethnicity data are key sources, in spite of their shortcomings, as are the national surveys for population-based cancer risk factor data (on smoking, drinking, diet, etc.). There is, too, substantial current under-recording of ethnicity in cancer registry databases (the process of cancer registration in England is conducted by nine regional registries which collect and collate data on cancer incidence, prevalence and survival). The Cancer Registration Dataset Project is implementing a mechanism by which information can be recorded and consolidated that will address issues of ethnicity. There is also negligible ethnically coded primary care data on consultation rates, prescribing and treatment. This is being addressed by the provision of the Primary Care Cancer Dataset, which includes a wide range of demographic information (including ethnic category and religion), as well as data items on risk factors, symptoms, screening, tests, diagnosis, treatment and family history.

Diabetes

In addition to those sources mentioned so far – ONS mortality data, HES statistics and national surveys – there is only limited additional data. The Practice-Based Register Datasets now being implemented include diabetes and an ethnic category field, so systematic data should accrue in time. The main sources on the prevalence of diabetes by ethnic group remain the 1999 Health Survey for England and local surveys such as the Coventry diabetes (Simmons *et al.* 1991) and London (Brent) (Chaturvedi *et al.* 1993) studies, both of which have been used to develop the PBS Diabetes Population Prevalence Model (PBS DPPM) (Yorkshire and Humber Public Health Observatory 2005). As with the other NSFs, there are supporting datasets in development for diabetes. The Diabetes User Dataset – containing 'ethnic category', 'religion', and 'main language' – will form the basis of a Core Diabetes Dataset to be used in conjunction with some 14 additional extension datasets to meet the needs of information sharing at each point in the care pathway. The core dataset on people with diabetes contains information on patient demographic factors, providers of services, patient diagnostic data, laboratory data, details of eye and foot examinations, diet, physical activity, smoking, care plan details, current medication and personal medical history.

Mental health

The main source of ethnic information on users of mental health services is HES data. There are, however, a number of specific collections relating to both treatment settings and type of care that yield ethnically coded data. First, ethnicity data are collected on those detained under the Mental Health Act, although the proportion of the returns with 'ethnicity not known' has fluctuated, falling from 6.7 per cent (1996/7) to 3.3 per cent (1998/9), rising to 11.2 per cent in 1999/2000, but falling to 3.3 per cent in 2000–2001 (Mental Health Act Commission 2001, 2003). Further, these data are collated from voluntary returns, with 269 establishments out of a possible 281 (95.7 per cent) completing them in 1999/2000. Second, some data are also voluntarily collated on use of Second Opinion Appointed Doctors and requests for private meetings with a Mental Health Act Commissioner. Third, a major census of Black and ethnic minority patients was conducted in 2005 and provides a baseline of information against which to measure future changes in care.

With respect to suicide, data deficiencies include the lack of recording of ethnic data on UK death certificates and the fact that verdicts of coroners' inquisitions do not currently include ethnicity of the deceased (NIMHE 2003a). Country of birth data has been widely used as a proxy for ethnicity in reporting suicide rates, but is now of diminishing value. This makes it difficult to establish the suicide rate by ethnicity, although the Department of Health is working towards collecting information on ethnicity by coroners (Department of Health 2003b) and changes to civil registration *might* result in the collection of ethnicity data at birth and death. Some estimates based on ethnicity have been undertaken by the National Confidential Enquiry team, but only for those in contact with mental health services in the year before death (Hunt *et al.* 2003) and the data are subject to confidentiality constraints.

Sexually transmitted infections

Until recently there has been a paucity of ethnically coded data on sexually trans- mitted infections (STIs). STI data are collected on the central statistical returns, but there has been a lack of demographic, socio-economic and sexual behaviour data. Only in Scotland are data collected in disaggregate form, the dataset containing infor- mation on demographic and behavioural variables including ethnic origin. The Department of Health (England) has recently introduced a Programme for Enhanced Surveillance of Sexually Transmitted Infections, a disaggregate dataset from GUM clinics similar to the Scottish system, which began in 2001 as a pilot (PHLS, DHSS and PS 2002). The programme was expanded so that by mid-2003 all computerised GUM clinics in England were included. The Gonococcal Resistance to Antimicrobials Surveillance Programme (GRASP) is a surveillance system for monitoring gonococcal antimicrobial resistance in England and Wales that has reported annually since 2000 (PHLS 2002). Gonorrhoea is the second most common bacterial STI and dispro- portionately affects the Black population. GUM clinics provide demographic and behavioural data, which includes ethnic background, for each GUM patient included in the GRASP collection. Finally, the Enhanced Laboratory Surveillance for Infectious Syphilis was established in August 2001 in all GUM clinics in the London region and was extended to the rest of England and Wales in 2002, the demographic and behavioural data collected including ethnic background.

These developments are in accord with the recent Department of Health (England) strategy for combating infectious diseases, which recommended the mandatory collec- tion of detailed data with all laboratory diagnoses, including ethnicity and source of report. Such laboratory surveillance now includes genital HSV infection and measure- ment of the impact of chlamydial screening. Indeed, one of the Minimum Data Set Core Items for the wider Chlamydia Screening Programme Roll Out is 'Ethnicity'. The justifications given for its inclusion are that ethnicity is an 'important determinant' of chlamydia infection, the data will assist in evaluating inequalities in sexual ill health, and it will provide the evidence base to develop targeted interventions, improved services, and monitoring of their impacts (Department of Health 2003d). For reasons of confidentiality, the research community's access to these datasets is restricted to the commissioning of more detailed tabulations that do not breach such constraints.

Different collections are involved for HIV/AIDS. Ethnicity was not collected for laboratory reports of HIV infection prior to 1995. Since 1995 the Surveys of Prevalent HIV Infections Diagnosed (SOPHID) have provided data across the United Kingdom for HIV infected individuals by year of diagnosis and ethnicity and these data are routinely reported: the SOPHID surveys continue to provide the only national measure of individuals with diagnosed HIV infection accessing HIV-related care. Initially, rates of incompleteness of ethnicity data were high. However, data for the most recent year, 2003, show that only 3.0 per cent of 34,103 patients in England had ethnicity 'not known' (CDSC [HPA] 2004). One of the drawbacks of the reported data for research purposes is the aggregation of some groups ('Indian/Pakistani/Bangladeshi') and the use of the non-standard category 'Other Asian/Oriental'.

Children and young people

The Social Services Inspectorate (SSI) reported in 2002 that information on children's cultural characteristics was poorly monitored. Of 394 files read, only 71 per cent had the ethnicity of the service user recorded, just over a half (51 per cent) had a record of their first language, and under a third (only 31 per cent) recorded their religion (Cooper 2002). However, the most comprehensive data collection on children, the annual Children in Need (CiN) Census, shows better results with 8–10 per cent of cases not having ethnicity recorded. This source relates to those who are in touch with ('on the books' of) Local Authority Social Services and approximates to the number of open 'Children in Need' cases at any one time. The census is undertaken in a 'typical' week of each year and three censuses (2000, 2002 and 2003) have now been undertaken (National Statistics and Department of Health 2000, 2002, 2004). A wide range of data items is covered, including demographic data on the child (age, gender, ethnicity, and whether the child is asylum-seeking), characteristics of children in need (need category), information on the hours and type of service received for children looked after and those supported in families or independently, and financial information. Coverage in 2003 was substantially complete, ethnicity not stated comprising 8 per cent of children in need and the authorities making returns accounting for 97 per cent of the 0–17 age group in England. Moreover, subject to confidentiality constraints, the data can be accessed.

While the Children in Need Census is probably the main *routine* source of ethnically coded data on health and social care for this population segment, local child health computer systems may also yield such information but the lack of routine reporting presents a barrier. An increasing body of data is now also becoming available through surveys, including the children and young people boosts of the Health Survey for England and surveys of smoking, drinking and drug use among young people.

Maternity services

Among key areas lacking comprehensive ethnicity data collection are maternity services. Although the Maternity Care Data Dictionary identifies a data item on the ethnicity of the mother, this standard has not yet been adopted (NHS Information Authority 2003). Indeed, with respect to maternity information systems, a recent Commons report found data collection at all levels to be 'seriously impaired' by inadequate or nonexistent data systems and by a lack of information technology (House of Commons 2003). The policy and associated research need for this information has been highlighted in a number of reports. Research evidence shows that women from ethnic minority groups are more likely to book late for antenatal care (Rowe and Garcia 2003, Department of Health 2003e) and that late bookers (including a disproportionate number from ethnic minority groups) comprised a fifth of maternal deaths (Drife 2003). Although there is a dearth of good quality evidence on ethnic inequalities in attendance for antenatal care, all four studies reported in a recent systematic review (Rowe and Garcia 2003) found that women of Asian origin were more likely to book late for antenatal care than White British women. An analysis of Hospital Episode Statistics by the Department of Health (2003e) similarly showed that women from ethnic minority groups were twice as likely to book later than 20 weeks gestation. The reasons for late booking are likely to be complex, including language and other barriers to access, significantly higher mobility among some groups (especially the Black African population), and migration during pregnancy. Comprehensive ethnicity data collection is required to systematically explore such factors. Finally, the five yearly infant feeding surveys include data about ethnicity and social class.

Health and lifestyle issues

Data are available on smoking prevalence by ethnic group from the large-scale national (PSI Fourth National Survey and 1999 Health Survey for England) and ad hoc (e.g. SmokeFree London's telephone survey of 10,000 Londoners) (London Health Observatory 2003) surveys. In the four years (2000/1–2003/4) since the Department of Health established smoking cessation services, information has been available by ethnic group for those setting a quit date, but only using a limited classification (White, Mixed, Asian, Black, Other, Not Stated). In the current (2004/5) year the full Census classification has been used. Incompleteness of ethnic coding has ranged from 2–5 per cent and the data do not separately identify pregnant women, nor are data collected by social class (Department of Health 2004). One of the drawbacks for researchers is the lack of compatible denominator data for smoking prevalence (the 1999 Health Survey for England used different ethnic categories).

Data on alcohol consumption and cessation by ethnic group are much more limited. The Department of Health's statistical *Bulletin* (Department of Health 2003f) relies on the 1999 Health Survey for England and most other sources that address ethnic differences focus on particular cities (such as the London Household and Greater Glasgow surveys (Bakshi *et al.* 2002)).

With respect to illicit drug use, ethnic group data were first collected on Regional Drug Misuse Databases from April 1996, although these have not been reported because 21 per cent of the data in 1999 and 14 per cent in 2000 were uncoded (Department of Health 2000). The system underwent a review and was revised in April 2001 as the National Drug Treatment Monitoring System (NDTMS), the latest results showing ethnicity missing for around 15.6 per cent of first contacts with large regional variations. There are few other sources of ethnically coded data. The British Crime Survey has a self-completion drugs module, that for 2001/2 providing data on a sample of over 24,000, of whom around 4,000 were from ethnic minority groups (Aust and Smith 2003). The London Health Observatory, the Imperial College Centre for Research on Drug and Health Behaviour, and the Greater London Authority joined forces in 2002 to establish the London Drug Indicators Project. The project monitors, collates and analyses information about drug use in London and reports on, for example, ethnic differentials in drug use and access to treatment (London Health Observatory 2003).

Patients' experiences of health services

A range of ethnically coded administrative data is potentially available to assess patients' experiences of health services and the quality of their care, although this falls substantially short of providing a comprehensive picture. In 2001 the Department of Health took its first steps to obtain information to be held centrally on the ethnic category of complainants (patients) and the ethnic category of staff complained against (NHS Information Authority 2001), although to date there has only been limited reporting of the data locally.

The main body of comprehensive information on the patient experience comes from the regular 'NHS Surveys of Patient Experience'. The current suite for 2004/5 comprises acute trusts (including a young patients survey), Primary Care Trusts (PCT), mental health trusts, ambulance trusts, accident and emergency departments and out-patient services. The surveys ask those who have recently used the specific services what they think about the care and treatment they have received along a number of dimensions: promptness of access and waiting times, coordination of care, information and education, environment and facilities, involvement and choice, physical and emotional needs, and respect. In the two most recent (2004/5) surveys of emergency departments and out-patients, ethnicity was missing in 1.4 per cent and 1.0 per cent of responses, respectively. In addition, a programme of Personal Social Services User Experience Surveys was initiated in 2000 that included ethnicity, those for 2000/1 and 2001/2 focusing on newly assessed social services clients, followed in subsequent years by user experience surveys, elderly home care users, physically disabled or sensory impaired users, and children in need and families.

Secondary analysis of data sources produced for research

As we have seen, administrative and routine sources of data frequently have limited utility and, in some case, validity for studies of ethnicity and health, as they were designed for administrative and policy purposes. Some deficiencies in these sources have been addressed by social and health surveys produced by Government and research bodies and these will continue to be a key source of information on the health and health care of ethnic minority groups.

Research data sources

Most social and health surveys fall within the set of continuous or regularly repeated household surveys commissioned by Government departments and which generally use harmonised concepts and questions. The primary harmonised variable, ethnic origin, was adopted before 1996/7 in the Health Survey for England (HSE), Labour Force Survey (LFS), and Scottish House Condition Survey (SHCS), in 1996/7 in the Expenditure and Food Survey (EFS), Family Resources Survey (FRS), General Household Survey (GHS), and Survey of English Housing (SHE), in 2001 in the National Travel Survey (NTS), in 2000/1 in the Omnibus Surveys, in 2002/3 in the English House Condition Survey, and in 2003 in the Welsh Health Survey. There is no current plan to introduce a harmonised ethnic origin variable in the Scottish Health Survey (SHS) and the Continuous Household Survey (CHS) (Northern Ireland). Other ethnically coded large-scale and regularly repeated surveys include the British Crime Survey, the Dental Surveys, and there are yet others designed to meet specific needs and commissioned by a range of departments, such as the Home Office Citizenship Survey.

The main national dedicated studies of the health of the ethnic minority population in recent years have been the Policy Studies Institute (PSI)'s 1994 Fourth National
Survey (FNS), the 2000 EMPIRIC survey of psychiatric morbidity in the community
(on Irish, Black Caribbeans, Indians, Pakistanis, Bangladeshis and White British),
the 1999 HSE, and the Health Education Authority (HEA)'s first (1991/2) and second
(1994) health and lifestyle surveys. Both these focused on African-Caribbeans,
Indians (including African Asians), Pakistanis and Bangladeshis, and a health and
lifestyle survey on the Chinese was undertaken by the HEA in 1998. The FNS
collected data on the White, Caribbean, Indian, African Asian, Pakistani, Bangladeshi,
and Chinese groups and 1999 HSE the Irish, Black Caribbean, Indian, Pakistani,
Bangladeshi, and Chinese groups. The 2004 Health Survey for England, to be published in 2006, includes Black Africans alongside the same groups as in the 1999
survey.

Other sources of data include the Annual Local Area Labour Force Survey
(a sample of around 384,000 adults, including 25,000 from ethnic minority groups)
and the (Quarterly) Labour Force Survey (138,000 adults per quarter, including 9,800
adults from ethnic minority groups), reporting labour market, education, training and
demographic characteristics; the Family Resources Survey (a sample of 25,000 households, including 1,600 households from ethnic minority groups), reporting on income,
savings and wealth; the British Crime Survey (30,000 core sample of adults, including
2,000 from ethnic minority groups, plus an additional ethnic minority boost sample
of 3,000 adults), focusing on crime and victimisation; the Home Office Citizenship
Survey (a 10,000 core sample of adults and an additional ethnic minority boost of
5,400 adults) addressing such issues as family and parenting, people and their neigh-
bourhoods, community participation, and racial prejudice and discrimination; and
the Millennium Cohort Study (19,000 families interviewed, covering 19,000 children
born in 2000/1, including around 3,000 children from ethnic minority groups),
reporting on child health and development and family circumstances, including
fathers' involvement in childcare and development.

Additionally, there are two sources of data relating to children and young people
(besides the England, Wales and Scotland Pupil Level Annual Schools' Censuses
(PLASCs) which collect data on eligibility for free school meals, school exclusions,
special educational needs and first language): the Youth Cohort Study (a sample of
17,000 16–19 year olds, including an ethnic minority group sample of 2,000), reporting
on GCSE and A level qualification attainment, participation in full-time education
and training, and employment circumstances after leaving school; and the Longitudinal
Study of Young People (a sample of 20,000 13–14 year olds, including an ethnic
minority group sample of 5,000), focusing on education, training and employment,
family and relationships, leisure activities and interests, and health and lifestyle.

Among these surveys and censuses, a number have a longitudinal focus, short-
term in the case of the Annual Local Area and Quarterly Labour Force Surveys
(annually over four years and quarterly intervals up to five, respectively), but long-
term for the Millennium Cohort Study, PLASC (which, although cross-sectional,
offers a longitudinal perspective via unique pupil identifiers), Youth Cohort Study,
and Longitudinal Study of Young People. In some their usefulness for the analysis
of ethnic minority groups may be limited by small sample size. Another key longitudinal dataset is the ONS Longitudinal Study (LS), containing linked census

(from the 1971, 1981, 1991 and 2001 Censuses) and vital event data (births, deaths and cancer registrations) for one per cent of the population of England and Wales.

Secondary analysis of such sources

Secondary analysis of data may be defined as use of data for a purpose other than that for which the original data were designed. Such analyses may be descriptive or analytic, hypothesis-generating or hypothesis-testing, cross-sectional, longitudinal, or involve the analysis of trends over time. The attraction of secondary analysis is that it does not incur the high costs and resources necessary to operationalise a new survey or data collection, including the lead-in time. Consequently, it can offer a lower cost and more timely research method. Moreover, developments in computer technology and statistical software tools, including online access to datasets, has substantially facilitated this approach. Where datasets or the sampled population are large and include many variables, there is often scope to explore complex causal relationships and to produce generalisable findings or the derivation of reliable estimates.

However, there are also limitations that need to be considered. A researcher may not have access to all of the data items needed, while others may have been collected in a suboptimal way or in less depth than desired. There is sometimes a lag between data collection and release of the data and the actual procurement of the data may be bureaucratically complex and lengthy, as in the case of confidential HES data items. Frequently, some aggregation of categories or geographical codes is necessary to protect respondent confidentiality. Moreover, although some national datasets may contain large numbers at the population level, the sample size may still be insufficient to study particular ethnic groups. As has been seen, lack of ethnic coding, problems of non-response, and selective attrition of cohort members can all introduce bias in these sources. Finally, the way a survey or database is designed, including sampling frame, sample methods, question wording, and timing of data collection may all constrain use of the data for research purposes.

Some of these problems can be minimised by adopting valid approaches to analysis, notably, the use of well-defined research questions, testable hypotheses and the use of appropriate conceptual models, as opposed to data-dredging and evidence from post hoc analysis (Bierman and Bubolz 2004). Often the available data may require modifications to the research questions, so a comprehensive evaluation of all data sources is needed. Particular attention needs to be accorded to the variables required for the analysis, including confounding variables such as social class, as well as dependent and independent variables, and this may involve combining variables or otherwise deriving new variables. As we have seen, some datasets may lack crucial variables, for example, personal social class on the HES dataset, so robust evaluation is a priority, using sources such as the Question Bank (Social Surveys Online)[3] and the Economic and Social Data Service Archive,[4] which can be used to identify ethnically coded data sources. Many of the individual surveys and sources will also offer comprehensive information on survey design, survey instruments, codebooks and dataset acquisition. These sources should also provide information on the number of achieved responses to the survey. It will be important initially for the researcher to identify whether there are sufficient data in the candidate sources to make reliable estimates about the particular subgroups of interest and to test the study hypotheses.

Adequate sample size is needed to minimise the risk of incorrectly rejecting a null hypothesis when it is true (a 'type I' error) or of accepting the null hypothesis when it is false ('type II' error). Power calculations can be undertaken using statistical software applications.

The survey or database design and the sampling frame used are of crucial importance in secondary analysis. Clearly, some datasets, such as HES or cancer registries, endeavour to provide information on all users, but surveys (apart from the decennial census) employ sampling strategies. Nationally representative samples or those drawn to represent the target population of interest may be obtained via a mix of random sampling, cluster sampling and multistage sampling. As described in Chapter 8, ethnicity surveys usually have complex sample designs, including clustering, stratification, multiple stages of selection and disproportionate sampling. The researcher must take account of the sampling method in the analysis and this is best done by using specific statistical software designed for this purpose. Researchers will also need sample weights to derive population estimates from the survey sample. In the case of ethnicity analyses, these will need to reflect the probability of being sampled, adjustments for non-response, and the matching of ethnicity subgroup distributions with a source such as the decennial census. Some surveys will supply documentation on estimation weights and in other cases technical guidance. Secondary analyses need to take into account the potential design effects of differing sample strategies. The sampling frame used may consist of individuals or households ('community surveys') and the population of interest may be persons living in households (for example, the EMPIRIC survey on psychiatric morbidity) or institutions (for example, the 2005 mental health census) or household/family units. Mode of survey administration will also be important, affecting responses and comparability of surveys. Methods include face-to-face interviews, increasingly using Computer Aided Personal Interviewing technology; telephone; and mail. Some of these methods may contain their own biases, for example, telephone surveys frequently use listings in telephone directories that may have incomplete coverage, in part because of the spread of cellular phone technologies. Regardless of mode, the respondent may be a mix of the subject or a proxy (as in PLASC data). In order to make inferences from the data the researcher must know how the population has been defined and accessed and which groups have been excluded, both by design and inadvertently.

Perhaps the greatest challenge to researchers in secondary analysis is understanding and taking account of potential sources of error over which the researcher has no control. This is particularly important in the case of ethnicity analyses as the population subgroups of interest often represent only a small fraction of all respondents or data subjects. Many types of error are common to all surveys – such as survey non-response, item non-response, measurement error, instrument error, interviewer error and respondent (and proxy response) error – but are frequently more problematic in some ethnic groups because of language and communication difficulties. These include issues of 'cultural nonequivalence' (Stewart and Napoles-Springer 2000), where concepts in surveys may have several referents and are not uniformly interpreted across different ethnic groups.

Missing data are a pervasive problem in secondary analyses, yielding bias, reducing sample size, and affecting tests of significance. As we have seen, significant levels of uncoded data characterises most of the ethnicity data collected, placing a priority on preserving sample size. The standard method is to restrict the analysis to subjects with complete data on the relevant variables, but such estimates can be biased if included subjects are systematically different in some way from those excluded. This approach also limits the use of multivariate regression that requires complete information on the variables used in the model. Alternative approaches include: weighting subjects who are included in the analysis to compensate for those who were excluded; multiple imputation where missing values are replaced by plausible values; and constructing the likelihood based on the incomplete observed data (Raghunathan 2004). Again, software packages are available for analysing incomplete data.

In conclusion, databases and survey datasets can provide a valuable and readily accessible resource for secondary analyses. However, when used to explore ethnic differentials, the frequently small number of cases or records, differential non-response by subgroup, cultural non-equivalence and related measurement issues, and often high levels of missing data, all constrain the utility of this approach. With careful attention accorded to choosing the appropriate data source to answer the research question, involving a consideration of design, capacity and limitations of the source, secondary analysis is a valuable research method.

Future opportunities

There are currently a number of developments under consideration that may lead to improved access to ethnic data in the future or to wider exploitation of such data. Some relate to possible new administrative collections arising from the Government's modernisation programme and others to generic developments in the NHS information infrastructure, notably the implementation of electronic care records. In addition, the development of standardised datasets for the NSF areas offer the potential of much richer data in these key health areas as cases accrue. The populating of these administrative and routine data sources with the patient's NHS number will facilitate the production of integrated datasets achieved through record linkage and extension to new data collections as and when established. However, a key challenge that will remain is the reconciliation of ethnicity as a self-ascribed measure that changes over time (as reflected in revisions to the classifications in the decennial census) with central patient databases that embed such classifications and are not always responsive to such changes.

Civil registration procedures

The possible addition of ethnic group data to the items collected at birth and death registration has been the subject of a detailed consultation process and is currently under consideration by Government (Aspinall *et al.* 2003). Such data are collected in the US, Australia, New Zealand, and selected provinces/territories of Canada. The addition of ethnic group at death registration is likely to lead to the immediate accrual of data which, as for other variables, have been demonstrated to be of utility in research studies. Recording the ethnic group of a baby at birth registration would address the substantial lack of such data in current collections. For example, ethnic group of newborns in not a mandatory item in the HES data collection. Although this data item will be collected on the Birth Notification Dataset (linked to the NHS Numbers for Babies Project), there is currently no basis for assessing the quality of the data.

Opportunities offered by record linkage

The populating of central administrative registers and other data collections with the NHS number of the patient raises substantial potential via record linkage for the research community. A pilot study has been undertaken linking maternity records from the HES system with the corresponding birth records used by ONS. Pilot work is also under way on building a national linked file of HES records and ONS mortality records that could be used for the development of health outcome indicators. Recently, ONS has proposed the development of a UK-wide integrated population statistics system that links census, survey and administrative data, to be developed over the next decade or so.

The ONS Longitudinal Study (LS) has demonstrated the utility of such an approach for the study of mortality by ethnic group, including differences by generational status. The linkage of the LS to 2001 census data has substantially increased its potential. The LS should over the next decade or so substantially enhance our abilities to examine mortality differentials by ethnic group, although there will be continuing problems with sample size in the early stages of further accrual.

Populating of central administrative registers with ethnic group

In the past there have been a number of suggestions and proposals to populate a range of central administrative records with ethnic group. The RoBIN review (a strategic review of business information needs for race equality data) (Stroud 2000) identified the National Strategic Tracing Service (NSTS) – a national tracing system for the NHS which contains no clinical data but is used to verify personal details (such as name and address) from the NHS number – as a possible long-term alternative to collecting ethnicity information at source as part of a patient profile. Under this proposal an ethnic data item would be included as part of the general demographic data, which would then be available to NHS organisations tracing a person referred to them. However, populating such a register would still need a source of ethnic origin information, the only candidate being Hospital Episode Statistics. Further, such a system, which is tailored to queries about individuals, would be difficult to utilise analytically for the entirely different function of population-based ethnic health research.

Electronic Patient Records and Electronic Health Records have frequently been suggested as a key source of ethnic/race information on the patient population. Given, however, that the highest possible levels of confidentiality will attach to care records, it is unlikely that these will yield a source for research purposes. While plans for Electronic Patient Records may lead in the long term to central reporting mechanisms for aggregated ethnic data, they are unlikely to be in widespread use for another five to ten years. The Department of Health has recently announced, for example, that every patient in England will have an individual electronic NHS Care Record (as it is now called) by 2010 (Department of Health 2003g). Progress on the development of this service is likely to be patchy in the early stages and the records themselves will need to be populated with ethnic group. The experience of other administrative systems such as HES indicates that this is likely to be a protracted process.

Conclusions

The currently limited extent to which the research community has been able to draw upon administrative and routine sources of data has been a consequence of the history of ethnic monitoring in health and social care settings: one of fragmentary and patchy data collection, yielding data of low coverage and questionable quality that is little used even by the services collecting the data. In the last decade, however, developments in the UK in clinical governance, performance management and equal opportunities have created a need for quality ethnic monitoring data to inform policy development and evaluation, leading to a commensurate increase in the amount of ethnicity data collected with potential for use in other research. More recently, the Macpherson inquiry report (Macpherson 1999) and the Race Relations Amendment Act 2000 which followed, have placed race equality at the centre of the policies of government and the Department of Health. However, there continues to be a lack of emphasis on ethnicity issues in the Performance Assessment Framework (whereby information is compiled on performance in health and social care areas against sets of indicators to which overall individual performance is measured) and associated indicator datasets. Undoubtedly, one of the key reasons for this is the poor quality of ethnic data in the core collections, such as Hospital Episode Statistics, general practice/PCT databases, disease registers, and cancer registry datasets. Further, the lack of comprehensive information on the range of ethnically coded datasets available, their content, and how they can be accessed has been a barrier to secondary use.

This lack of completeness in administrative and routine data has undoubtedly been a constraint on their use in secondary analysis. Only recently have methods to assess the consistency of ethnic coding and analytical approaches capable of overcoming some of the data limitations (such as proportional mortality and admission ratios) been used on the core datasets. Other technical guidance has been sparse. Further, given the strong evidence that socio-economic position has an important effect on ethnic/racial disparities, empirical research needs to be undertaken on what are the best geographical proxy measures of socio-economic position and at what spatial scale of analysis. However, some use of the data has resulted from the wider dissemination of methods such as health equity audit, health impact assessment, and Policy Appraisal for Equal Treatment (PAET) (developed within the Government's Cabinet Office).

In the next decade the amount of ethnically coded administrative data that is of quality is likely to increase substantially, especially from core collections such as Hospital Episode Statistics where completion rates among some trusts have risen substantially. This should enable the routine and continuous examination of ethnic disparities in access to and use of services and in the type of care and treatment received. Moreover, the potential of new collections and those still subject to review – such as the birth notification process and the collection of ethnic group in civil registration – offer major opportunities, such as accurate fertility estimates by ethnic group and ethnically stratified mortality statistics. Similarly, the new datasets linked to the National Service Frameworks have the potential to transform our understanding of patterns of disease frequency, care pathways and service use. Finally, as the Longitudinal Study expands, a better understanding is likely to emerge of the relationship between socio-economic position and poor health in ethnic minority groups through exploration of a life course perspective.

However, the extent to which such potential is realised will, too, depend on the response from government and collaborative working with the research sector on analytical issues. A programme of development of analytical tools to assist the research and practitioner communities in the analysis and interpretation of race equality data in all current sources is urgently needed. This is beginning to be addressed with good practice examples for the analysis of health inequalities provided by the addition of funnel plots (Spiegelhalter 2002), Shewart's control charts (Mohammed *et al.* 2001), and spider diagrams (as in the Health Poverty Index Chart[5]) and generic toolkits in development. Further, there is scope for developing the capacity of ethnic communities themselves to utilise the data, through access to data, guidance on evidence-based policy making, and representation at board level on statutory bodies and committees.

Notes

1   In this chapter the term 'ethnic group/origin' is used in preference to 'race', except when the context is specific, for example, the Government and Commission for Racial Equality frequently use the term 'race' in the context of 'race equality' policies, often as a shorthand for broad pan-ethnic groupings such as 'White', Black', and 'Asian'. The term 'race' carries much ideological baggage and scope for misinterpretation and has been eschewed here for the more widely accepted term 'ethnic group/origin'.
2   For full details see: Approved Central Returns from the NHS, www.ic.nhs.uk/rocr/approved.
3   http://qb.soc.surrey.ac.uk/
4   www.esds.ac.uk/
5   www.hpi.org.uk/index.php

References

Abubakar, I. and Kanka, D. (2002) 'Access to invasive procedures can be audited by ethnic group', *British Medical Journal*, 324: 1454.

Airey, C., Bruster, S., Erens, B. *et al.* (1998) *National Surveys of NHS Patients: General Practice 1998*, London: National Centre for Social Research.

Alexander, Z. (1999 September) *The Department of Health: study of Black, Asian and ethnic minority issues*, London: Department of Health.

Aspinall, P.J. (1995) 'Department of Health's requirement for mandatory collection of data on ethnic group of inpatients', *British Medical Journal*, 311: 1006–1009.

Aspinall, P.J. (1999) 'Ethnic groups and our healthier nation: whither the information base?', *Journal of Public Health Medicine*, 21(2): 125–132.

Aspinall, P.J. (2000a) 'Asking a question about religion in the 2001 British census. A public policy case in favour', *Social Policy and Administration*, 34(5): 76–92.

Aspinall, P.J. (2000b) 'The mandatory collection of data on ethnic group of inpatients: experience of NHS trusts in England in the first reporting years', *Public Health*, 114: 254–259.

Aspinall, P.J. (2000c) 'The new 2001 Census question set on cultural characteristics: is it useful for the monitoring of the health status of people from ethnic groups in Britain?', *Ethnicity and Health*, 5(1): 33–40.

Aspinall, P.J. and Anionwu, E. (2002) 'The role of ethnic monitoring in mainstreaming race equality and the modernization of the NHS: a neglected agenda?', *Critical Public Health*, 12(1): 1–15.

Aspinall, P., Jacobson, B., Klodawski, E. and Polato, G.M. (2003) *Missing Record: the case for recording ethnicity at birth and death registration*, London: LHO.

Aust, R. and Smith, N. (2003) *Ethnicity and Drug Use: key findings from the 2001/2002 British Crime Survey. Findings 209*. London: Home Office.

Aveyard, P. (1998) 'A fresh look at proportional mortality ratios', *Public Health*, 112: 77–80.

Bakshi, N., Ross, A. and Heim, D. (2002) 'Drug and alcohol issues affecting Pakistani, Indian and Chinese young people and their communities: a study in Greater Glasgow', Glasgow: NB Associates & Human Factors Analysts.

Bardsley, M., Hamm, J., Lowdell, C. *et al.* (2000) *Developing Health Assessment for Black and Minority Ethnic Groups: analysing routine health information*, London: Health of Londoners Project and NHS Executive (London).

Bhopal, R.S. (2004) *Concepts of Epidemiology*, Oxford: Oxford University Press.

Bierman, A. and Bubolz, T. (2004) 'Secondary analysis of large survey datasets', in M.B. Max and J. Lynn (eds) *Symptom Research: methods and opportunities*, Bethesda, MD: National Institutes of Health.

CDSC (2003) *AIDS/HIV Quarterly Surveillance Tables: cumulative UK data to end September 2003. No. 60: 03/03*. November 2003. Health Protection Agency, SCIEH and Institute of Child Health.

CDSC (HPA) (2004) *Survey of Prevalent HIV Infections Diagnosed (SOPHID)*. Regional data for 2003, London: CDSC (Health Protection Agency).

Chaturvedi, N., McKeigue, P.M. and Marmot, M.G. (1993) 'Resting and ambulatory blood pressure differences in Afro-Caribbeans and Europeans', *Hypertension*, 22: 90–96.

Cooper, P. (2002) *Delivering Quality Children's Services: inspection of Children's Services. [CI(2002)19]*, London: Department of Health.

Cornish, J. (1993) 'National experiences in the measurement of ethnicity: Australia', in *Challenges of Measuring an Ethnic World: Science, Politics and Reality. Proceedings of the Joint Canada–United States Conference on the Measurement of Ethnicity*, Washington, DC: US Government Printing Office.

Department of Health (1997) *The Caldicott Committee. Report on the Review of Patient-Identifiable Information*, London: Department of Health.

Department of Health (2000) *Statistics from the Regional Drug Misuse Databases, Bulletin 2000/13* (June) [and *Bulletin 2001/18* (June 2001)].

Department of Health (2003a/May) *Review of Central Returns: dealing with race information in the ROCR approval process*, London: Department of Health.

Department of Health (2003b/October) *Delivering Race Equality: a framework for action. Mental Health Services*, London: Department of Health.

Department of Health (2003c/May) *NHS Maternity Statistics, England: 2001–02. Bulletin 2003/09*, London: Department of Health.

Department of Health (2003d) *Chlamydia Screening Programme Roll Out. Data Manual*, London: Department of Health.

Department of Health (2003e/10 July) *Select Committee on Health Written Evidence. Memorandum by the Department of Health (MA1)*, London: Department of Health.

Department of Health (2003f/Ocotber) *Statistics on Alcohol: England, 2003. Bulletin 2003/20*, London: Department of Health.

Department of Health (2003g) 'Every patient to get electronic patient record', *Press release notice 2003/05/02*, London: Department of Health.

Department of Health (2004) *Statistics on NHS Stop Smoking Services in England, April 2003 to March 2004. Statistical Bulletin 2004/18*, London: Department of Health.

Department of Health. HES website, *Data Quality Indicator Report, 2002/03: Components & Fail Counts*: www.dh.gov.uk/assetRoot/04/08/37/68/04083768.xls. Last accessed 28 January 2005. Data relate to records with valid codes (those missing, not stated, or coded to the 1991 Census ethnic classification are counted as invalid).

Drife, J. (2003) 'Appendix 33', Memorandum by Professor James Drife, Medical Director, Confidential Enquiry into Maternal Deaths (MS 40). Select Committee on Health.

Erens, B., Primatesta, P. and Prior, G. (eds) (2001) *Health Survey for England: the health of minority ethnic groups 1999, Vol. 1: Findings. Vol. 2: Methodology & Documentation*, London: The Stationery Office.

Feder, G., Crook, A.M., Magee, P. *et al.* (2002) 'Ethnic differences in invasive management of coronary disease: prospective cohort study of patients undergoing angiography', *British Medical Journal*, 324: 511–516.

Fitzgerald, C. (2004/May) 'How good is HES ethnicity coding and where do the problems lie?' (Ethnicity category: coverage report), London: Department of Health (HES).

Gill, P.S., Kai, J., Bhopal, R.S. and Wild, S. (in press) 'Health care needs assessment: black and minority ethnic groups', in J. Raftery, A. Stevens and J. Mant (eds), *Health Care Needs Assessment: the epidemiologically based needs assessment reviews*, 3rd series, Abingdon: Radcliffe Medical Press. Available at: http://hcna.radcliffe-oxford.com/bemgframe.htm (accessed 11 March 2006).

Hansell, A. and Aylin, P. (2000) 'Routine data and health impact assessment – a review of epidemiological studies of socio-economic influence on health and evaluation of outcome indicators derived from routine health data for health impact assessment', Report to the Department of Health, London: Imperial College School of Medicine.

Haskey, J. (ed.) (2002) 'Population projections by ethnic group: a feasibility study', Studies on Medical and Population Subjects No. 67, London: The Stationery Office.

House of Commons Hansard. Written Answers for 3 April 2002 (col. 1050W).

House of Commons Hansard. Written Answers for 4 July 2003 (col. 537W).

House of Commons. *Health Committee. Fourth Report of Session 2002–03. Vol. 1. Report and Minutes. HC 464-I*. London: The Stationery Office, 2003 (June).

Hunt, I.M., Robinson, J., Bickley, H. *et al.* (2003) 'Suicides in ethnic minorities within 12 months of contact with mental health services. National clinical survey', *British Journal of Psychiatry*, 183: 155–160.

Karlsen, S. and Nazroo, J.Y. (2004) 'Fear of racism and health', *Journal of Epidemiology and Community Health*, 58: 1017–1018.

Karlsen, S. and Nazroo, J.Y. (2002) 'Relation between racial discrimination, social class, and health among ethnic minority groups', *American Journal of Public Health*, 92(4): 624–631.

Klodawski, E. (2003) *Fertility of Ethnic Groups in London. DMAG Briefing 2003/19*, London: Greater London Authority.

Krieger, N. (2002) 'Geocoding state data and establishing collaborations', in *National Committee on Vital and Health Statistics, Department of Health and Human Services, Meeting of: Subcommittee on Populations*, Fairfax, VA: CASET Associates.

Krieger, N., Waterman, P.D., Chen, J.T. *et al.* (2003) 'Monitoring socioeconomic inequalities in sexually transmitted infections, tuberculosis, and violence: geocoding and choice of area-based socioeconomic measures – the public health disparities geocoding project (US)', *Public Health Reports*, 118(3): 240–260.

London Health Observatory (2003) *Diversity Counts: ethnic health intelligence in London. The story so far*, Report, London: London Health Observatory.

Lowdell, C., Evandrou, M., Bardsley, M. *et al.* (2000) *Health of Ethnic Minority Elders in London: reporting diversity*, London: The Health of Londoners Project.

McCormick, A., Fleming, D. and Charlton, J. (1995) *Morbidity statistics from general practice. Fourth national study 1991–1992*, London: HMSO.

McKenzie, K. (2003) 'Racism and health: antiracism is an important health issue', *BMJ*, 326: 65–66.

Macpherson, W. (1999) *The Stephen Lawrence Inquiry: report of an inquiry by Sir William Macpherson of Cluny*, London: The Stationery Office.

Mental Health Act Commission (2001) *Ninth Biennial Report 1999–2001*, London: The Stationery Office.

Mental Health Act Commission (2003) *Tenth Biennial Report 2001–2003*, London: The Stationery Office.

Mitchell, R. (2004) *A Review of Race Relations (Amendment) Act Implementation by NHS Organisations within the North Central London Sector – September 2004*, London: North Central London Strategic Health Authority.

Mohammed, M.A., Cheng, K.K., Rouse, A. and Marshall, T. (2001) 'Bristol, Shipman, and clinical governance: Shewart's forgotten lessons', *Lancet*, 357(9254): 463–467.

National Statistics and Department of Health (2000) *Children in Need in England: first results of activity and expenditure as reported by Local Authority Social Services' Children and Families Teams for a survey week in February 2000*, London: Department of Health.

National Statistics and Department of Health (2002) *Children in Need in England: preliminary results of a survey of activity and expenditure as reported by Local Authority Social Services' Children and Families Teams for a survey week in September/October 2001*, London: NS and Department of Health.

National Statistics and Department of Health (2004) *Children in Need in England: results of a survey of activity and expenditure as reported by Local Authority Social Services' Children and Families Teams for a survey week in February 2003*, London: NS and Department for Education & Skills.

Nazroo, J. (1997) *The Health of Britain's Ethnic Minorities*, London: Policy Studies Institute.

NHS Executive (1994/30 September) *Collection of ethnic group data for admitted patients. (Letter EL(94)77)*, Leeds: NHS Executive.

NHS Information Authority (1999) 'NHS Number for Babies', Autumn 1999 Seminars: Questions & Answers. NHS Number Programme (ref. doc. 1999–1A-162), Exeter: NHS Information Authority.

NHS Information Authority. Maternity Care Data Dictionary: Data Item Definitions and Category Values within Entity. Version 3.0 (updated 03.09.01). www.nhsia.nhs.uk/mcd/pages/data_dictionary.asp. Last accessed 19.11.03.

NIMHE (National Institute for Mental Health in England) (2003a) *Engaging and Changing: developing effective policy for the care and treatment of Black and minority ethnic detained patients*, Leeds: NIMHE.

NIMHE (2003b) *Inside Outside. Improving Mental Health Services for Black and Minority Ethnic Communities in England*, London: Department of Health.

Office for National Statistics (2003) *Ethnic Group Statistics. A guide for the collection and classification of ethnicity data*, London: ONS.

Office of the Deputy Prime Minister. Indices of Deprivation, 2004: www.odpm.gov.uk/stellent/groups/odpm_control/documents/contentservertemplate/odpm_index.hcst?n=4610&l=3.

PHLS (2002) *GRASP: The Gonococcal Resistance to Antimicrobials Surveillance Programme. Annual Report, Year 2001 Collection*, London: PHLS.

PHLS (2002) (England, Wales and Northern Ireland), DHSS and PS (Northern Ireland) and the Scottish ISD(D)5 Collaborative Group (ISD, SCIEH and MSSVD). *Sexually Transmitted Infections in the UK: new episodes seen at genitourinary medicine clinics, 1991–2001*, PHLS, DHSS and PS, and ISD(D)5 Collaborative Group.

Raghunathan, T.E. (2004) 'What do we do with missing data? Some options for analysis of incomplete data', *Annual Review of Public Health*, 25(1): 99–117.

Rainford, L. (1997) *2001 Census Testing Programme: report on the ethnic group and reli-gion question test carried out in March 1997*, London: Office for National Statistics.

Rowe, R.E. and Garcia, J. (2003) 'Social class, ethnicity and attendance for antenatal care in the United Kingdom: a systematic review', *Journal of Public Health Medicine* 25: 113–119.

Shah, R., McNiece, R. and Majeed, A. (2001) 'Socio-demographic differences in general prac-tice consultation rates for psychiatric disorders among patients aged 16–64', *Health Statistics Quarterly*, 11: 5–10.

Simmons, D., Williams, D.R. and Powell, M.J. (1991) 'The Coventry Diabetes Study: preva-lence of diabetes and impaired glucose tolerance in Europids and Asians', *Quarterly Journal of Medicine*, 81: 1021–1030.

Simpson, L. (2004) *Quantifying Stability and Change in Ethnic Group*, Manchester: Cathie Marsh Centre for Census and Survey Research, University of Manchester, 2004: www.iser. essex.ac.uk/seminars/mondays/2004/autumn/papers/simpson.pdf.

Spiegelhalter, D.J. (2002) 'Funnel plots for institutional comparison', *Quality and Safety in Health Care*, 11: 390–391.

Stewart, A.L. and Naploes-Springer, A. (2000) 'Health-related quality-of-life assessments in diverse population groups in the United States', *Medical Care*, 38(9 Suppl.): II 102–124.

Stroud, J. (2000 November) *Strategic Review of Business Information Needs (RoBIN): Race Equality Review – Final Report*, London: Department of Health.

Sutton, G.C., Storer, A. and Rowe, K. (2001) 'Cancer screening coverage of south Asian women in Wakefield', *Journal of Medical Screening*, 8(4): 183–186.

UK Parliament *Written Answers for 7 Jan. 2004 (pt. 14)*. Col. 398 w. Ethnic monitoring in 2002–03. [145081]. Ms Melanie Johnson.

Unal, B., Critchley, J.A. and Capewell, S. (2003) 'Missing, mediocre, or merely obsolete? An evaluation of UK data sources for coronary heart disease', *Journal of Epidemiology and Community Health*, 57: 530–535.

West, R., McNeill, A. and Raw, M. (2003) *Meeting Department of Health Smoking Cessation Targets. Recommendations for Primary Care Trusts*, London: Health Development Agency.

Yorkshire and Humber Public Health Observatory (June 2005) PBS Diabetes Population Prevalence Model – Phase 2, Briefing Document, York: YHPHO.

Chapter 11

Making sense of research in multicultural societies

Melba Wilson

The gap between good intentions and actual practice in research – especially as it relates to multicultural societies – threatens to remain wide and unbridgeable. This volume sets itself the task of identifying the discrepancies and anomalies that exist and which serve to militate against an ethnically and culturally appropriate context to research; and offers solutions for bringing about constructive change.

An underlying theme is that one of the main reasons for 'doing research' (in particular research to do with ethnicity and race) is to effect change and contribute to improving the status quo – in this case change in health and social care service provision – for those who use services and for those who provide them. These end users – people from ethnic minority communities (as well as other communities of diversity) and service providers (in the UK setting, National Health Service trusts, including primary care trusts who have responsibility for providing a wide range of hospital and community services) – have a symbiotic relationship that is not always clearly defined or understood. It is this relationship that research, conducted within an inclusive frame of reference, can attempt to positively influence.

The volume is concerned with highlighting issues relating to research in multicultural societies, with considering the social and political context within which such research is conducted, as well as offering an examination of the implications of these for best practice. A number of unifying and interrelated themes emerge. These relate to issues of context in relation to: (1) *exclusion and inclusion* or what Irena Papadopoulos defines as: 'culturally competent research ... that both utilises and develops knowledge and skills that promote the delivery of health care that is sensitive and appropriate to individuals' needs, whatever their cultural background' (Chapter 6, p. 82); (2) an examination of the *effectiveness and (therefore) relevance of research techniques* that do not take as their starting point an awareness or acknowledgement of the pivotal role of ethnicity in research design and analysis; and (3) a discourse on the importance of understanding the *political and ethical dimension* of data collection and the implications for improving health and reducing health inequalities. These themes are addressed below in turn.

Shifting from exclusion to inclusion

Chapters 2, 4, 6, 8 and 9 are useful in this discussion. Karlsen and Nazroo firmly set the tone in their chapter, arguing that there is an imperative for a clear basis for measuring ethnicity and race in the face of misleading and unclear information, including a lack of an objective discussion on racism. The significance of this in policy and practice terms is that it helps to show how the argument of a colour-blind approach in service delivery is not only flawed, but disingenuous and unhelpful. Their starting point is the 'socially contingent nature of ethnicity' and the acknowledgment that 'ethnicity is strongly related to social circumstances and economic position' (Chapter 2, p. 20, see also Chapter 1). A key premise within this is that to a certain extent people choose what characteristics with which to define themselves, which may or may not have recourse to ideas of colour, language, history or ancestry. This needs to be better understood by those who plan and deliver services in a society that is multicultural. It is important and necessary because this sharpened awareness about who is presenting for care and treatment; within what circumstances; and with what factors to be borne in mind, must always be integral to decision-making in relation to how those services are constructed. Increasingly, this means that the old, neat categories with which ethnicity is classified no longer suffice (if they ever did). Instead, there is now a pressing requirement – felt at least by people from ethnic minority communities – to re-draw the boundaries of what is regarded as relevant information. This will have far-reaching consequences for policy and practice development.

Given the current global context, there is added impetus to reconsider the ethnic categories we use. It is useful here to refer to Sarfraz Manzoor's (2005) discussion of the increasing tendencies of many who have been described as 'Asian' in Britain to define themselves by their religion (Sikhs, Muslims, Hindus). He notes that the term 'Asian', had its origin as 'a bureaucratic classification, [which] was promoted to a cultural term' and that 'It took a catastrophe to remind us that the word obscured as much as it illuminated and to expose just how much it hid' (p. 22). This unlayering of identity has resonance with the themes explored in this text. The issues have relevance because they address the need to develop a workable, as well as acceptable, understanding of what constitutes modern multicultural societies. Thus, the key role of research is to provide the reader with a language and a discourse that sets this in context and, indeed, unpacks it.

Among the current mantras in health and social care, within the UK at least, are choice and the requirement to treat people with dignity and respect. The danger, with regard to people from ethnic minority communities, is that this can end up being just another set of words that carries little meaning in terms of how they experience services. This is quite often because their needs are excluded or obscured through a failure of providers and commissioners of services to understand culture, ethnicity, heritage and race. It is the role of research in this context to inform policy and practice so that it is possible to decipher, translate and transfer the knowledge in relation to multiculturalism.

An important and allied point is that this is not just about Black people. Karlsen and Nazroo rightly note that 'Being "white" is as much a definition of ethnicity as being "non-white"' (Chapter 2, p. 22). This is a huge point, because unless and until there is a shift in the mind set which implicitly perceives mainstream services as those that equate to provision for the majority 'White' communities, and non-mainstream as relating to everyone else or 'the other', nothing will change. In this regard, American academic Patricia J. Williams has noted: 'Perhaps one reason that conversations about race are so often doomed to frustration is that the notion of whiteness as "race" is almost never implicated.'

Again, a key role for research on ethnicity and race is to help provide an evidence base that challenges this orthodoxy. One particular area I would highlight in this regard is the need to undertake research about the identities, needs and complexities associated with the growing numbers of people of mixed heritage in Britain. They are likely to be one of the main beneficiaries in service provision terms of a discourse on multiculturalism.

The inclusion theme is developed further by Johnson (Chapter 4) and Papadopoulous (Chapter 6) in their complementary discussions on the importance of identifying and understanding the user perspective; and also of involving them effectively in the design and evaluation of research. Johnson outlines the imperatives and the pros and cons for user involvement in research. Everyone, he states, is a potential user, including researchers themselves, and this has implications for the 'interests' they may themselves inject into their work (see also Scambler and Nazroo's discussion in Chapter 3). In addition, he argues, there is a compelling case for a strong community base for health research, and it is important for researchers to take issues of diversity, sensitivity, access, language, expectation, profile and sustainability on board when conducting research involving a community of users – in particular those from multicultural communities. To ignore this dimension, he argues, is to ignore the potential significance that research performed from an 'ethnic minority' perspective has for also meeting the needs of the majority 'white' populations.

One need look no further than the area of mental health and race for an understanding of why this is so important. The wariness and fear with which many ethnic minority service users approach mental health services is well documented (see, for example, DH 2005, Wilson 2003, Sainsbury Centre for Mental Health 2002). Part of this frustration lies with the misinterpretation and misappropriation of their views. In an attempt to address this anomaly, the Department of Health, the governmental department that sets policy and practice by which the National Health Service in England is governed and operated, has underscored its commitment to better quality and more intelligent use of information to improve services and equity in outcomes and to develop new strategies and services particularly when it comes to Black and minority ethnic communities (DH 2005). Other research from the Sainsbury Centre for Mental Health (2002) has stated:

> There is a need to shift the priorities of research, away from the traditional hospital-based epidemiological studies, towards both qualitative and quantitative community studies in which the hospital is not the sole sampling frame. We are particularly interested in 'intervention studies' which aim to comparatively evaluate outcomes from . . . innovative services provided by Black voluntary agencies alongside traditional statutory services.

Similar sentiments were echoed in a new report published by the Greater London Authority (Chouhan and MacAttram 2005). This outlined the importance of the Black community and voluntary sectors in meeting the needs of ethnic minority service users – viewed as successful because of their ability to relate more directly with and to empathise with ethnic minority service users.

Thus, it is clear that if research is to be believable and add value, it must take seriously its responsibility to work in partnership with service users – understand their viewpoints, accurately record their message, and agree an interpretation with them that reflects rather than clouds the issues, as well as helps to identify an acceptable and mutually agreed way forward for improving services.

Papadopoulos develops the theme further by stating that 'irrespective of the scale of the research projects – international, national or local – researchers need to understand the world views of their collaborators and target populations' (Chapter 6, p. 82), if they are not to run the risk of getting it wrong. And she goes on to say that 'researchers need to overcome the existing indifference and superficiality of treatment of ethnicity and culture, and must at least be convinced of the centrality of culture when developing their research programmes' (Chapter 6, p. 82–83). Crucial to this is an acknowledgement that 'we are all cultural beings' and that culturally competent research is not (or should not be) aimed at solely researching the health needs and problems of minority ethnic groups. This reflects Karlsen and Nazroo's (Chapter 2) comment on the need to move away from viewing people from minority ethnic groups as 'other' while the 'white' majority is regarded as mainstream.

Papadopoulos further argues that the lack of good culturally competent research and the failure by health researchers to produce information based on the values, health needs, disease patterns, health behaviours and religious practices of people from different cultural and ethnic groups, along with the failure to acknowledge problems such as the socioeconomic inequality and racism experienced by them, has contributed to the persistence of health inequalities. This has major implications for a health service that is meant to develop in a public health context. Extending this into work at the coal face, it is possible (and necessary) to argue for more action research that allows communities to work in partnership with primary care and other NHS trusts to deliver health care that has meaning and relevance. In mental health policy and practice, for example, many service users have grown wary of the usefulness of research in improving the care and treatment they receive. Many now refuse to participate in research, which they regard as changing nothing where it really counts – in their experiences on acute psychiatric wards, in engagement with community mental health teams, and in their lack of access to good psychiatric care and treatment in primary care services (general practitioners, community services) and in prison.

The Department of Health, in the *Choosing Health* White Paper (DH 2004), outlined its commitment to ensuring communities – with particular reference to ethnic minority communities as a priority – have clear and accessible information in order to understand the issues and engage in action to improve health:

> We will develop a standard set of local information that can be linked to other local data sets for publication. Public Health Observatories will produce reports designed for local communities at local authority level which will support Directors of Public Health in promoting health in their area.

Importantly, however, in the context of the imperative for 'standard' information, Papadopoulos sounds a note of caution to researchers and argues that in working with ethnic minority communities, there is a strong case to be made for 'researchers examining and challenging their own personal value bases and understanding how these values are socially constructed' (Chapter 6, p. 85). This is a welcome note of caution.

Papadopoulos' recognition of the pitfalls that occur as a result of these missed connections is reinforced in her conclusion and admonition to sceptics, that far from this being a discussion about political correctness, on the contrary everyone loses because research that is culturally incompetent is 'wasteful, dangerous and unethical'. Communities lose because their needs are not appropriately interpreted and this contributes to the lack of a useful reference point for practice to identify next steps. Likewise, the costs for service providers – opportunity, human, financial – when they get it wrong or only have part of the picture contribute both to a sense of impotency and a view that they cannot get it right because they don't know where to start, and to piecemeal or ad hoc practice that fails to address systemic shortcomings in a comprehensive or joined up way.

Karl Atkin and Sangeeta Chattoo (Chapter 7) build a good argument on how to avoid wastefulness and bankruptcy in research by effectively capitalising on the richness that can flow from involving diverse communities in qualitative research. They raise some important issues that are worth exploring here. First, it is important to make an up-front acknowledgement that much existing research has served to 'reinforce essentialised notions of "the other" and fail to deal appropriately with ideas about equity and access" (Chapter 7, p. 95). Second, they argue that difficulties in including ethnic minority communities, because of the need to ensure the robustness of methodology (for example, having to take account of obtaining interpreters or obtaining adequate samples and mix), has led to the marginalisation of ethnic minority communities in clinical and qualitative studies (see also the discussions in Chapters 8 and 9). Finally, they make a case for applying more rigorous methods in order to try and ensure that 'qualitative research methods might contribute towards positive change in policy and practice in terms of addressing issues of diversity, inequalities and discrimination at a collective level' (Chapter 7, p. 95–96).

This requires not only a statement of the needs of ethnic minority people, but also effective *translation* of what is said to enable good service delivery. The authors describe in detail the components required to bring this about in the context of qualitative research. They contain few surprises, for example, better and more effective language support and incorporating an understanding of the context in which the research is undertaken in terms of ethnicity, socioeconomic status, age and gender. This latter point needs constant reinforcement, as too often service providers tend to lump communities together using what are increasingly outmoded terms and categories. Again, with reference to the earlier discussion of the need to unlayer the complexities contained within communities, it is important to state the role that research can play in contributing to the evidence base. Take, for example, a current hot topic in health care provision in the English NHS – the value of patient profiling, as opposed to the simple arithmetic of ethnic monitoring. Patient profiling refers to the gathering of information to understand the nature of the patient population in order to provide a systematic approach to assessing need and resources, and information to plan services that are responsive to the community's needs. Belman (2004) notes that patient profiling helps to:

- identify differences in health patterns;
- enable people to access services appropriately and effectively;
- influence policy and planning;

- deliver health services and promote health;
- meet the requirements of the Race Relations (Amendment) Act 2000.

Atkin and Chattoo's focus is on the 'significance of qualitative strategies within the broader context of making "meaningful" observations about the experiences of ethnic minority people . . . and providing explanations that will add to our current understanding' (Chapter 7, p. 95). And for this, it could be argued, having in-depth knowledge about those communities should be a minimum prerequisite. They also, however, make the important point 'that in some ways ethnic minority populations may not be all that different from the general population [and] that every significant finding from the data might not necessarily relate to a participant's ethnic background – [rather] the challenge is to know when ethnicity makes a difference and when it does not' (Chapter 7, p. 109). This underscores the importance of moving beyond ethnic monitoring to understand the nuances of getting service delivery right for a particular population. Simply knowing the numbers is not sufficient to ensure that, for example, primary care trusts (which are responsible for all first line services relating to general practice and community nursing, as well as acting as gatekeepers to secondary care provision) in the UK are delivering services appropriately. It is perhaps fair to say that the presence of a large percentage of ethnic minority people in the local population doesn't *necessarily* justify an automatic assumption that patients are denied access to treatment. What is required is an assessment of the figures in the context of demographic particularities, which then give a fuller picture of how or whether services that are being provided are, indeed, accessible and appropriate for their needs. This is the domain in which sensitively conducted research can make a difference.

Atkin and Chattoo build upon this discussion by noting, however, that 'an analysis of the problems facing ethnic minority populations is one thing: doing something about it is another' (Chapter 7, p. 109). This gap between research and policy and practice goes some way towards explaining (though not excusing) why provision of appropriate care to diverse communities, based upon the huge evidence base provided by existing research and methodologies, still means that health service providers continue to fail to meet the expectations that the research engenders. Atkin and Chattoo note:

> Professionals need to listen carefully and ask sensible questions in order to provide appropriate support. This requires health and social care professionals to constantly evaluate and reflect on their practice and focus on the *context of need.*
>
> (Chapter 7, p. 110, their emphasis)

And:

> Research itself must be seen as part of a broader political process and can also be used as a means of empowering ethnic minority populations to realize their citizenship rights.
>
> (Chapter 7, p. 110)

Finally, within this vein of inclusion/exclusion, Oakley (Chapter 9) moves the discussion forward by discussing the consequences of exclusion in health research. In the context of exploring 'the treatment of ethnic minority people in health intervention evaluation research as part of a general phenomenon of social exclusion' (Chapter 9, p. 143), she argues that 'questions about the *outcomes* assessed in the evaluation of interventions need to be supplemented by others relating to the *processes* involved in the design, implementation and evaluation of health-related interventions' (Chapter 9, p. 143). Oakley contends that the need for sound evaluation design, raises the question of whether ethnic minority people are included in such studies as often as majority populations. Inclusivity matters in research trials because heterogeneous research samples allow us to explore the possibility of differential outcomes for different population sub-groups, with the reasonable hypothesis that there will be differential impact on the basis of socioeconomic differences, or differences in geographical location, as well as cultural (or genetic) differences.

An inclusive process towards research matters because without such differentiation in research trials, the complexities of providing services aimed at ensuring equitable and appropriate access to diverse communities may be lost. Oakley makes this point in her discussion about the context of health need. She notes:

> Evaluation research in health and social care takes place in a context in which people from ethnic minorities are not treated equally. Patterns of health service use show problems of access to primary care and a lower incidence of referrals to secondary and tertiary care.
>
> (Chapter 9, p. 155)

Appropriately targeted and directed research, however, can do much to address these differentials in health care access.

Work under way in Wandsworth Primary Care Trust (PCT) provides one example. Wandsworth is one of the 32 PCTs in London that are responsible for purchasing and/or providing health and community services for the capital's diverse population. Twenty-three per cent of Wandsworth PCT's client population comes from an ethnic minority community. It is about to undertake an action research project to look at the usage by people from ethnic minority communities of the Accident and Emergency department at its main acute hospital provider. The aims are to identify: whether it is higher than the norm; what factors contribute to higher access of services at a secondary rather than primary care level; and what initiatives need to be put in place to help ensure that primary care service providers are more readily able to meet these needs. The Wandsworth approach is an example of how baseline information can be obtained through directly involving a specific client community in order to determine how services should be planned and delivered. If the research confirms a higher usage of emergency services by ethnic minority communities, the PCT aims to creatively work with local community groups to provide better information, skills development to enable people to better articulate their needs; and to offer programmes that help communities to become more familiar with the health services that are available. The PCT also aims to work with primary care providers to put into place appropriate, relevant and accessible services for ethnic minority users, including assessments of language support needs. This is the kind of inclusive approach that must be made integral if health disparities are to be efficiently and effectively addressed.

Oakley notes that: 'people have an equal right to take part in research designed to inform public policy . . . if such research is not democratic in its methods, it cannot be democratic in its conclusions' (Chapter 9, p. 145) and as such represents a form of institutional racism. An extension of this argument is that people have a right to participate in research that is designed to influence service delivery. This has import-ance, too, for service providers who maintain that they operate a 'colour-blind' service and therefore do not accept the label of being institutionally racist. Such an approach can at least give a steer in helping them to address the gaps and inadequacies in the services that are provided. Oakley cites the UK Race Relations (Amendment) Act 2000 as placing a duty on public authorities to work towards the elimination of such discrimination. This is, indeed, a powerful tool, and one whose implications are only slowly coming to be understood in the context of ensuring service providers take seriously the nuances of race, culture and ethnicity in planning, developing, commissioning and delivering services.

In my view, this is another suitable area for building up a research evidence base, one that focuses on assessing the impact – in race equality terms – of service provi-sion. And here, Peter Aspinall's chapter (Chapter 10) underscores the point by arguing that 'the implementation of race equality policies and assessment of their outcomes can only properly be undertaken if such policies are linked to appropriate ethnic data collection, making the mainstreaming of ethnic monitoring a logical extension of mainstreaming race equality' (Chapter 10, p. 165). In order for this to be effective, he notes, it is necessary for a more systematic approach to data collection.

Effectiveness and relevance of interventions

The second key theme identified in this text concerns the extent of the effectiveness and relevance of the process of research to health outcomes. Nazroo (Chapter 1), Grewal and Ritchie (Chapter 5), Atkin and Chattoo (Chapter 7) and McManus, Erens and Bajekal (Chapter 8) all tackle the issues of research and its relevance to outcomes.

Nazroo argues that research studies that fail to take account of racism, or to acknow-ledge that socioeconomic inequalities are an important dimension when ethnicity/race is considered, are only capable of offering flawed interpretations which, in turn, help to perpetuate flawed interventions in health care. Similar conclusions are evident in the *Health in London Report* (London Health Commission 2004) which reviews the health of Londoners, with a focus on ethnic minority communities, against specific indicators that include: unemployment; educational attainment; proportion of homes judged unfit to live in; domestic burglary rate; air quality indicators; road traffic acci-dents; life expectancy at birth; infant mortality rate; and proportion of people with self-assessed good health. Among its conclusions were the need to recognise the importance of addressing diversity and reducing health inequalities through main-stream services and programmes and the need to acknowledge the complexity of the relationship between ethnicity and health.

The report further notes (along similar lines to Nazroo in Chapter 1) that:

> The link between racism and health inequalities has been poorly studied in the UK and Europe [though] some evidence from the USA and New Zealand has made a link between a health outcome such as high blood pressure, stress and living in racist environments.
>
> (London Health Commission 2004: 34)

(See also Karlsen and Nazroo 2002.) It can be argued that this is precisely the kind of information that primary care and other NHS trusts will need to develop, understand and *demand* of research if it is to be relevant to meeting the needs of diverse local populations.

As part of this, Grewal and Ritchie (Chapter 5) make the case for ethnic and language matching to be extended beyond the data collection stage to the design and analysis of research. This seems almost to state the obvious, but the authors note that little consideration has been given to matching in design and analysis. As Papadopoulos does, they highlight the need for social policy research to adopt the idea of cultural competence or an approach that:

> advocates that all researchers need to be culturally aware (conscious of how the cultural backgrounds of the researcher and the respondent interrelate); culturally knowledgeable (understanding of similarities and differences in order to avoid essentialism); and culturally sensitive (which may involve language matching and ethnic matching alongside the awareness that there are other factors such as gender and socio-economic status at play).
>
> (Chapter 5, p. 78)

McManus, Erens and Bajekal (Chapter 8) take the discussion a step further in discussing issues concerned with quantitative surveys with a representative sample of ethnic minority groups in Britain. This chapter is concerned with the practicalities of categorising ethnic minority groups, translating questionnaires, fieldwork issues and analysis and sample weighting. Their aim is to offer useful tips to make the research practical and efficient, while maintaining the representativeness and quality of results. Again, the importance of this lies in the need to ensure that the demographics of a given population are understood by health and social care providers and are able to be acted upon in a coherent and systematic fashion.

Politics and ethics

Chapter 3 and Chapter 9 are concerned with the politics and the ethics of doing research, respectively. Scambler and Nazroo's (Chapter 3) discussion concerns the value judgements that researchers bring to their work; and they lament the fact that in social research this often – whether by ignorance or design – goes unrecognised or unacknowledged. The accepted wisdom has been that scientific research must take pains to 'exclude all intrusions of matters of value, whether moral or political, and remain strictly neutral when doing research' (Chapter 3, p. 40). The view is that it is then the job of politicians and policymakers to make use of that research, outside the bounds of scientific enquiry, and within a context of a wider public engagement and debate.

This supposed view of scientific neutrality is the one that broadly governs research today. However, Scambler and Nazroo rightly argue that:

> no social research is conducted independently of value reference, and the values most likely to inform personal and collective research interests at any given time

are those broadly compatible with the vested interests of the wealthy and powerful. The wealthy and powerful are of course overwhelmingly White males.

(Chapter 3, p. 46)

Few would argue with this premise, given the vested interests that fund research and, also, the need to satisfy academic research assessment exercises for the all-important research ratings for universities in the UK context. What is important is that there must be a critical mass of researchers who will continue to hold the mirror to themselves (and hopefully others) so that those of us who rely on the conclusions they draw can take a greater degree of comfort in the findings – even if they are limited.

I have discussed Oakley's input in the context of the practicalities of evaluating research. The other key aspect of her work is that she places this firmly within a context of issues of science and ethics. She notes:

The importance of rigorous intervention evaluation research means that there are critical issues, not only about the extent to which such evaluations have been carried out, but about who takes part in evaluation research: how 'representative' are the samples included in such studies, and why does representativeness matter?

(Chapter 9, p. 142)

She identifies the barriers to inclusiveness and representativeness – additional costs of including people from ethnic minority communities in research (for example, translation, gaining a good sample size, etc.). Oakley concludes, however, that ethically, 'research funders should *require* inclusivity unless there are sound scientific reasons for an exclusive approach' (Chapter 9, p. 158) and that this should include funding additional costs. McManus, Bajekal and Erens indicate the significance of the need for this additional resource when designing a survey. The importance of such a statement in policy and practice terms is that it strengthens the evidence for removing race and culture from the realm of 'the other' and serves to make legitimate the view that to do otherwise is to discriminate as well as exclude.

Conclusion

This volume provides a practical guide to the conduct of research in the multicultural societies of the developed world. In addition, and importantly, it is placed in the context of theoretical and ethical discussions around the nature of ethnicity, the inequalities faced by ethnic minority groups, and the purpose and ethics of health and social care research. As such, it should be an integral part of the toolkit for those concerned with commissioning, conducting, evaluating and using research in health and social care. It provides guidance for good and useful research, research that aims to provide a strong evidence base for improving health and reducing health inequalities from the point of view of incorporating a sound ethical and political base – one that respects and values the lives and contributions of diverse communities in modern multicultural societies.

References

Belman, J. (2004) *Black and Minority Ethnic Communities and Primary Care*, London: Voluntary Service Council.

Chouhan, K. and MacAttram, M. (2005) *Towards a Blueprint for Action: building capacity in the Black and minority ethnic voluntary and community sector providing services*, Greater London Authority/African & Caribbean Mental Health Commission.

Department of Health (2004) *Choosing Health – making healthy choices easier*, p. 83.

Department of Health (2005) *Delivering Race Equality in Mental Health Care: an action plan for reform inside and outside services and the Government's response to the independent inquiry into the death of David Bennett*, p. 65.

Karlsen, S. amd Nazroo, J.Y. (2002) 'Agency and structure: the impact of ethnic identity and racism in the health of ethnic minority people', *Sociology of Health and Illness*, 24(1): 1–20.

London Health Commission (2004) *Health in London – Review of the London Health Strategy high level indicators*.

Manzoor, S. (2005) 'We've ditched race for religion', *The Guardian*, 11 January, p. 22.

Sainsbury Centre for Mental Health (2002) 'Breaking the Circles of Fear', Executive Briefing No. 17.

Williams, P. (1997) The Reith Lectures: *Seeing a Colour-Blind Future: the paradox of race*, London: Virago Books, p. 4.

Wilson, M. (2003) 'The mental health of Black and minority ethnic people', *The Mental Health Review*, 8(3): 7–15.

Index

Please note that page references to non-textual data such as figures are in *italic* print; references to footnotes are followed by letter 'n' and note number, while references to boxes are followed by the letter 'b'.

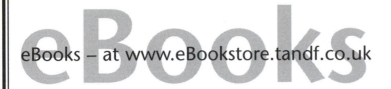

eBooks – at www.eBookstore.tandf.co.uk

A library at your fingertips!

eBooks are electronic versions of printed books. You can store them on your PC/laptop or browse them online.

They have advantages for anyone needing rapid access to a wide variety of published, copyright information.

eBooks can help your research by enabling you to bookmark chapters, annotate text and use instant searches to find specific words or phrases. Several eBook files would fit on even a small laptop or PDA.

NEW: Save money by eSubscribing: cheap, online access to any eBook for as long as you need it.

Annual subscription packages

We now offer special low-cost bulk subscriptions to packages of eBooks in certain subject areas. These are available to libraries or to individuals.

For more information please contact webmaster.ebooks@tandf.co.uk

We're continually developing the eBook concept, so keep up to date by visiting the website.

www.eBookstore.tandf.co.uk